12.12.78

CRISIS IN HEALTH CARE

THE OATH OF HIPPOCRATES

∴

I SWEAR BY APOLLO THE PHYSICIAN·
AND AESCULAPIUS· AND HEALTH· AND ALL-HEAL· AND ALL THE
GODS AND GODDESSES · THAT   ACCORDING TO MY ABILITY AND
JUDGMENT · I WILL KEEP THIS OATH AND THIS STIPULATION—
TO RECKON HIM WHO TAUGHT ME THIS ART EQUALLY DEAR TO ME
AS MY PARENTS· TO SHARE MY SUBSTANCE WITH HIM · & RELIEVE
HIS NECESSITIES IF REQUIRED · TO LOOK UPON HIS OFFSPRING IN
THE SAME FOOTING AS MY OWN BROTHERS· AND TO TEACH THEM
THIS ART · IF THEY SHALL WISH TO LEARN IT · WITHOUT FEE OR
STIPULATION · AND THAT BY PRECEPT · LECTURE · & EVERY OTHER
MODE OF INSTRUCTION· I WILL IMPART A KNOWLEDGE OF THE ART
TO MY OWN SONS· AND THOSE OF MY TEACHERS· AND TO DISCIPLES
BOUND BY A STIPULATION AND OATH ACCORDING TO THE LAW OF
MEDICINE· BUT TO NONE OTHERS·· I WILL FOLLOW THAT SYSTEM OF
REGIMEN WHICH · ACCORDING TO MY ABILITY AND JUDGMENT · I
CONSIDER FOR THE BENEFIT OF MY PATIENTS · AND ABSTAIN FROM
WHATEVER IS DELETERIOUS AND MISCHIEVOUS ·· I WILL GIVE NO
DEADLY MEDICINE TO ANYONE IF ASKED· NOR SUGGEST ANY SUCH
COUNSEL · AND IN LIKE MANNER I WILL NOT GIVE TO A WOMAN A
PESSARY TO PRODUCE ABORTION ·· WITH PURITY & WITH HOLINESS
I WILL PASS MY LIFE & PRACTICE MY ART I WILL NOT CUT PERSONS
LABORING UNDER THE STONE · BUT WILL LEAVE THIS TO BE DONE
BY MEN WHO ARE PRACTITIONERS OF THIS WORK ·· INTO WHAT-
EVER HOUSES I ENTER · I WILL GO INTO THEM FOR THE BENEFIT OF
THE SICK · AND WILL ABSTAIN FROM EVERY VOLUNTARY ACT OF
MISCHIEF & CORRUPTION · AND FURTHER · FROM THE SEDUCTION
OF FEMALES OR MALES· OF FREEMEN AND SLAVES ··WHATEVER · IN
CONNECTION WITH MY PROFESSIONAL PRACTICE· OR NOT IN CON-
NECTION WITH IT · I SEE OR HEAR · IN THE LIFE OF MEN · WHICH
OUGHT NOT TO BE SPOKEN OF ABROAD · I WILL NOT DIVULGE AS
RECKONING THAT ALL SUCH SHOULD BE KEPT SECRET ·· WHILE I
CONTINUE TO KEEP THIS OATH UNVIOLATED · MAY IT BE GRANTED
TO ME TO ENJOY LIFE AND THE PRACTICE OF THE ART · RESPECTED
BY ALL MEN · IN ALL TIMES· BUT SHOULD I TRESPASS AND VIOLATE
THIS OATH · MAY THE REVERSE BE MY LOT

CRISIS IN HEALTH CARE

JORDAN BRAVERMAN

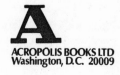

ACROPOLIS BOOKS LTD
Washington, D.C. 20009

ACROPOLIS BOOKS LTD.
Colortone Building, 2400 17th St., N.W., Washington, D.C. 20009

Printed in the United States of America by
COLORTONE PRESS, Creative Graphics, Inc.
Washington, D.C. 20009

Library of Congress Cataloging in Publication Data

Braverman, Jordan.
    Crisis in health care.

    Bibliography: p.
    Includes index.
    1. Medical care—United States. 2. Medical
economics—United States. I. Title.
RA395.A3B7   362.1'0973   78-6701
ISBN 0-87491-217-2

DEDICATION

To my parents,
Morris and Molly Braverman,
who educated one son to be
a physician and another son
to write about the coming
revolution in American
medicine under which his
brother will one day practice.

Contents

Figures

Acknowledgments

I would like to express my appreciation to my publisher, Mr. Al Hackl, for his patience; Ms. Janice Knestout, assistant editor, for her sharp editorial pencil; Sidney Friedman of New York, attorney-at-law, for his constructive comments in reviewing the manuscript; David Greenburg, Executive Director of the National Health Lawyers Association, Washington, D.C., for allowing me access to his organization's resources; Casey Crawford, Washington Editor of *Health Information Services,* for past considerations; and to my editor, Sandy Alpert, who showed an author what an editor does when she does it very well.

Photo Credit:
Author's photograph by Doug Bandos
Washington, D.C.

Preface

THE CHARGE

"I know that doctors care very seriously about their patients, but when doctors organize into the American Medical Association their interest is in protecting the interests not of patients but of doctors. They have been the major obstacle to progress in our country in having a better health system in years gone by."

President Jimmy Carter
Spokane, Washington
May, 1978

THE RESPONSE

"Surely there have been few times in our history when the problems of health have been so complex and pressing. It is unfortunate that the good faith of the medical profession should be impugned at this point when cooperation and understanding between the public and private sectors is so essential to the solution of our commonly apprehended problems."

Frank J. Jirka, Jr., MD
Vice Chairman, Board of Trustees
American Medical Association
Chicago, Illinois
May, 1978

THE GENERAL SERENITY prevailing in our country today is nothing but a deceitful illusion within organized medicine. Today's physician is on the threshold of a decision-making process whose outcome will materially affect his profession for many generations to come. That decision is whether the physician will survive to practice medicine as he always has and in the manner he deems best; or whether he will practice his art in a way elements outside of the medical profession deem appropriate.

The crises presently faced by the physician as well as other health providers have many names and beseige them on many fronts. The nomenclature is diverse—*health planning, national health insurance, health maintenance organizations, Professional Standards Review Organizations, drug substitution laws, antitrust investigations, public fraud* and *abuse, medical malpractice lawsuits professional image problems,* and many more. The ultimate aim of those in our society challenging the physician is simple—to exert control over the practice of medicine so as to bridle out-of-control health care costs while improving the quality of health services.

This book intends to give the reasons behind what is happening to your personal physician and the health system through which you receive your care. It will show you how events affecting your doctor will influence the kind of treatment you receive as his patient, and will demonstrate that health care is not an isolated system within our society, but rather part of an integrated whole affecting all of us. It will give an overview of America's health problems as a whole, and of its interrelated parts, and arm you with knowledge to become an active participant in solving our health problems. By exploring the merits and demerits of proposed alternatives for solving our health care crisis, it will show how you can reduce and control, to some extent, your personal medical expenses including the cost of health insurance and drugs, while improving the quality of care you receive. This is what the book is all about—American medicine as it exists today and how today's events will affect it tomorrow and all the tomorrows that follow.

Jordan Braverman

Washington, D.C.
September 1978

Introduction

THE STATUS OF AMERICAN HEALTH CARE is said to be in "crisis"- a word used so frequently it is almost a cliché. Yet, that word aptly summarizes the severe economic, social and political problems affecting us in terms of our personal health care. We have many questions about the health care dilemma but very few answers. Some of the questions raised today include: *Can I afford to become sick? Why doesn't my high priced health insurance pay for a routine checkup? Why must Congress increase my Social Security taxes? Why does a stay in a hospital cost more than $100 per day when a hotel room costs only $40? Why does my doctor order tests that I think are not necessary? Why does my health insurer require me to pay higher and higher premiums to protect my employees with less and less benefit coverage? How can I make sure that my surgery is necessary? Why am I hearing so much about physician fraud and abuse under Medicare and Medicaid? Why is there a call for national health insurance?*

This book attempts to answer the crucial questions affecting you medically as a patient and financially as a consumer, in view of the problems within our health care system. In bringing together the different major issues in health care today, the book explains and describes, in practical terms, not only what is happening to American medicine and why, but also why the richest country in the world has a health system that is literally bankrupting the financial health of its citizens.

FOR THE PATIENT ● The book explains:

● why doctor bills, hospital bills and health insurance premiums are rising so rapidly in cost and what measures have been proposed to curb their increase;

● how to purchase private health insurance;

● how drug substitution of the medicine your physician prescribes may save you money;

● how to participate in planning your community's health facilities;

● what is the meaning of national health insurance for tomorrow's medical system;

● how new special health groups called health maintenance organizations are being developed to provide comprehensive care at lower costs;

● why more and more tax money goes for public medical care programs for which many people do not qualify;

● how medical malpractice suits can affect patients and potential plaintiffs.

FOR THE DOCTOR ● The book tells:

● what has happened to his professional image and why;

● what his potential role is under national health insurance;

● how physicians contribute to high health care costs;

● what the impact of medical malpractice suits is on professional practice and physicians' solutions;

● what the significance of PSROs, HMOs, and health planning is to medical practice;

● what the implication of government intervention and investigations is on professional status including such areas as surgery, advertising, and third party reimbursement;

● how and why government programs alter the prescribing of medicine.

FOR BUSINESS COMMUNITY ● The book describes:

● what the impact of health costs is on the private insurance industry;

● what effect health insurance expenses have on private business and the reasons behind their rapid rise;

● which methods corporations use to reduce their health insurance expenditures;

● why it is difficult to know which kinds of health insurance best meet individual business needs.

FOR GOVERNMENT ● The book explains:

● what the government's role is in the rising costs of health care;

- how the legal system has helped create a medical malpractice crisis;
- how government may alter the profit and distribution structure of the American pharmaceutical industry;
- what success and failure government has experienced in altering the cost and quality of health care;
- how government allows incompetent physicians to continue their medical practice;
- why fraud and abuse exists in public medical care programs and what measures government has taken to correct the situation.

By examining these and other issues, this book presents a picture of where American medicine stands today and where it is likely to be tomorrow. American medicine can deliver the highest quality of health care at reasonable and equitable costs, or it can devour the fabric of its citizens' physical and financial well-being. Understanding our present health system enables the consumer-patient to contribute solutions to the crisis, solutions affecting, in a positive sense, the cost and quality of health care in future years. It is the author's hope that the book, together with its glossary of health care terminology, will add to the mutual understanding of the physician and the patient.

CHAPTER 1

Health Care in America: Why It Costs So Much

IT IS THE MOST VALUABLE POSSESSION we have. It is with us every moment of our lives. We enact laws to protect it. We cannot buy it. We cannot sell it. But we can inherit it and pass it on. We spend billions to keep it, billions to improve it, and billions to find it when it is lost. It is valued and accepted; it is ignored and abused. As a science it is glamourized; as an art it is criticized; as an issue it is politicized. It affects the private purse of each of us. It affects the public purse of the entire nation. Some enrich themselves from it. Some are impoverished by it. It is the core of our soul, our essence, our well-being—*it is our health.*

Health care in America today is a kaleidoscope—a composite of programs, acronyms, and issues. It is HSAs, HMOs, PSROs, MACs, and CATs. It is Medicare, Medicaid, and medical malpractice. It is private health insurance, social health insurance, and national health insurance. It is abuse of drugs, abuse of patients, abuse of doctors and abuse of government. It is defensive medicine and preventive medicine. It is necessary surgery and unnecessary surgery. It is nursing home care and home care nursing. It is hospitalization and monopolization. It is accusations and investigations. It is charges which are rising and rising to different charges. It is considered a right and not a privilege but some use the privilege and abuse the rights. It is the desire to keep everything as is. It is the desire to change everything from that which is. It is the crisis in health care today!

The status of American health care was well summarized in 1969 by Dr. James H. Cavanaugh, a former assistant in the U.S. Department of Health, Education, and Welfare, in terms which are still applicable:

"The delivery of health services is faltering so badly that we will have to shake the present system literally to its foundations . . . . revolutionary changes are needed . . . . the nation must have new careers, new professions, new kinds of manpower; and we do not have thousands of years, perhaps not even thousands of days to lose . . . . we will have to question every cherished belief about how health care ought to be provided—that the physician must always be the first line of health manpower; that a stay in the hospital at $100 a day is the best way to deal with serious health problems; that prepaid group practice is somehow second-rate medicine."[1]

The irony of this statement is that it is made in an era when America's capacity for the cure and prevention of illness and disease has never been greater. In the past century, the life expectancy of Americans has been lengthened from about 50 years to about 70 years. In cardiovascular diseases more progress has occurred in the past 20 years than in all recorded history. Cancer research has allowed more than one million Americans who have had a major form of cancer to lead productive, happy lives. Significant declines occurred in infant mortality, diseases of early infancy, maternal mortality and tuberculosis between 1965 and 1975. There has also been a decline in the number of mental hospital patients. At the same time, new drugs, new laboratory techniques, organ transplants as well as new immunological techniques have been developed. As a further example of the progress made in the health care field, legislation has been enacted since 1965 in such areas as health care financing for the aged and indigent, health manpower, and planning and construction of health care facilities.

Yet, something has gone wrong. Our ability to deliver needed health services at a reasonable cost and to provide for the basic physical needs of our society is in doubt. Anxiety over providing quality health care to every American is now prevalent and is termed the "health care crisis." It is the purpose of this chapter to examine this crisis, and to explore how this nation arrived at so paradoxical a stage. Despite all of its great technology and resources, the United States now finds itself in the position where a breakdown of its health delivery system is predicted unless immediate and concerted preventive action is taken by government and the private sector of society.

Evolution of Health Care Services

The crisis in health care besets a nation whose public and private spending in this area approximated $163 billion during fiscal year 1977. It vexes a nation which employs 4.7 million people in this field. The institutions and organizations which constitute the health care industry include hospitals, nursing homes, clinical laboratories, an insurance and pharmaceutical industry, academic health institutions, health maintenance organizations and government health agencies on the local, state and federal levels. The health problems appear in many guises: a breakdown in the delivery of health care services; smog enveloping our cities; chemicals and sewage polluting our rivers; high mortality from lung cancer, chronic respiratory disease and coronary heart disease; severe discrepancies in health between different social classes living in the same cities; and a deteriorating physical environment as reflected by housing which is of substandard quality in many areas.

The question is how we reached such an unfortunate position when logic indicates that the reverse should be true, especially in view of the long history of federal commitment to health programs. In fact, the involvement of the federal government can be traced as far back as 1798 when the Public Health Service was created to ensure that the health needs of merchant seamen, moving from port to port throughout the world, were met. During the 19th century, the federal government assumed responsibility in the control of communicable disease, first through quarantine and then through the application of the newly developed science of microbiology at the turn of the 20th century. The federal health effort changed in the 1930s, when the Public Health Service launched its programs of grants to states to assist them in attacking specific disease problems. After World War II, the Hill-Burton Act brought the federal government into partnership with the states for hospital construction. Then, in the 1950s, came rapid advances into bio-medical research and development, with fast growing support in this area.

While spectacular federal support for research was undertaken to develop weapons to combat disease, a controversy developed over another social demand—high quality health care as a right for all citizens. Today, federal activities provide direct health care to veterans, servicemen and their dependents, retired military personnel and other beneficiaries. We award grants to health services and hospitals for rehabilitation, vaccination, technical assistance and research, as well as grants for specific diseases. We support programs for mental health, child health, migrant health and Indian health. We now have major health service payment programs such as Medicare and Medicaid as well as physician peer review programs called Professional Standards Review Organizations and new health delivery systems called health maintenance organizations.

Between 1960 and 1977, federal health expenditures increased from $3.5 billion to about $46.5 billion.[2] The reason for this enormous growth in federal spending is found in the activities of the 88th, 89th and 90th sessions of Congress, which passed more significant health legislation than all other Congresses combined. During the Johnson Administration, the U.S. Department of Health, Education, and Welfare enumerated 102 pieces of legislation, many health-related, which were enacted into law. Some of this legislation may radically alter, if not revolutionize, existing concepts of health care. The programs which these laws created include health planning, Medicare, Medicaid, and the neighborhood health centers. In addition, legislation was passed to stimulate the development of various health professions. The implications of these programs are so far reaching that their impact on society is only now being measured. Will Rogers once said that everytime Congress makes a law it becomes a joke and everytime Congress makes a joke it becomes a law. But there is nothing humorous about the economic impact of these and other health-related laws. For example, between 1965 and

1975 federal health spending as a proportion of our total national health expenditures jumped from 12 percent to 28 percent while the national expenditures themselves rose from $38.9 billion to $122.2 billion during this same period of time.[3] Hence, one issue is quite clear. Health care is a basic human right. By setting up special mechanisms to support that tenet, the Johnson Administration sparked a social revolution. These health reforms are taxing to the severest limits the ability of our system to deliver quality services at reasonable costs and fulfill the purposes for which these laws were enacted.

Origin and Elements in Health Care Crisis

The crisis in health care is only one aspect of the complex problems of American life which embrace such issues as racial, urban, hunger, welfare, population, and poverty. As health is inextricably linked with all these concerns, fundamental progress in health care depends upon solving these other national problems as well.

Dr. Lester Breslow, a past President of the American Public Health Association, commented on the origins of the health crisis as follows:

"One element in its origin was the failure to comprehend that long-term adverse health effects can result from the application of certain technological innovations. An outstanding example is cigarette smoking. Machine production of a novel, attractive form of tobacco early in this century led to the expansion of an industry that had been highly profitable but which has taken its toll in the lives of millions of consumers. We did not even recognize the consequences until four decades had passed, and it has taken us another three decades to reach the point of taking action.

"A second element in the health crisis is the continuing reliance on industry to find simple technological solutions to problems that are identified. If cigarette smoke is harmful, so the argument runs, simply find the harmful ingredient and remove it. If automobile exhaust results in smog, find the specific chemical responsible and remove it by changing gasoline composition or the engine.

"The other and unspoken side of this argument is the dangerous one: namely, while searching for the technological solution, do not interfere with the industry. Production and its profits must continue, whatever the cost in health. Just let industry alone to find the technological solution ... This blind faith in industrial technology as the only path to solution is increasingly unjustified, especially when damage to health and life as a whole lies in the balance.

"A third and perhaps more pervasive factor in the health crisis is that we have not yet developed adequate social mechanisms for the control of current health problems. This failure is manifest with respect to the environment; it is also evident in medical care."[4]

However, these comments on the origins of the problem do not effectively convey the urgency which exists in resolving it. Its consequences include long hours incurred in the "waiting room," hurried and impersonal attention once assistance is received, difficulty in obtaining night and weekend care, reduction of services because staff is not available, and gaps in insurance coverage or higher taxes by government to pay for the increasing costs of health services. More specifically, the following are some of the outstanding reasons for our nation's inability to control health care costs in such areas as institutional care:

- There is a duplication of some high cost hospital services in various geographic areas, with consequent idle capacity, as a result of improper community planning of health facilities.

- Prevailing health insurance reimbursement plans provide little incentive for efficiency and economy of operations and few disincentives for unnecessary utilization.

- There are shortages and maldistribution in less costly alternatives to hospital care such as outpatient care, home health services, nursing homes and extended care facilities.

- There are inadequate incentives to use paramedical personnel and shared services.

- Although the nation has made many advances in medical science, it has only recently begun to focus its attention on improving the system through which the benefits of these scientific achievements are delivered.

● Health manpower is in short supply in various parts of the nation, due, in part, to the maldistribution of health care personnel.

● The administration of many public medical programs is weak, and their services are fragmented and lack coordination.

These are but a few of the problems which plague our nation in terms of health care. As examples, they dramatically illustrate the multi-faceted aspects of the crisis which this nation must solve. If we do not solve the problem we may face a situation which forever denies access of adequate health care to growing numbers of Americans.

Health Care Costs

When the health care crisis is examined in detail, one issue surfaces more quickly than any other, namely, that of costs. This factor becomes relevant whether these costs are incurred in the training of health manpower; the funding of public programs which pay for the care of particular groups; the funding of research for curing disease; the costs involved in purchasing health insurance; or the funding of public programs such as comprehensive health planning. The issue of cost underlies many of the problems besetting the health care field. Consequently it is necessary to examine the issue as well as the ancillary ones which emanate from it.

Increasing medical care costs are not a new dilemma. For more than a decade, these costs have been climbing more swiftly than other cost-of-living components. The roots of the problem are complex and intertwined. For example, the multi-billion dollar-a-year health care industry has been slow in adjusting to the increasing demand by the public for its services. This demand has grown, suddenly and immensely, by the establishment of Medicare and Medicaid. But these programs are not the only explanation for rising costs. The industry's scientific advances have outpaced its management capability. Physicians and hospitals can accomplish much more than they once could—but they continue to be impeded by a lack of adequate space, personnel and equipment. Additionally, rising incomes and the prevalence of private health insurance increase the ability of the public to pay for the health care they desire. Thus, the demand for health services far exceeds the nation's capability to provide them.

Nation's Health Bill

The fact that the demand for health care services has grown far more rapidly than the source of supply is clearly reflected in our nation's health bill which is illustrated in Figure 1. In 1950 the nation spent only $12 billion for health care services. By 1960 this dollar amount doubled. By 1970 the total expenditures almost tripled over the figure of 1960. At the present rate of increase economists predict that by 1980 we will be spending almost $230 billion for health care services—more than three times the amount spent a decade earlier. This country now spends for this single service more of its Gross National Product (the total market value of the nation's output of goods and services) than any other country in the world. Our health care expenditures are so huge that during fiscal year 1977 as a nation we were spending $737 for every man, woman and child—almost a fourfold increase in only a decade since Medicare and Medicaid became law.[5] According to the Social Security Administration, this per capita amount is still rising. These costs increases are so significant that Senator Edward M. Kennedy stated that Americans must work more than one full month of every year just to pay for health care, of which two weeks wages pay for hospital costs. According to Senator Kennedy, if health care were not so expensive, workers could take home higher wages and have better pensions.[6]

The strike of the United Mineworkers Union during 1977-1978 illustrates the importance of this situation. The key bargaining disputes of this strike were not centered solely on higher wages but rather on better pensions and health benefits. As a result of the length of the strike, various states whose industries were dependent upon coal as a primary energy source began to suffer economic paralysis with subsequent employee layoffs. The strike illustrates how one group's personal disenchantment with the economic impact of a social issue, such as health care, ultimately can have a direct effect and impinge upon the well-being and livelihood of other groups in our society who are not even a party to the problem. As John Donne wrote more than three hundred years ago, "No man is an island, entire of itself; every man is a piece of the continent, a part of the main..." When the coal miners went out on strike, partially to keep their free health care system, millions of Americans found the miner to be *indeed* "a part of the main."

Hospital Costs

Hospital care is the greatest contributing component in health care. In fact, 40 cents of every dollar spent for health care in this country is for hospital services. In fiscal year 1977, Americans spent $65.6 billion for hospital care. Hospital prices—as measured by semi-private room charges—have been rising at an annual rate of 15.5 percent since price controls over the health care industry, including hospitals, ceased when the Economic Stabilization Program ended in April, 1974.[7]

The meaning of these statistics to the patient-consumer is quite significant. First, the cost of hospital care is increasing twice as fast as all other goods and services. Second, the amount of money which this nation spends for hospital care has been doubling at a rate of every five years since 1965 when Medicare and Medicaid became law. Thus, at the present rate of increase economists predict that the American people will be spending $110 billion for hospital care alone by 1981 unless measures are taken soon to slow down this rise. On a more personal level, these statistics mean that the average cost of a day's stay in a hospital has risen more than 1000 percent since 1950—from $15 per day to today's daily average of $176. The cost of an average hospital stay has skyrocketed in the last decade from less than $300 to more than $1,300.[8]

Thus, the question arises—why is there such an explosion in the costs of hospital care? There are a variety of factors which have contributed to the significant rise in these institutional charges and costs, but two of these determinants are unique. The first is that 90 percent of all hospital costs are paid by someone else other than the patient—otherwise known as the "third party"—such as Blue Cross, Medicare, Medicaid, other insurance carriers or public programs. In fact, some patients may not even know the cost of their own hospital stay because of this situation. The second reason is that hospitals are presently reimbursed on the basis of the costs of the services which they provide. The budget is open-ended and there is no incentive to hold down expenses. This reimbursement system tends to encourage hospitals to add expensive facilities and technologies like the computerized axial tomography (CAT) scanner, a technological miracle which combines a computer with an X-ray machine to produce super-detailed, three-dimensional views of any cross section of the human body. The problem with the machine is that it may cost between $400,000 to $700,000 to purchase and about $300,000 annually to operate. But under the prevailing reimbursement system these costs are included in the hospital's charges to the third party after the costs are incurred. The third parties pay these bills from revenues which come mainly from the premiums which the American public pays at ever increasing rates. The hospital may attempt to add equipment such as a CAT scanner, even if it is not needed, or underutilized, or already present in other hospitals in the community. The hospital will do so because technologies such as CAT scanners not only may yield large operational profits to the medical institution but also the availability of such advanced technology will enable the hospital to compete with other institutions, attract doctors to its staff, patients to its beds and thus stay or advance in business.

In addition to technological advances which have led to the use of expensive equipment, there are other contributing factors to the increase in hospital charges. These include the following:

- The prices of goods and services purchased by hospitals have been subject to inflation.
- Payroll costs, which have lagged behind other industries, have been catching up.
- The demand for hospital services has necessitated the hiring of additional staff.
- New approaches to less expensive health care methods have been tried on too limited a scale.
- Health insurance coverage has been tied too closely to the requirement that the patient be hospitalized for treatment rather than on coverage for preventive care. Coverage for preventive care would pay for treating the patients outside of the hospital in order to ward off or detect any illness in its incipient stages before it becomes worse.

But what do these statistics and reasons mean in the everyday world of hospital care? The following excerpt of a letter from a constituent to her Congressman, as published in 1977 in the *Congressional Record,* illustrates what happens when statistics and reasons begin to merge. The incident referred to in that letter should not be interpreted as being representative of all hospitals or all patients in the country. But, it applies to other hospitals and patients where you as a consumer-patient have had similar experiences;

"I was recently hospitalized for 10 days. I am a heart patient and have been in several times so I know something about hospital policies. I must say they are just awful now. My bill was over $3,300 when it used to be about a thousand. If you ever are going to bring down health care costs, you should start with the hospitals! I know some doctors overcharge, but I haven't had that experience—it's the padding of bills and if you dare question them, they get awfully mad. They are a mean bunch and immediately go on the defensive which shows they know they are wrong. Put a ceiling on what they can charge. I will not name the hospital but the doctors seem to have no control on how much they will run up a bill. They gang up together and all do the same thing. For instance, I had to have a PT each day, a simple blood test for the clotting of the blood. That was because of my heart. I have no blood trouble, and my laboratory bill should have been no more than $110. But they billed me for $599—making tests costing $40 and $50 that I didn't need. They said Medicare paid it, why are you kicking? I told them because it wasn't right. I didn't need it. They got mad at me.

Then I asked for a heating pad for neuralgia in my leg one night. I supposed they would just loan it to me for a while, but they left it down there 6 days, part of the time it was hanging on the wall. When I got my bill, I found they charged me $8.95 a day rent for it, or over $50.00. You can buy a good new one for about $12.00 that will last for years. Wish I had taken mine along but they probably wouldn't have let me use it. Also, the doctor ordered 2 pairs of elastic stockings for me and they charged me over $40.00 for them. You can get them for about $5.00 a pair in a store that sells these things. These things I know were padded—altogether my bill was at least $700.00 more than it should have been. They charged me over a hundred dollars for medicines when I could have bought them and taken them myself for 3 or 4 dollars! Your real "rip-off" is from the hospitals. There is no end to what they will charge and the Congress should put tight controls on them."[9]

The federal government apparently thought along the lines of the last statement of the patient's letter. Early in 1977, the Carter Administration introduced a Hospital Cost Containment bill designed to curb the rate of hospital cost increases nationally but on a transitional basis, until longer-term control measures could be fashioned by the Congress and the executive branch of government. The proposed legislation would limit the rate of increase of hospital revenues, with certain exceptions, from all public and private sources to 1½ percent of the economy's annual inflation rate or about 9 percent for the 1978 fiscal year. The proposed bill also would place a limit of $2.5 billion nationally—about one half of what was spent in 1976—for hospital capital expenditures. This was partly because HEW has estimated that this nation has an excess of 100,000 hospital beds, which cost all of us over $2 billion a year. The excess is said to result from improper community planning of health care facilities. But by the time the second session of the 95th Congress began in the winter of 1978, the measure was still languishing in Congressional committee.

The proposed legislation met vigorous opposition from the medical profession and hospital industry for a variety of reasons. One of the main criticisms was that the bill would place controls over a hospital's annual income without placing similar controls over costs for goods from outside suppliers, such as energy, or for services of its employees, such as wages. Under this situation more and more of a hospital's controlled income would be absorbed in purchasing non-medical goods and services at increasing costs because of inflationary pressures operating within the general economy. As a result, the proportion of a hospital's income available for providing medical care services could decline over a period of time. The consequences of such a scenario are summed up by Dr. William R. Felts, immediate past President of the American Society of Internal Medicine and Professor of Medicine at George Washington University:

"... it will lead to: battles between physicians and hospital administrators, physical deterioration of hospitals, attrition of medical research, increased medical school tuition, a "dumping" of chronically ill patients by hospitals and doctors, much heavier expenses for increasing numbers of seriously ill people treated outside institutions, and an irreversible administrative bureaucracy. The bottom line has to be the rationing of services and care for patients."[10]

Backing up Dr. Felt's observations, in part, was the 1977 findings of a poll commissioned by the American Hospital Association. The survey showed that two out of three hospitals believe that they would be forced to reduce or eliminate "certain patient services" if revenue limits are put into effect. Leading the list of services to be trimmed back were X-rays, diagnostic laboratory services and hemodialysis.[11]

Would such events ever come to pass if the Carter program for hospital cost containment became law? No one knows for sure. The government states that about 22 percent of the hospitals in this country already operate under the revenue limitations which the Carter Administration seeks to impose without any deterioration in either the quality of their administration or the care which the institution delivers. Such economies of operation are said to be achieved by various management techniques including more ambulatory surgery; closing down beds; reduction of personnel; better money management; more efficient use of energy; economies in purchasing; more preadmission testing; and tighter utilization review. The question the government now asks is why can't the remaining hospitals in the country do the same? (A question, according to the bill's proponents, which is still begging an answer.) However, whatever the answers may be, hospital costs, despite their rapid rise, are not the sole factor which is contributing to the inflationary spiral besetting medical care services in the nation.

Physician Services

Prices for services of physicians have behaved similarly to those for hospital care. Like hospital services, the amount of money which Americans have been spending for physician care has been doubling at a rate of every five to six years since Medicare and Medicaid became law in 1965. In fact, since price controls over the health care industry ended in April, 1974, physicians' fees have been increasing at an average annual rate of 12.6 percent—almost twice the rate of the 1966-1971 period which preceded the establishment of the Economic Stabilization Program in August, 1971.[12] This growth rate is reflected in the $32.2 billion spent on physician services in fiscal year 1977—2½ times the amount of 1970 and 4 times that of 1965.

There are a variety of reasons for the rapid rise in the doctors' fees. Some patients might say, "you show me a rich physician and I'll show you a doctor with a healthy respect for money." However, it should be noted that before Medicare and Medicaid became operational in 1966, many physicians reduced their customary fees for persons with low incomes. But now physicians can, with good conscience, charge Medicare and Medicaid patients the same amount they ordinarily charge other patients. In addition, population increases, more widespread insurance and increasing awareness of the benefits of medicine have contributed to the growing demand for physician services by all segments of society without a corresponding increase in the supply of physicians.

Whereas 40¢ of every dollar was spent for hospital care in fiscal year 1977, only 19¢ of that same dollar went for physician care.[13] The reason for this situation relates to the changing character of the American population. As the number of older people in our society increases, more monies are spent on institutional services provided by a hospital or nursing home. The monies which are being spent by or on behalf of the elderly has had a profound effect on the rise of health care expenditures within recent years.

The Elderly

Over the years government has established many programs to help the elderly through the financial trauma of what should be their "golden years." But, unfortunately, for many of the aged the "golden years" are a time when low incomes must be budgeted to meet high personal expenses because of circumstances such as ill health. Within recent years government has established two programs—Medicare and Medicaid—which have brought financial relief to the elderly in at least one area of their lives—their personal health expenses. The necessity for such social programs is underscored by the following fact. In fiscal year 1976, we, as a nation, spent $120.4 billion to meet our personal health needs. Of this total amount, the elderly, who represent only 10 percent of our nation's population, accounted for 29 percent of the expenditures.[14]

The reasons for their large medical expenses are varied:

- The average elderly person has more and costlier illnesses than the average person under 65 years of age.
- Aged persons are more than four times as likely to have their activity limited by chronic health conditions than are those under age 65.
- The elderly are hospitalized at 2½ times the rate for persons under age 65, and their length of stay is almost twice that of such persons.
- An older person, on the average, uses physicians to a far greater extent than a younger individual.[15]

As a direct result of the Medicare program, the financial burden of high costs on the elderly for hospital and medical care has been substantially reduced. In the year prior to Medicare's enactment, $7 out of every $10 of the elderly's medical bill was paid privately. In fiscal year 1976, only $3 out of every $10 came from private funds. The enormity of the elderly's need for some kind of assistance by government can be appreciated from figure 2. In fiscal year 1976, the medical care bills for the average aged person was more than six times ($1,521) that of young person under 19 years of age ($249) and almost three times ($547) that of a person between the ages of 19-64.[16] The elderly's need is partially reflected in the continuing necessity by Congress to increase the wage base and tax rate of the Social Security program to prevent the program from becoming bankrupt. For Medicare, together with the other Social Security programs, pass on their respective cost increases to the taxpayer, whose annual Social Security taxes may be higher now, in some instances, than his yearly income taxes. But these increasing costs not only affect those under 65 years of age, but also the elderly who must assume a greater and greater share of their own medical expenses under Medicare compared to a decade ago.

But excessively high inflation is not the only reason why Medicare, together with the other programs within the Social Security system, have been subject to financial problems. Unemployment has also plagued the Social Security system and has caused the

Social Security trust funds to suffer a financial shortfall. Because unemployment has been higher in the past few years than originally anticipated, fewer people than expected have been contributing Social Security taxes to the trust funds; more have retired or claimed disability insurance. Another major cause stems from 1972 when Congress enacted a cost-of-living adjustment to raise Social Security benefits automatically as the Consumer Price Index increases. Thus, as a result of high inflation, Social Security benefits have been automatically increased to a greater extent than projected a few years ago.

Additionally, a severe long-range deficit in the program compounded these short-range problems. The deficit resulted from the changing economic and demographic assumptions which were used originally in 1972 when the long-term projections of the solvency of the Social Security trust funds were made.[17] These assumptions related to fertility and mortality rates in our society as well as the annual percentage increases both in the Consumer Price Index and in the average wages in this country. Consequently, because of external economic forces beyond the capability of our government to manage or foresee, the American public must assume a greater and greater financial burden to protect itself and its future generations from the financial ravages accompanying aging. These can be expressed, for example, in an individual's need for disability income or the need for financial assistance under the Medicare program.

Health Insurance

Today the costs of health care have jumped so high that other groups are beginning to demand the kind of protection which programs such as Medicare provide the elderly. Room and board in New York City and Boston, for example, is $140 or more per day. The average hospital stay costs over $1,300. With daily hospital charges this high, even the relatively affluent in our society can have their savings and other assets wiped out by a single catastrophic or chronic illness. As costs of health care soar, wide gaps still exist in insurance coverage. Private insurers have increasing difficulty keeping up with rising service charges as they attempt to cover needed health services. As additional benefits are provided, the costs of insurance are inflated even more. Increasingly, requests by health insurers from state insurance commissions for rate increases are meeting more and more resistance. In fact, some decisions as to the relevancy of such increases are being brought into courts of law for review. As a result, health insurance prepayment plans, commercial insurance companies and some state governments are beginning to support the concept of a federal national health insurance mechanism to replace, wholly or partially, private health insurance programs.

Today, the working man is not only confronted by escalating private health insurance rates, but he is also faced with:

● Increased state and local taxes to pay for Medicaid.
● More of his federal tax dollar going to the federal share of Medicaid and Medicare costs.
● More out-of-pocket costs to cover his co-insurance portion of higher and higher medical charges.
● More out-of-pocket costs for rapidly rising charges for largely uninsured health services such as dental care.

Beseiged with all these demands on his tax dollar, and with so many separate health insurance plans, how can an individual determine which plan offers adequate coverage, which is commensurate with his earnings, and which meets *his* particular needs. This is especially true since private health insurance does not provide complete coverage. Although private health insurers often cite the extensiveness of their coverage and the fact that the number of insured persons is constantly growing, it is important to bear in mind the limitations of the coverage. Large categories of medical expenses such as drugs, dental care and non-hospital "ambulatory" office visits are still excluded from many basic policies.

As an example, let us illustrate why a physician's-out-of-hospital office visit is not usually covered by private health insurance policies.

If non-hospital visits to a physician's office were to be covered by private health insurance, insurers believe this might encourage patients to see their doctor for all kinds of ailments and complaints for which the patient would not ordinarily make an appointment. Such a result is feared because another party, the private health insurer, would be paying the bill. It would mean health insurers would have to process even more claims than they handle at present. These administrative costs, in addition to physician payments, would cause an increase in the costs of health insurance premiums. Thus, by not providing out-of-hospital coverage for physician office visits, the insurers believe a deterrent is created. Patients will only visit a doctor's office when they feel it is medically necessary since the patient himself must pay for the visit. Unfortunately, if a doctor must perform a procedure which can be easily carried out in his office, but is covered by the patient's health insurance policy only when it is performed in a hospital, then the physician may admit the patient to the hospital so the patient himself would not have to pay for the cost of the procedure. This situation adds to the cost of hospital care which is reflected in the increasing cost of health insurance which the insurer charges the consumer. So the question arises, can these hospital costs be reduced by providing coverage for non-hospital "ambulatory" visits to a physician's office? There is no definitive answer. Tentative evidence from health maintenance· organizations seem to indicate that such a benefit would reduce the cost of hospitalization. However, the private health insurance industry has not introduced such coverage on a broad population basis. Thus, no one knows whether patients will visit their physicians for the most minor ailments and thereby overburden the physician's office consequently increasing the costs of health care.

Meanwhile, the costs of hospital care continue to rise and efforts to control their increases seem fruitless. Needless to say, this kind of policy exclusion becomes even more critical at a time of inflationary medical care prices. And the situation is many times worse for the poor, the black, the itinerant and the self-employed.

These groups are on the outer-fringes of the health care system, not only in terms of health insurance protection, but also in terms of their accessibility to and availability of health care services. In fact, it is estimated that in fiscal year 1978, about 26 million Americans approximately 12 percent of the U. S. population) will have no insurance coverage through private insurance or public programs such as Medicare and Medicaid. However, an estimated 8 million of the uninsured have other sources of aid such as through the Veterans Administration. Thus, 18 million people in this country can be considered totally unprotected against the costs of ill health or the consequences which may flow therefrom. The following case illustrates the problem.[18] In February, 1978, a jury in Florida, which was urged by the plaintiffs' attorney to return a judgment that would serve as a warning to the medical field, awarded $950,000 to the heirs of a meningitis victim. The prospective patient died after she was turned away from one hospital and sent to another because of her poverty.[19] An extreme example, perhaps, but the event did take place in America—the richest nation in the world.

Medicare and Medicaid

Although the government, principally through Medicare and Medicaid, has ventured into paying some of the medical bills of those least able to pay—the elderly and the poor—many problems remain for those groups in terms of obtaining the quality of care they deserve. Since these programs are concerned with different groups and have different administrative structures—which together cost the federal government about $30 billion in fiscal year 1977—Medicare and Medicaid have had dissimilar records, (with Medicare considered more of a success and Medicaid more of a failure.)[20] In spite of their different histories and structures, both programs have a common weakness, shared also by private insurance carriers. They allow money to providers of care, without giving any incentive to the providers to lower their rates. Critics consider this lack of providing incentives as one of the primary reasons for the inefficiency of health care delivery and for the inflationary cost spiral. In addition, Medicare now only covers about 38 percent of the total health bill of individuals over 65, compared to about 47 percent of the bill back in 1970. As health care costs rise, the Medicare program is able to purchase less and less services with its medical care dollar.[21] Also, Medicare reimburses physicians on the basis of "reasonable" charges—meaning whatever physicians feel is the prevailing community rate, nature of service and self assigned value to their time. Medicaid permits the state to choose its own financing system but recommends Medicare-style financing. Thus, physicians set the fees and the government pays for them. One example of how completely physicians control their income is revealed in a study which used the Medicare data of the Social Security Administration for fiscal year 1975. The study showed that geographic differences in surgical fees could not be explained by differences in the cost of living, professional expenses (including malpractice insurance premiums) or the quality of care. For example, it could have cost Medicare $1,000 for a gall bladder removal in New York City, and $290 for the same operation in Findlay, Ohio—a difference of 245 percent. Yet, the cost of living was only 37 percent higher in New York City. A cataract operation in Beverly Hills, California would cost $1,000 some 270 percent more than its maximum of $375 in rural Nebraska, despite the fact the cost of living was only 11 percent higher in Beverly Hills.[22] Thus, the difference in fees is not due so much to differences in the cost of living between the areas as it may be due to the personal standard of living a physician wishes to maintain. And the physician's standard of living is determined in part from the income of his medical practice which results from the fee levels the physician establishes as being the value of his service. The annoyance American society may feel toward the different monetary values which surgeons place on the same procedure may well be summarized by the comments of George Bernard Shaw. Shaw wrote in *The Doctor's Dilemma:* "That any nation, having observed that you could provide for the supply of bread by giving bakers a pecuniary interest in baking for you, should go on to give a surgeon pecuniary interest in cutting off your leg is enough to make one despair of political humanity."

Thus, in an attempt to put a brake on rising physician charges, Congress put a provision into Public Law-92-603, the Social Security Amendments of 1972. The provision was intended to limit the annual increases in a physician's prevailing fees to an amount reflecting increases in the costs of practice and earnings in an area. This provision, aimed at Medicare and Medicaid programs, took effect on July 1, 1976. Whether the stipulation will have any impact on physician fee increases remains to be seen, but one fact is certain, until now physician fees have been rising faster than the Consumer Price Index and more rapidly than they had prior to the enactment of Medicare and Medicaid in 1965.

But physician fees are not the only culprits in the inflationary rise of health care costs. Medical prices, in general, have consistently outpaced the prices of all the goods and services which the Consumer Price Index measures. These other indices include food, apparel, housing, transportation, recreation, and other goods and services. In fact, one of the primary reasons why mandatory price controls were placed upon the health care industry under the Economic Stabilization Program was due to medical care prices rising 50 percent faster than all other consumer prices between 1965 and 1970. Under the Economic Stabilization Program, however, medical care prices only rose at two thirds the rate of all other consumer items. Since controls were lifted in 1974, medical care prices once again have begun to outgain those of all other goods and services, registering a 10 percent increase in 1976 compared to a 6 percent gain for the other consumer items in the Index.[23]

In order to bring some kind of cost control to and, hopefully, reduce over time, the public expenditures of Medicare, Medicaid and other public social programs, HEW Secretary Joseph A. Califano, Jr. announced on March 8, 1977 a major reorganization of the health care, social service, student aid and income assistance programs involving about one-third of his department's $145 billion budget. One aspect of this entire reorganization, projected to save the government at least $1 billion through 1979 and $2 billion annually by 1981, was the establishment of a new Health Care Financing Administration. Five major HEW units constitute the new financing agency. They include the Bureau of Health Insurance, which administered the Medicare program in the Social Security Administration; the Medical Services Administration, which administered the Medicaid program in the now abolished Social and Rehabilitation Service; the Bureau of Quality Assurance, responsible for the Professional Standards Review Organization program, originally in the Health Services Administration; the office of Long-Term Care formerly in the assistant secretary for health's office; and the enforcement offices of Long-Term Care Standards originally in each of HEW's ten regional offices. Thus, for the first time since their enactment, both Medicare and Medicaid will be administered by a single agency which reports directly to the Secretary of HEW.

Medicare is one example of the impact that increasing health costs have on publicly-sponsored programs. This program consists of two parts. Part A uses payroll taxes to cover the costs of hospitalization for those in our population who are 65 years of age or older. Part B is the voluntary medical insurance portion which pays part of the physician's fees at a monthly premium cost to the elderly. When Medicare began in 1966 these Part B premium payments were set at $3 per month. By July 1, 1978 the same premium payments had risen over the twelve year period to a level of $8.20 per month or almost three times the premium costs of a decade earlier. The slowly escalating costs during this twelve year period seems to indicate that unless health care costs, especially for the elderly, are brought under control and soon, even a program as publicly-spirited and publicly-minded as Medicare may become too expensive for those in our society who need it the most and who can afford to do without it the least. This is one way in which inflationary health care costs eat away at the very fabric of our well-being and standard of living. This is especially true for those in our country who, like the elderly, must live mostly on fixed incomes and cannot cope with inflationary pressures which affect the quality and status of their personal health. Regardless of age, people become sick in good times and bad. An unemployed worker can defer the purchase of a new car, but he cannot defer an appendectomy if his appendix bursts. Moreover, many Americans have come to regard health care as a necessity, not as an optional expense. A solution of this health care cost problem is needed and needed quickly before government takes the kind of action which many segments of the health care field may regret one day, especially when they had the opportunity to police their own house, but failed to do so partly in the name of personal economic gain.

Manpower

Today the demand for health services, which far exceeds the supply of manpower, is another of the factors influencing the rising costs of medical care. Yet, there are some who disagree as to whether or not a manpower shortage really does exist in some of the 200 odd health categories—from nurse's aide to physician—some of which are noted in figure 4. In fact, it is suggested that the public policies of the 1960s and 1970s, which increased the number of physicians in this country are potentially cost-enhancing. This is because great numbers of physicians can generate higher rates of utilization and higher total expenditures for health in the 1980s and beyond. For example, it has been calculated each additional physician conservatively adds $250,000 to the amount of health care provided either by himself directly or by others whose services he prescribes. One federal official deeply concerned about these economic implications for the health field is Robert A. Derzon, Administrator of the Health Care Financing Administration in the U. S. Department of Health, Education, and Welfare:

"By 1980 we will have 200 physicians per 100,000 population and the ratio will still be climbing. . . . over a lifetime a doctor will add more than $9 million to health care spending."[24]

But HEW is not alone in being alarmed by this implication. In 1976, the Carnegie Council on Higher Education warned that "we are in the serious danger of developing too many medical schools."[25]

Rather than stating that larger numbers are needed to solve the manpower problems, critics point out that present medical manpower is utilized in a wasteful manner. They feel it is poorly organized and it is impossible for anyone other than physicians to climb the health career ladder, resulting in many in the lower echelons simply dropping out. It is also stated there are health personnel in training who often find family responsibilities and financial hardships insurmountable. Thus, they are not able to complete their training, with the result that the nation is deprived of needed additional manpower. It is also claimed the medical profession has allowed itself to become so fragmented that certain specialties, rather than the profession as a whole, have been allowed to determine who of their number will practice what kind of medicine. Dr. John Knowles, President of the Rockefeller Foundation and former Director General of the Massachusetts General Hospital, has been highly critical of a system which permits the certifying boards of the various medical specialties "to function in glorious isolation without moral commitment to larger social and economic issues." He said this produces too many of certain kinds of doctors—notably surgeons—and not enough of others, such as pediatricians.[26] To try and correct some of these problems, the Health Professions Educational Assistance Act of 1976 was enacted (P. L. 94-484). Among the key provisions of the Act is one whereby medical and dental students, for example, can receive financial assistance for school, provided they are willing to repay the subsidy by practicing for a period of time in a medically underserved area through the National Health Service Corps which is massively expanded under the Act. Another important aspect of the law is the emphasis it gives to the training of primary care physicians. As a condition for capitation aid, medical schools must have in 1978 at least 35 percent of their filled first-year positions in direct or affiliated residency training programs in primary care, defined as family medicine, general internal medicine and general pediatrics. This percentage rises to 50 percent by 1980. But will increasing the number of physicians within the various medical specialties through the financial stimulus of Congressional enactment solve the manpower problem within the medical field? This health manpower question was examined thoroughly several years ago by a distinguished Presidential Commission, the National Advisory Commission on Health Manpower. It found that the inadequacies in health manpower could not be successfully tackled outside of reform of the institutional framework within which the manpower is utilized. The Commission reported:

"There is a crisis in American health care ... the crisis, however, is not simply one of numbers. It is true that substantially increased numbers of health manpower will be needed over time. But, if additional personnel are employed in the present manner and within the present patterns and systems of care, they will not avert or even perhaps alleviate the crisis. Unless we improve the system through which health care is provided, care will continue to become less satisfactory, even though there are massive increases in costs and numbers of personnel ... Medicine has participated in the general explosion of science and technology, and processes cures and preventives that could not have been predicted even a decade ago. But the organization of health services has not kept pace with advances in medical science or with changes in society itself. Medical care in the United States is more a collection of bits and pieces (with over-lapping, duplication, great gaps, high costs, and wasted effort) than an integrated system in which needs and efforts are closely related."[27]

Similarly, Walter McNerney, President of the Blue Cross and Blue Shield Association stated that "we would get more bang for the buck if we put relatively more emphasis on organization, financing, and design of the health system than simply producing professional manpower. In short, we are faced with an economic problem of organization."[28]

Resolving the Health Care Crisis

Recognizing the need for resolving the many health care problems which beset the nation, the federal government in the first half of the 1970s proposed and enacted into law various health programs dealing with diverse issues. These included Professional Standards Review Organizations in 1972, health maintenance organizations in 1973, and Health Systems Agencies in 1974. Even on the state level, commissions are being established by law to control hospital costs and to have rate making authority for various public programs within the jurisdiction. Some of these states include Maryland, Connecticut and Massachusetts. The establishment of these rate setting commissions reaches the heart of the health care cost issue, according to some critics—the basic philosphy of maintaining the traditional free enterprise system of American health care versus total government regulation, whether this control emanates from the federal or state governments. This issue underlies today's health problems because some groups feel the conditions which led to the regulation of other industries now exists in the health system. It is their contention that the medical system is not competitive; hospitals generally are not operated for profit and have little incentive to keep costs down; and that there is little price competition among physicians. In fact, Joseph A. Califano, Jr., Secretary of HEW, has been quite specific in his analysis of the non-competitiveness of the health care field. According to Secretary Califano, the non-competition has the following characteristics:

● "The patient may select his family doctor . . . but he does not select the services he is told he needs. The physician is the central decision-maker for more than 70% of health care services.

● "Ninety percent of the hospital bills are paid by third parties.

● "These reimbursement mechanisms usually operate on a cost-plus or fixed fee-for-service basis, the most expensive and least efficient way to function.

● "Most public and private benefit packages are heavily biased toward expensive in-patient care.

- "The unavailability of price and quality information keep the patient dependent on the decisions of the health care provider ... whose financial well-being is determined by the price charged.

- "The ability to restrict access to competitors—hospital credential committess that can deny or delay privileges to health maintenance organizations, for example—provide special layers of market control."[29]

Secretary Califano has concluded that "doctors, hospitals, pharmaceutical companies—all the inhabitants of this non-competitive, free-spending third-party world—act exactly as the incentives motivate them to act: conscious of quality but insensitive to cost. As a result, health care resources are neither well distributed nor efficiently organized."[30] Reinforcing Secretary Califano's view of the lack of competition in the health care industry is Senator Edward M. Kennedy who has said:

"I start from the belief that health care is not like most other industries where free market competition operates. The consumer is not, and cannot be, fully informed. Risk of illness is randomly distributed, and risk of the cost of health care is not uniformly borne by the population. The economic injunction that more is better does not work well in health care; more may be detrimental to health. Too many surgeons in an area, competing with each other, produce more and more surgery and higher and higher fees, not lower ones. Too many hospital beds in a community means too much hospitalization, not lower hospital rates. Too many insurance companies in an area mean not better competition with premium prices, but higher premiums because no one insurer can control the costs of the system."[31]

In other words, the present character of the health care system fosters the direct opposite of competition.

In order to avoid a direct confrontation on this issue, many groups are seeking alternatives. One example is promoting the idea of a national health insurance plan under which the federal government would pay hospitals and nursing homes to run themselves, using incentives and disincentives to promote efficiency. Accordingly, various groups in the private sector who may be most affected by proposals such as national health insurance are trying to experiment with their own sponsored systems to reduce health costs. For example, the commercial insurance industry and Blue Cross plans are sponsoring the development of health maintenance organizations since these plans have generally demonstrated cost saving potential in delivering health care.

Consequently, what is seen today is a variety of proposals and experiments, advanced by public and private groups to resolve the problems which have brought the present system to its current state. Some of these actions embrace the concepts of control by the private sector, quasi-public controls, while others imply total government control. The question arises as to what kind of future lies ahead for American society with respect to a system which must continue to meet the health care need of an ever growing nation?

The Future

Despite the many problems which beset this nation today, the future resolution of these issues can be considered optimistically. Society is aware of the problems, is debating the most feasible solutions for them, and realizes that in health care, whether it be in the medical or environmental sense, what is at issue is the survival of society itself. A 1977 Louis Harris poll revealed that the high cost of medical and hospital care was of deep concern to the American people.[32] Thus, looking into the future, it may not be long until this nation will have a national health insurance program in which all of its population, generally, will be protected against the costs and incidence of ill health with the dissolution of such ineffectual public programs as Medicaid. The health care professions will enlist the assistance of paramedical personnel in increasing numbers. These personnel will be authorized to provide simple diagnosis, prescriptions and prevention of disease. These new types of practitioners will have training which lies somewhere between the training of physicians and the training of nurses.

Prepaid group practices will continue to grow, being stimulated by public funding and the support of the private health insurance industry, as ways are sought to reduce costs and bring a greater efficiency and coordination into the health care system. These plans will not only care for those who are seriously ill but also will provide preventive care programs to discern the initial phase of any illness. As these prepaid group practices grow and health planning becomes more prevalent, strengthened by legal enforcement, more physicians will be practicing in clinics or prepaid groups with the subsequent decline of the solo practice of medicine.

Alternatives to hospital care, such as home care services, will continue to expand. Emphasis will be on the continuing development of such institutions as extended care facilities and out-patient or ambulatory clinics. Many inpatients requiring attention in the major care hospitals will be sent to these less expensive centers for their initial and perhaps complete care, if their physical status so warrants. Care will continue to expand through such organizations as neighborhood health centers and community mental health centers and reach those who require but cannot find health services. These are not all the changes which will occur nor will this system suddenly develop. Health care, both in concept and practice, is an evolutionary process. But the public conscience that health care is a right and not a privilege has been awakened. An enlarging society demands that this basic right be applied in fact rather than in theory. Individuals now find themselves affected by health care problems whether it be in requiring assistance in the payment of bills they cannot afford, or the purchase of health insurance beyond their economic grasp, or in the elimination of deteriorating environmental conditions which lead to ill health, or obtaining medical assistance when needed rather than when the first opportunity is available to receive it. If the present battle for maintaining this society in as good a state of health as possible is lost, either in the physical or environmental sense, then society will have lost the basic element for its future existence, namely, a healthful life itself.

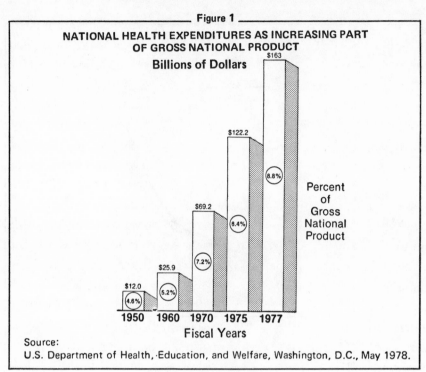

_____ Figure 1 _____

**NATIONAL HEALTH EXPENDITURES AS INCREASING PART
OF GROSS NATIONAL PRODUCT**

Billions of Dollars

Percent of Gross National Product

Fiscal Years

Source:
U.S. Department of Health, Education, and Welfare, Washington, D.C., May 1978.

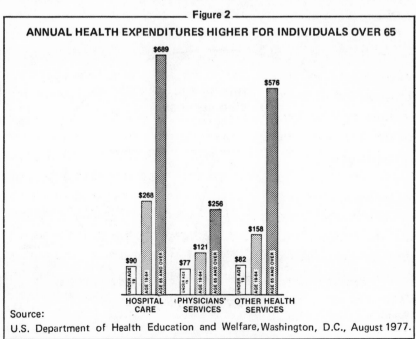

_____ Figure 2 _____

ANNUAL HEALTH EXPENDITURES HIGHER FOR INDIVIDUALS OVER 65

HOSPITAL CARE   PHYSICIANS' SERVICES   OTHER HEALTH SERVICES

Source:
U.S. Department of Health Education and Welfare, Washington, D.C., August 1977.

Note: The category "other health services" includes such items as dentist and other professional services, drug and drug sundries, eyeglasses and appliances, nursing home care, and other services.

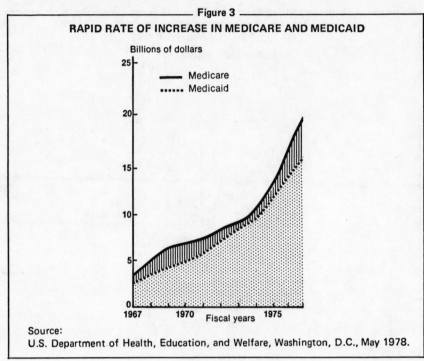

Figure 3

RAPID RATE OF INCREASE IN MEDICARE AND MEDICAID

Billions of dollars

—— Medicare
····· Medicaid

1967   1970   Fiscal years   1975

Source:
U.S. Department of Health, Education, and Welfare, Washington, D.C., May 1978.

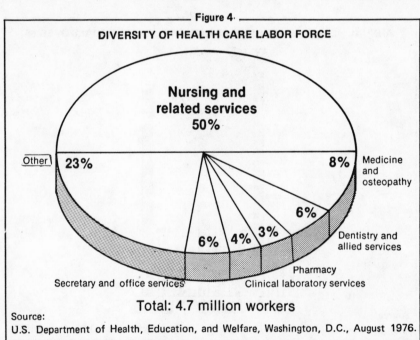

Figure 4

DIVERSITY OF HEALTH CARE LABOR FORCE

Nursing and
related services
50%

Other 23%

8% Medicine
and
osteopathy

6%

Dentistry and
allied services

6%   4%   3%

Pharmacy

Secretary and office services

Clinical laboratory services

Total: 4.7 million workers

Source:
U.S. Department of Health, Education, and Welfare, Washington, D.C., August 1976.

CHAPTER 2

The American Physician:
A Tarnished Halo

THE RINGING INDICTMENT by one of our nation's leading newspapers is that the phrase, "physician heal thyself," now seems to mean "physician get thyself well-heeled."[1] The media is filled with revelations of physician fraud and corruption. The American doctor and his manner of practice are being attacked today as never before. Though still ranking high in popularity polls relative to other professions, the physician's popularity has been slipping from an approval rate of 72 percent in 1966 Harris poll, to a figure of 43 percent in a 1976 Harris poll.[2] However, in December 1977 the same poll showed a reversal in the approval rate when 55 percent of the public expressed confidence in the medical profession. But the public's vote of confidence has yet to attain the level of 1966.

The physician's decline in public esteem seems to have paralleled the decline of the American presidency. The office of the presidency has declined from the lofty Democratic ideals of Thomas Jefferson to the statement of former president Richard Nixon "I am not a crook." Similarly, the physician seems to have lost the idealism of the oath of Hippocrates.

Everywhere the physician looks someone is either investigating the way he practices medicine or endeavoring to change the manner by which he delivers his services. Thus, the U.S. Congress enacts a Professional Standards Review Organization law in 1972, a Health Maintenance Organization law in 1973, and a new health planning law in 1974—all of which impinge upon or will change, in some respect, his manner of medical practice. In August 1976, the U. S. Department of Health, Education, and Welfare establishes a new drug program called Maximum Allowable Cost. This program influences the drugs the physician prescribes to patients who qualify for such public programs as Medicaid. At the same time states are repealing their drug antisubstitution laws. In addition, insurance companies are dropping the physician's malpractice insurance, partly, because he is being sued by his patients in ever increasing numbers. This situation makes it very difficult for the doctor to practice at all. Meanwhile, agencies such as the Federal Trade Commission are investigating his manner of practice. The physician is accused of defrauding Medicare and Medicaid out of greed; he is accused of performing unnecessary surgery out of greed; he is accused of acting out of greed in overprescribing drugs which may result in needless patient's deaths or dependency, due to the alleged influence of drug industry advertising, and the list goes on. These charges are being made even though most physicians are highly ethical practitioners and polls reveal most patients are satisfied with their own doctor. However, exposure of unethical practices among a small minority of doctors can plant suspicions in the public's mind that such accusations are true for other physicians it does not personally know.

What has happened to American medicine? How did the image of the noble doctor, the saviour of life and healer of the sick, reach such a state that the physician is under the microscope of public scrutiny? Why is he beset with so many problems? How are all these public and private activities affecting the practice of medicine? When the practice of medicine is affected so is the delivery of health services. When that happens the general public and the individual patients who constitute that public pay the price. However, before discussing these issues, it is worthwhile to examine the profile of the American physician around whom these controversies swirl.

Physician's Profile

As of December 31, 1974, there were 379,748 physicians in the United States or one for every 566 persons. About 79 percent of the number of physicians were classified as active and involved in providing direct patient care as their primary activity. The remaining

21 percent were involved in a myriad of activities including hospital and medical administration, research, medical education as well as private business such as being employed in the pharmaceutical and insurance industry.

While the solo practitioner still delivers a substantial portion of the nation's health care, medical group practice is growing significantly. As of December 31, 1975, about 23.5 percent of the active physicians in the private sector were providing health care through a group delivery mode.   2032124

As studies exhibit, the availability of physicians varies widely throughout the country. The site of their medical practice is influenced by such factors as the number of hospital beds, average income and population size of the area. In 1973, about 86 percent of the physicians who provided patient care practiced in metropolitan areas. The greatest concentration of physicians is found in the northeastern part of the country, such as Connecticut, Massachusetts, and New York and in the west, as in California. The lowest concentration of doctors is found in the rural south such as Arkansas, Mississippi and Alabama as well as in rural western states such as North and South Dakota, Wyoming, Idaho and Alaska.[3]

Expenditures for physician services has grown enormously over the years. In 1950, only $2.7 billion was spent for physician care. But by 1977 after the advent of such public programs as Medicare and Medicaid, and the continuing expansion of private health insurance coverage, physician income had risen to $32.2 billion. The estimated average net income of physicians reached the sum of $51,224 in 1974. When examined by professional specialty, net income averaged the highest for surgeons ($60,031) and the lowest for psychiatrists ($39,997) in that year. Today doctors earn more than five times as much as the nation's average wage earner and twice as much as lawyers.

Clearly, physicians represent an affluent professional class within our society. Despite the protests of organized medicine against the enactment of Medicare and Medicaid during the early

1960s, the American doctor has not suffered financially from the establishment of these programs. In fact, the impact of these and other government programs has been to increase the physician's income. In 1965, for example, only 6 percent of the physicians' $8.4 billion income came from public programs. In 1975, these programs accounted for 27 percent of their $22.1 billion income.[4] In other words, the income of physicians from government programs rose from about $500 million to almost $6 billion—an increase of 1200 percent in only ten years.

Yet, despite the ability of more people to pay for their medical care either tnrough the availability of public programs or private health insurance coverage, the nation has not been able to induce physicians to practice in areas of the country where there is still a need for medical services, particularly general practitioners. The irony of the situation is that despite the need, the number of physicians who now elect to be general practitioners has been a declining proportion of the total physician population. In 1968 general practitioners represented 23 percent of the total doctors in this country and in 1974 they accounted for only 18 percent of the profession. This trend does not appear to be reversing itself in the immediate future. Such is the paradox of America. While we remain the wealthiest nation in the world, 16 million Americans—7 million of whom live in our inner cities and the remainder in rural areas—still dwell in communities which the federal government designated as having a doctor shortage during 1977.

Potential Scandals

As the previous figures show, the health care field has grown very rapidly in the past quarter century, especially in terms of the amount of money which is being expended not only for physician care but also the other services which presently constitute the multi-billion dollar health care industry. Where money abounds, scandals also tend to appear.

Former Senator Frank Moss, testified in 1976 before the Senate Finance Committee that doctors, laboratory owners, nursing home operators, and others cheated the Medicare program out of $1.5 billion or 10 percent of the $15 billion the government spent on Medicare that year. In other words, 10 percent off the top went for fraud. Senator Moss cited various examples of fraud including a laboratory owner making kickbacks to a doctor who sent him business, a doctor removing warts and charging for the removal of cancerous lesions, and a doctor who walked through a nursing home once a month and filed claims for alleged visits to patients. As bad as abuses were under Medicare, Senator Moss indicated that the fraud perpetuated in the Medicaid program was even worse. "Medicare," he said, "is light years ahead of Medicaid from the point of view of fiscal integrity. Medicaid is almost completely without controls."[5] Another report, issued by the General Accounting Office (GAO), the official watchdog agency of the U. S. Congress, in the summer of 1976 described price gouging by physicians on laboratory tests for Medicare and Medicaid patients. The GAO's sampling in four states showed that three-fifths of the doctors reviewed were adding markups of 100 percent to 400 percent to commercial laboratory charges. In one case cited, a Florida doctor charged Medicaid $20 for a test for which he paid the laboratory only $4. The physicians apparently were ignoring an American Medical Association resolution declaring that "any markup, commission or profit by doctors on outside laboratory tests amounts to exploitation of the patient." Also, it appears that few of the abusers are ever punished. Senator Moss noted that of 9,907 physician-related fraud cases in Medicare since 1971, only 400 were referred to the Justice Department. Fewer than 60 were convicted. Only 15 served time in jail, Senator Moss stated, and only two have had their medical licenses suspended. "The message we give to physicians," Senator Moss said, is: "Go ahead and steal. The worse thing that can happen to you is that you will be asked to pay some money back. The odds are you will never get caught." But Senator Moss also stated that of the 250,000 doctors participating in Medicare, *only 4 percent* have committed fraud-involving each year about 10 percent of the $3 billion in

Medicare physician payments—while *another 6 percent* have abused the program since 1971. Abuse is a wide variety of program violations, excessive services and improper practices not involving prosecutable fraud.

According to Senator Moss, the most common kinds of Medicare fraud and abuse practiced by some physicians are the following:

- Charging for services not rendered.
- Charging for work performed by others unqualified to receive Medicare payments.
- Soliciting, offering or receiving kickbacks.
- Upgrading of claims, that is, charging for major surgery when minor work was done.
- Unnecessary surgery.
- Gang visits to nursing homes—walking through a facility and billing every patient in the home for a visit and examination.
- Overutilization, that is, bringing patients back to the office again and again though there is no medical necessity for the visit.
- Brokering or laboratory procedures—billing as if laboratory tests were performed personally and by hand when, in fact, they were performed at an automated laboratory for a fraction of the cost.
- Charging patients for service after accepting Medicare assignment.

Given the variety of abuses, why are so many cases declined for prosecution by the Department of Justice? According to Senator Moss, U.S. Attorneys refuse to take Medicare cases for many reasons, ranging from a heavy workload to the difficulty of transporting witnesses to and from court. The principal reason seems to be that the beneficiaries who complain are the key witnesses in the case against physicians who are generally well thought of in the community. Also, Medicare by definition is limited to the aged and disabled. Quite often, beneficiaries are ill or have died before the cases can be prepared. But according to Senator Moss it appears that U.S. Attorneys and their staff do not regard Medicare cases as glamorous and dealing with the elderly is viewed as difficult.

Some of the reasons for declining cases, as viewed by Senator Moss and his staff from the files, include:

- "The witnesses are elderly. They make poor witnesses. They can't remember the exact nature of services they received."
- "The witnesses are aged and senile. They are at a disadvantage in testifying against articulate and well educated physicians."
- "The lawyers the physician has hired are strong and there is little likelihood we can win the case given the current nature of our proof."
- "There is no way to disprove the diagnosis which prompted the doctor's treatment. We can't find anyone who will question his medical judgment."
- "The medical profession is held in high esteem. To overcome a doctor's favorable image, in a passive crime such as this the case must be fairly aggravated, which is not shown in this case."
- "There is no evidence the physician is continuing to engage in fraudulent practices."

Under these circumstances, Senator Herman Talmadge sponsored a bill in 1976 to correct abuses under the Medicare-Medicaid programs. The measure died as Congress adjourned for the 1976 elections. However, the legislation was not a total loss. One section of the bill was hurriedly attached to an unrelated bill which was enacted into law. The final result was an amendment which created within HEW an Office of Inspector General with a special Medicare-Medicaid investigative unit to oversee program abuses. When Congress reconvened in January 1977, Senator Herman Talmadge reintroduced a bill to bring about administrative and reimbursement reforms to correct program abuses in Medicare and Medicaid. The bill, the Medicare-Medicaid Anti-Fraud and Abuse Amendments, was passed by Congress and signed into law by President Carter in October 1977. In addition to other provisions, the law toughens penalties for doctors and pharmacists who defraud the government's Medicare and Medicaid programs. The legislation makes such an act a felony subject to a maximum sentence of five years in prison, a $25,000 fine, or both. The bill apparently became law just in time. A few weeks later in November 1977, HEW computers, examining the bills paid by the Medicaid program for 1976, buttressed the necessity for the law and confirmed Senator Moss's worst fears about the programs. By using a series of computer "screens," which identify questionable billing, HEW spotted initially 47,000 cases. Of these, about 2500 cases—1400 physicians and 1100 pharmacists—appeared to contain some form of "blatant abuse." Some examples which were found include the following:

- A doctor presented bills for performing three hysterectomies in one year and was paid. According to the bills, the hysterectomies were performed on the same woman.

- A pharmacist billed Medicaid for 478 prescriptions in one year, all for the same person.

- A doctor was paid for making 33,918 home visits to Medicaid patients in 1976. That is roughly one visit every 15 minutes, assuming the doctor worked a 24-hour day, 365 days a year.[6]

Fifty cases, 25 of them involving possible fraud by physicians and 25 involving pharmacists, have been sent to prosecutors. In March 1978, HEW's Inspector General reported that fraud, waste and abuse had cost Medicaid between $2.3 billion and $2.6 billion and Medicare about $2.2 billion in fiscal 1977. That amounts to about one out of every five dollars for Medicaid and one in ten for Medicare. Is it any wonder that Congress deems it necessary to pass laws which make fraudulent delivery of health care services an offense punishable by imprisonment under specified circumstances.

Federal Trade Commission Investigations

Congress is not alone in investigating the medical profession. The executive branch of the federal government also is beginning to investigate organized medicine. In December 1975, the Federal Trade Commission (FTC) began to take action to remove some of the mystery from medicine by allowing doctors to provide information about their fees, qualifications and services to potential patients. The federal agency moved in this direction by charging that the American Medical Association's ban against physician advertising violates the antitrust laws and illegally stabilizes or fixes fees for doctors' services. Specifically, the FTC filed a complaint attacking a section of the AMA's Principles of Medical Ethics which prohibit doctors from soliciting business through such means. The FTC contends the prohibition against advertising stifles competition between doctors in the provision of services, deprives patients of the benefits of competition and of the information which is pertinent to selecting a physician. An FTC official refused to speculate whether advertising would drive down medical fees, or at least slow their rapid rise. However, he did say that should the FTC's action be successful it would have a substantial effect on the medical profession. "We would hope, at the very least, that the public would be made aware of the prices doctors are charging for specific services, the qualifications of doctors, which medical schools they attended, their specialties and the honors they have received. This information, according to the FTC official, should provide the public with a decisional basis for selecting a doctor."[7]

However, the Montgomery County Medical Society in Maryland is not awaiting any Federal Trade Commission decision in this regard. The society has initiated a program called the Montgomery County Patient Advocacy Referral Service. The kind of problems which the program handles includes patients who need transportation to get to a doctor, individuals who cannot speak English in seeking medical care, individuals who are not satisfied with the patient care they presently are receiving, people who do not know how to find a doctor, and others who have difficulty in explaining their needs to a physician and need someone to do it for them. The service lists about 570 physicians all of whom are members of the county medical society. The program also has a quality control system. Patient complaints are referred to the medical society. The idea of the service is to tailor the doctor to the individual's needs and offer the person a choice of several doctors. The prospective patient will ask for a certain kind of doctor who has a particular specialty and skills. The medical society maintains such information. The service also follows up difficult cases. Patients are encouraged to call the service and let the program know if they have obtained care. If they do not call back, then the service will call the patients within a day or two to make sure they received help. The program has been so successful that other counties and cities around the country are using it as a model. Perhaps, the Montgomery County Medical Society has implemented a concept which will resolve one of this nation's most vexing health care problems—how do you find a qualified physician when you need medical care and do not know where to look. Perhaps, your own county medical society also can help you in this regard. You should ask and find out.

Aside from county medical societies, other sources exist for finding a physician. If you are moving from one location to another, your present physician, pharmacist, friend or family member may know of doctors in your new area in whom they have confidence. In addition, local accredited hospitals or a medical school, if one is located near your community, can assist you in finding the kind of specialist you seek. In case of emergencies, the most convenient source of assistance in any urban or suburban community, if you cannot reach a physician, is the local police or fire department. There even might be a volunteer ambulance corps available in your community which provides emergency transportation to a hospital. Also, remember hospitals maintain emergency facilities which are staffed 24 hours per day. Finally, ask the local or state medical societies whether physician directories exist in your community which list a doctor's education, training, board certification, if any, hospital affiliations, fees, whether he makes house calls and is a member of the local medical society and other information which profile his professional qualifications and manner of medical practice. Although these directories are not yet commonplace, some medical societies have begun to develop such publications. It is to your advantage to find out if your community has such information.

But until such directories become nationwide in scope the Federal Trade Commission believes it is necessary to institute action to help bring physician information to the patient-consumer.

The Federal Trade Commission files a complaint when it has a reason to believe the law has been violated. The complaint, adopted by a unanimous vote, is only the first step in a series of long proceedings. In the fall of 1977, a hearing began before an FTC administrative law judge, whose initial decision may be appealed to the commission. If the panel decides against the American Medical Association, the organization may challenge that ruling in the courts. Although the AMA's Principles of Medical Ethics do not act as an ironclad ban on advertising by physicians, the ethics are considered by the FTC to constitute an agreement resulting in a restraint of advertising and, therefore, restrictions on free trade.[8] The FTC position is that medicine is a trade or a business like others and should be subject to regulation to permit free competition without restrictions on prices or availability of service. The AMA's response to the Federal Trade Commission's action was quite direct. According to former AMA Board Chairman Raymond T. Holden, MD, and former AMA President Max H. Parrott, MD, "Advertising by a professional is the very antithesis of professionalism. We think there is enough hucksterism in this country without hucksterism in medicine. And we are going to fight it."[9] How successful the American Medical Association will be in its fight may turn upon a decision handed down by the Supreme Court of the United States in June 1977. In that month the Supreme Court ruled in *Bates and O'Steen v. State Bar of Arizona* that advertising by an attorney as to his rates for routine services cannot validly be prohibited. The case applied to lawyers but possibly might be extended to physicians. The Supreme Court did not rule on the antitrust question because states are exempt from antitrust laws. But any private organization within a state which restricts advertising may be subject to freedom of speech and antitrust law violations.

Lawyers say that the FTC complaint arises from the Goldfarb

case of 1975 *(Goldfarb v. Virginia State Bar and Fairfax County Bar Association)* when the Supreme Court ruled that lawyers were not permitted to fix fees through local bar associations. Although the FTC complaint against the AMA does not exactly parallel the Goldfarb case, the real issue is whether the professions of law and medicine are subject to the same laws and regulations as other forms of private enterprise. The Goldfarb ruling, one lawyer pointed out, opened the door for federal antitrust action against the professions, including medicine.[10]

The dust had barely settled from FTC's dramatic announcement of investigating the ban of physician advertisements when the federal agency struck again two months later. In February 1976, the FTC announced it was investigating possible antitrust violations resulting from physician control of the Blue Shield plans. The investigation will examine the nature and extent of such control on 71 individual Blue Shield plans and on the National Association of Blue Shield Plans which had merged with the national Blue Cross Association, effective January 1978. The FTC stated in its announcement that the investigation does not imply that legal violations had occurred. According to FTC sources, the commission wishes to examine the effect the plan's reimbursement level has on local medical service rates. Consumer advocates charge that Blue Shield boards have been too lenient in setting their reimbursement rates and thus have contributed to the surging costs of medical care. An FTC staff member noted that physicians initiated the Blue Shield plans during the 1930's to help patients who could not pay their bills. He added that the local plans remain closely affiliated with local and national medical societies. The FTC has stated that about 40 percent of the population pays for physician services through Blue Shield plans. Thus, the policies and practices of the plans may affect fee levels and other forms of competition in the provision of health care.[11]

The medical community again was taken aback two months later. In April 1976, the FTC announced it had begun an investigation to determine whether or not the American Medical

Association may have illegally restrained the supply of physicians and health care services through activities relating to the accreditation of medical schools and graduate programs; definitions of fields of practice for physicians and allied health personnel; and limitations on forms of health care delivery consistent with a traditional fee-for-service approach.[12] Then, in the summer of 1976, the FTC announced still another investigation, this one possibly affecting the physician's prescribing practices. The agency stated the study will explore in connection with the sale of multi-source drugs whether consumers are being subjected to unfair or deceptive acts or practices anywhere in the United States, in or affecting commerce, including whether price competition or product information is unduly restricted by state or private action. The commission unanimously authorized the investigation to help answer such questions as:

Is it in the public interest to permit pharmacists to select less costly sources of prescription drugs prescribed by a doctor by brand name if the doctor does not object?

Would consumers actually save and if so, how much, if doctors delegate more authority to pharmacists to select less costly sources?

Is price competition unfairly impeded in the distribution of multiple source prescription drugs, due to state or private action?[13]

As always, the Federal Trade Commission stated that the investigation does not imply that violations of law actually occurred. What is being witnessed today is a more aggressive federal government taking steps to see why the costs of health care continue to skyrocket, what role, if any, the physician has in this escalation and what remedies can be adopted to slow down such increases. If physicians are committing fraud under public medical care programs such as Medicaid and Medicare, then the counterattack of the federal government, as exemplified in part by the FTC investigations, is of the physicians' own doing. The federal government dispenses billions of dollars through its various programs to help those in our society who cannot help themselves. But, the accompanying abuse, by those the government enlists to help those in need, may even cause the government to take away the privileges which it so accorded. When you add up investigations into the advertising ban on physician services, physician fee payments through third party organizations, medical education and physician prescribing habits, the government is now focusing on the very reason for the physician's being, namely the manner in which he practices medicine and what measures, if any, can be taken to alter it.

Prescription Drugs, Laws and Programs

Congress and the Federal Trade Commission are not the only governmental bodies investigating the way medicine is being practiced. Our state legislatures and the U.S. Department of Health, Education, and Welfare are also active in adopting measures affecting organized medicine. One of their activities relates to drugs and the way they are prescribed and dispensed. Since 1970 pharmacy groups have been lobbying for the repeal of state antisubstitution laws which, upon repeal, will give the pharmacist the right to substitute lower priced generically equivalent medication for the physician's recommended brand name item.

There has been a great deal of debate generated by those who advocate and those who oppose the repeal of drug antisubstitution laws. For example, *who* assumes the legal liability if a patient suffers an adverse drug reaction when drug substitution takes place? Some say it is the physician. Others say it is the pharmacist. Still others state it is both the pharmacist and the physician, depending upon the circumstances of the case. Another debated issue is whether a substituted drug product has the same bioequivalency as the drug product for which it is submitted. Bioequivalency is those chemical equivalents which when administered in the same amounts will provide the same biological or physicological availability as measured by such criteria as blood levels. A chemical equivalent drug refers to those multi-source drug products which essentially contain identical amounts of identical active ingredients, in the identical dosage forms and which meet existing physico-chemical standards in the official compendia.

While these debates continue, by the winter of 1978, thirty jurisdictions had repealed or at least modified their antisubstitution laws in some form or other. For example, in Florida the physician must write in his own handwriting "medically necessary" on his prescription if he wishes to stop substitution. In Alaska the doctor's prescription blank has two imprinted boxes. One box reads "dispense as written" (DAW) while the other allows for substitution. If the physician checks the DAW box, the pharmacist must follow his instructions. Several states, including Michigan, Oregon, and Arkansas, allow the physician's handwritten DAW to stand as a veto to the substitution. Not all the laws specify the substitution of a lower priced generic drug product.[14] Of all the states which allow substitution of generic drugs, only New York has a Food and Drug Administration approved list of some 2,000 generic drugs considered equivalent to brand-name products. The *generic* name is the established or official name given to a drug or drug product while the *brand* name is the registered trademark given to a specific drug product by its manufacturer. In terms of a pharmacists' liability the druggist is exempt from liability in making substitutions in such states as Florida, Oregon, California, Colorado, Rhode Island and the District of Columbia.[15]

However, regardless of the form the repeal or modification of the antisubstitution law may assume, the factor of drug product selection brings the pharmacist and the physician into closer partnership in regard to maintaining the patient's health and well-being. Repeal of antisubstitution laws also gives a boost to generic prescribing. If the substituted drug performs, from the physician's viewpoint, as effectively as the brand name product which he had prescribed in the past and if the physician had not used the generic drug prior to the pharmacists' substitution of it, then the physician may begin to prescribe the generic drug for his other patients as well. Thus, the physician may save the patient the difference in price between the generic drug and the brand name product. In addition, physicians collectively, through their drug prescribing, can alter the pattern of drug distribution and sales from brand name products to generic drug products. Anticipating that savings will accrue to the public from the substitution of a generic drug for a brand name product, consumer oriented groups have joined with pharmacy groups in seeking repeal of such antisubsti tution laws.

While antisubstitution laws are slowly being repealed by our state legislatures around the country, the U. S. Department of Health, Education, and Welfare took another step which will alter the physician's prescribing habits. In August 1976, a new program called Maximum Allowable Cost (MAC) went into effect. The program puts a price ceiling on prescription drugs whose patents have expired, which are produced by more than one company and which are covered by Medicare, Medicaid, and child health programs. Although the MAC applies to the three programs, government savings are expected to come almost exclusively from Medicaid. Medicare does not as yet cover out-of-hospital drugs and most hospitals enforce their own cost controls on in-patient drugs. In 1975, the American Medical Association, the Pharmaceutical Manufacturers Association and five doctors filed a suit against HEW in the Chicago Federal District Court. The American Medical Association argued that the MAC program would interfere with the traditional prerogatives of the physicians. The Pharmaceutical Manufacturers Association argued that the program would intrude on the professional perogatives of the doctor and the pharmacist, would disrupt pharmaceutical distribution patterns and possibly result in inferior drugs for Medicare and Medicaid patients. It should be noted that the program also could affect the profits of the $9.4 billion domestic pharmaceutical industry to an unknown degree. In March 1977, the Chicago Federal District Court dismissed the suit against HEW with a 74 page opinion which concluded that all of the objections to the MAC program were without legal merit.

In establishing the MAC program, HEW announced it will send

lists of drug price comparisons to physicians and pharmacists in order to encourage them to reduce patient costs. The significance of this announcement to the pharmaceutical industry is similar to the economic impact which the repeal of the antisubstitution laws creates. If a physician begins to prescribe a generic drug which is less expensive than a brand name product but one which he has not prescribed previously and if in his judgement the effectiveness of the generic drug is equal to that of brand name drug product in treating the illness at hand, then the physician could begin to prescribe the same generic drug for his non-Medicaid patients as well. In this manner the sales and distribution pattern of prescription medicine by the American pharmaceutical industry will be dramatically altered over time. Companies depending essentially on brand name drug sales could find their profits declining unless they can meet the price competition offered by generic drugs or unless they diversify into other health care areas such as medical devices or into non-health care business operations. As far as the U. S. Department of Health, Education, and Welfare is concerned, the MAC program is essential. It is one of the building blocks to control health care costs in the event of any national health insurance program.

The battle for and against the MAC program is deeply intertwined with repeal or modification of the antisubstitution laws. Those laws were originally passed many years ago to prevent the pharmacist from substituting home-brewed nostrums for doctor-prescribed patent medicines. Those who favor the creation of the MAC program state that the antisubstitution laws now function to support artificially high prices for brand name drugs. It is argued that physicians have become accustomed to prescribing the brand name products under heavy drug company advertising during the years of their patent protection. As a result of this situation, the proponents of the Maximum Allowable Cost drug program contend it is almost impossible to persuade the physicians to prescribe a less expensive generic drug product or even a competitive brand name drug. These advocates state the MAC drug program destroys this artificial support while permitting the physician to insist on a specific brand if he feels it is genuinely superior. HEW regulations provide for a notation by the physician requiring a specific brand without substitution. However, without a notation the pharmacist will telephone the physician for permission to substitute the MAC drug, thus forcing the physician to make a deliberate rather than an habitual choice.

But the opponents of the MAC program also have their arguments. They state that chemically identical prescription drugs are not necessarily bioequivalent, that is, they may not have the same curative effects. As already noted, this argument is also used in their battle against the repeal of state antisubstitution laws. In rebuttal, a Food and Drug Administration (FDA) official, who is associated with the MAC program, has stated that FDA rules will eventually eliminate variations in bioequivalency. Before a MAC limit is proposed, the drug will be studied by the FDA to assure that there is no unresolved quality or bioequivalency problems which would warrant delay in setting a MAC limit for that drug. Dr. Donald Kennedy, Commissioner of the Food and Drug Administration, stated in Congressional testimony during 1977 that:

"We find no evidence of widespread differences between the products of large and small firms or between brand name and generic drugs."[16]

Under regulations issued in preparation for the Maximum Allowable Cost drug program, manufacturers of generic drugs with known variations must match the effectiveness of the standard drugs or withdraw their drugs from the market. Meanwhile, HEW's Pharmaceutical Reimbursement Advisory Board will set MAC limits only for drugs of proven bioequivalency, eventually including up to 50 or more drugs which account for the majority of all prescriptions involving multi-source drugs. In October 1976, HEW's Pharmaceutical Reimbursement Advisory Board recommended a maximum allowable cost limit for ampicillin tryhydrate and ampicillin anhydrous. This was the first drug considered for the MAC limit. The Advisory Board recommended that a MAC be set at $7.25 per 100 capsules at 250 milligram strength and $13.90 per 100 capsules at

500 milligram strength. These are only recommendations to HEW. After the MAC for any drug is approved by the advisory committee, it must be published as a proposal in the government's *Federal Register*. This allows time for comments and hearings before the MAC limit becomes effective, should that prove to be the case. On June 27, 1977 the price ceiling for ampicillin went into effect. Should the price of a drug product, for which a MAC limit has been set, rise or fall in the market place due to an increase or decrease in its supply, then after appropriate review by HEW, the MAC limit can be adjusted upward or downward as the circumstances may warrant.

The impact of the MAC program will not be felt immediately. HEW expected only limited savings in the program's first year of operation. But a great deal of savings is expected in future years. An estimated $3 billion is involved in the cost of purchasing drugs as financed by Medicaid, Medicare and child health programs. However, pharmaceutical industry representatives are divided in their opinion as to the eventual impact of the MAC program. Some believe that generic drug manufacturers, bearing the cost of the research and development necessary to attain bioequivalency, will increase their product prices and brand name manufacturers will reduce their prices, or else lose a large part of their market. Thus, there would be a narrowing of prices between brand name and generic drug producers. Others state that lower industry profits may mean a curtailment of research due to a lack of money where the market for a particular drug may not be very large because of its specialized nature, or the uniqueness of the disease. Others say that research will not be affected because manufacturers will recoup their financial losses by charging more for their patented specialties and by increasing research on patentable drugs. Still others feel that nothing will happen in terms of prices because the price competition which HEW expects to take place has already occurred. This is because generic prescribing has been growing in the past several years and the manufacturers of brand names have had to review their price levels in view of the increase in generic prescribing. But whatever does happen in regard to prescription drug prices and the physician's prescribing habits, one fact is certain—government, both federal and state, is acting in many different areas of medicine to affect it in ways never before contemplated. Only time will permit ultimate judgement as to whether the American public will be the positive beneficiaries of such activities.

However, until that time arrives and regardless of the merits or the demerits of the debates taking place in the medical and pharmaceutical fields, be they for or against the repeal of antisubstitution laws, or the scientific discourse on the chemical and therapeutic equivalency of drug products, or the technicalities involved in establishing and administering a Maximum Allowable Cost drug program, one thought should be stressed. These discussions may be beyond the everyday interest of the ordinary citizen. But the outcome of these political, economic and scientific debates will become apparent when it comes time for the individual patient to pay for his prescription medicine. Regardless of whether scientists agree or disagree that generic drugs are inferior, equal or superior to brand name drugs, there is no disagreement that generic drugs are less expensive than their brand name counterparts. As a consumer and as a patient, you should be aware of the course and outcome of these debates as they indicate positive action you can take for your own benefit. The next time you obtain a prescription from your physician, you should ask your doctor if he knows of a generic drug product which can achieve the same medical therapy for which the brand name drug is being prescribed and what is the difference in price. If there is such a generic drug product available, find out if your state allows for its substitution and if your physician will recommend such a change. Also, ask your physician if he can recommend pharmacies in your local area which offer quality drugs at lowest cost. If you are able, shop around and compare the drug prices among the pharmacies since variations in price for the same brand can be very great. In addition, you may want to ask your physician if he has any prescription drug samples from the pharmaceutical companies. In this way, you do not have to purchase your initial supply. Also, you can test the medication for its effectiveness before you purchase a large supply. In addition, you have the opportunity to report your findings to your physician which will allow him to prescribe another medication which he may feel is more useful in alleviating your ailment. Also, ask your physician if you can save money by buying as large a quantity of a prescribed drug as will remain fresh at the rate you use them. In this way and with this knowledge you can control your personal drug expenses to some extent and perhaps reduce their costs.

Malpractice Insurance Crisis

The physician is not only under attack from government, but he is also encountering problems with those elements within the private sector, such as the commercial insurance industry, which also influence and affect his practice of medicine. Increasingly, private carriers have been cancelling their malpractice insurance coverage for practicing physicians. There are a number of reasons for this, including the rise in the number of malpractice suits filed against physicians, higher jury awards, and initial premium ratings which proved to be inadequate to cover losses incurred when judgements were rendered years after the suit was initially filed. But whatever the reasons may be, the impact on the practice of medicine is becoming very marked.

Some doctors, in seeking a personal way out of the malpractice mess, have left high insurance premium states such as California and New York and have relocated in less costly insurance states such as Indiana and Mississippi. Ironically, an unexpected and unintended by-product of the malpractice insurance crisis is the redistribution of medical manpower from highly concentrated areas to those parts of the country where there are physician shortages. Other physicians have found a haven in the federal service—the military, the Veterans Administration or the Public Health Service—or in an organization which pays their malpractice insurance premiums such as a health maintenance organization. Still other doctors have taken the offensive by establishing medical liability insurance companies in order to protect themselves financially against malpractice litigation. Some physicians even are beginning to countersue those former patients who they believe wrongfully have taken them to court. And more than a few doctors have left the practice of medicine altogether, either by quitting or retiring early. Those still in practice, who have lost their malpractice insurance coverage, have been forced to limit and modify their methods by practicing defensive medicine such as ordering extensive tests and X-rays. This is as much for their own protection as for that of the patient.

The reasons for the sudden emergence of medical malpractice into a national crisis, in addition to the reasons already mentioned, can be found in some of the statistics being published about the way medicine is being practiced today. During 1976, for example, the Subcommittee on Oversight and Investigations of the Committee on Interstate and Foreign Commerce of the U. S. House of Representatives held hearings on the subject of unnecessary surgery. The Committee report, entitled "Cost and Quality of Health Care: Unnecessary Surgery," alleged that 2.38 million unnecessary operations were performed in the United States in 1974 and resulted in 11,900 deaths and an expenditure of $3.92 billion dollars.[17] However, the American Medical Association disagrees with these findings and the procedures, data and definitions used, claiming data from limited regional studies were extrapolated to encompass all surgical procedures performed in the United States. However, some physicians believe there is unnecessary surgery in various areas, for example in tonsilectomies and hysterectomies. Dr. Edward Berman, past President of MEDICO and a former teacher at Johns Hopkins Medical School says:

"We know that there's a million and a half tonsilectomies done a year. I would say that if 25,000 are necessary, it's a lot. This has become a routine whereby the parents think there's something wrong with the doctor unless he takes the kid's tonsils out by the age of four or five. The other one is the hysterectomy and I've seen this with the professors in the medical schools down to the sleeziest abortionists. The easiest thing to do with a female's complaint—and females are the bulk of office visits—is to remove the uterus. There's always an excuse for it. First, sooner or later, it's going to get into trouble. The menopause will come anyway. While you're in the abdomen why leave in something potentially dangerous? Well, this is all baloney, you know. There is no reason for a uterus to come out anymore than a gallbladder to come out unless it's pathologic."[18]

And the Carter Administration has backed up the charges being made that excess surgery is being performed in this country. In the fall of 1977, Undersecretary of HEW, Hale Champion, praised the House Commerce Subcommittee for its focus on the unnecessary surgery issue:

"For three years, this subcommittee has tried to point out that there is too much unnecessary or inappropriate surgery in this country. For three years this subcommittee has been right ... While experts may argue over some of the data and exactly what it means, the evidence seems clear to me ... We have to recognize that there are many thousands more surgeons than we need, and cut back significantly on the number trained at public expense ... Surgeons, as you might expect, favor a surgical approach to medical problems. And the result is that excess surgeons lead to excess surgery."[19]

Consequently, in an attempt to reduce the amount of unnecessary surgery being performed in this country, the U. S. Department of Health, Education, and Welfare formulated a new policy in the fall of 1977. HEW plans to pay for any second opinion on an elective surgery which a Medicare or Medicaid patient seeks on a voluntary basis. This program has the following significance. If your doctor tells you that you require surgery you will be able to consult another physician for a second opinion to determine whether the operation is necessary. The government will pay for your visit under the Medicare and Medicaid programs. Eighty percent of the reasonable charge will be reimbursed under Medicare while Medicaid participation and payments are at the option of the state. Also, if you have a private health insurance plan such as Blue Cross or commercial health insurance, you should find out if your health insurance policy now includes a second surgical opinion as a benefit.

Remember, it is still your decision whether you want the operation. You are entitled to have your family physician and surgeon explain all the alternatives which may be available in place of surgery as well as all the complications which may result from an operation. In fact, a doctor who fails to inform you about the risks of surgery may himself be subject to a possible malpractice suit. Under the legal doctrine of informed consent, a patient who has not been fairly advised about the risks of surgery has not legally consented to it. He may, therefore, sue for malpractice any physician who operates on him without fairly disclosing the risks.

In the fall of 1977 HEW made a further attempt, aside from its second opinion surgery plan, to curb unnecessary surgery and place doctors who perform such procedures under even greater scrutiny of their physician peers. HEW ordered its agency which is responsible for the activities of Professional Standards Review Organizations (PSROs) to develop, with the advice of the National PSRO Council, criteria which operational PSROs throughout the country can use to determine whether a surgical procedure is necessary. HEW hopes that by the winter of 1979 criteria for 75 percent of most common surgical procedures within each surgical specialty will be developed—criteria which are specific and measurable and which can be applied by the local PSROs. Thus, the federal government has begun moving aggressively into the operating rooms of our nation's hospitals in an attempt to curb one aspect of medical practice which the government believes is being abused. At the same time, HEW, in promoting HMO development, has noted that surgeons in health maintenance organizations operate only half as much as those who are paid by fee-for-service. The question now arises as to what other medical procedures are being overutilized in the government's opinion to warrant its intervention into the practice of medicine.

But whether the physician is being sued on grounds of improper surgery or other grounds, there may be more behind the reasons for filing a malpractice suit than just a lack of skill or improper judgement at a particular moment. One important reason for a physician's improper performance is his failure to keep abreast of the latest developments in medicine. Patients also suffer at the hands of doctors who because of the generally permissive attitude of the medical profession are legally free to undertake procedures which they have not been trained to handle. Dr. Robert C. Derbyshire, a Santa Fe surgeon and an authority on medical licensing and the disciplining of erring physicians, has estimated that at least 5 percent, or more than 17,000, of the country's physicians are unfit to practice medicine.[20] Mechanisms of a sort do exist for calling to account a doctor who is dangerously incompetent or who blatantly overtreats his patients. In principle, if his transgressions are sufficiently flagrant, his license can be revoked. But few state licensing boards have the staff to carry out investigations on their own. They must therefore rely heavily on other physicians to build a case for suspending or revoking a doctor's license. But most doctors are unwilling to point an accusing finger at another doctor, especially in a public forum. A few years ago 214 doctors were asked hypothetically whether they would be willing to testify against a surgeon who had set out to remove a diseased kidney and had taken out the wrong one. More than two-thirds said they would not be willing to testify.[21]

In many states, the law provides that a doctor's license may be revoked only if he has been convicted of a felony or has violated narcotic laws or if he has been guilty of certain other specified transgressions. Dr. Derbyshire has pointed out that, appallingly, only 15 state licensing statutes enumerate professional incompetence as a cause of disciplinary action.[22] All of this can make it very difficult to put a doctor out of business even when there is overwhelming evidence as to his unfitness. Even if a doctor's license is revoked, he does not necessarily have to give up his practice of medicine. If he already has a license in another state, as many doctors do, or if he can obtain such a license, which may not be too difficult, the doctor can move to another state and start a new practice.[23] Perhaps, these conditions will be remedied one day by the National Commission for Health Certifying Agencies which was established in December 1977. Among its members is the American Medical Association and sixty-four other health and medical groups. One of the interests of the commission will be methods of assuring the continued competence of health professionals, including physicians whose professional competence can be difficult to determine. In addition, the American Medical Association states that it is firmly behind initiatives to reform medical licensing boards, having in fact published model legislation to that end.[24]

Although the AMA's Principles of Medical Ethics say a physician should expose, without hesitation, illegal or unethical conduct by his colleagues, the good physicians have failed to police the bad ones. The surgeon who performs unnecessary or inept surgery, or the doctor whose skills are failing with age or the doctor who is an alcoholic only tends to smear the whole profession—the bad as well as the good—and bring the government into the picture to clean medicine's house.[25] The fact that medicine is generally practiced in a highly ethical manner in this country allows such incidents to have a dramatic impact on the public's perception of the profession. The image of American medicine is not enhanced when United Press International reports in the spring of 1977 that a patient in the state of Alabama was awarded $5,000 in damages against a physician who removed fresh stitches from the patient's wrist because the patient could not pay $25 for his services. Such acts can unfairly impugn the professional integrity of most physicians who do not practice in this manner. Their everyday medical achievements in treating the sick are not newsworthy because such professional practice is common and expected and not sensational and unexpected. But as incidents such as this extreme case of physician malfeasance or fraud in public medical programs or other areas of medical abuse come to light, government, as the people's representative, begins to enact laws like Professional Standards Review Organizations. Hopefully, these programs will focus on the errant physician since they require a physician's colleagues to review his medical treatment of patients who qualify for certain public programs such as Medicare and Medicaid. Should PSROs prove effective in achieving their goals, then, perhaps there will be at least one national mechanism to correct certain of the deficiencies in medical practice today, especially should the program be incorporated into any national health insurance plan which becomes law. Doctors at that moment, finally, will not have to use the following rationalization for failing to discipline their colleagues: "There, but for the grace of God, go I. If I pick on this doctor, the next thing he'll be picking on me."[26]

Conclusion

American medicine is being stained today with a broad brush. The spectrum of the paint has changed over time from pure white to gray to a slight blackened coloring. The question may be raised as to why the doctor is being attacked today more than anyone else in the health care field. The physician is not alone—clinical laboratories, nursing homes and other elements within the health care industry are also being investigated and being charged with malfeasance. But the physician is the centerpiece of the health care industry. For when a patient sees a physician, it is the physician who decides how and when he comes back, what other medical services or medical specialists he requires, what drugs he needs, and whether he needs hospitalization or other institutionalization and for how long. Once a patient goes to the hospital, the insurance company picks up the bill and the patient does not usually feel its financial impact except for the increases in his health insurance premiums, which his employee benefits absorb. While these circumstances, in part, may expose the physician to charges of corruption, exorbitant income, unnecessary procedures, kick-backs and all the other accusations which have plagued medicine within recent years, the doctor's positive profile is often unheralded. For example, it has been estimated that of the many millions of visits each year 80 percent of the patients who have nothing wrong return to their doctor to maintain their good health through his preventive care checkups.[27]

Did the sign at the entrance of a medical museum accurately portray our longing for the past when it read: "See the re-enactment of a house-call—See the doctor answer the telephone—See the hospital bed you could stay in for only $10 a day."? Was this so long ago? In terms of time it was only yesterday. The image of scientific medicine and of the compassionate paternalistic physician confidante is now eroding in the public's conscience. The communication media's portrayal of American medicine as brilliant diagnosis, technological miracles, sympathy and endless hours of time for the care of each patient does not match the reality of events for many people. Today, many patients expect very high medical bills, care whose quality may be questionable, physicians who are perceived as impersonal and uncaring and who have subdivided the human body into specialized areas of treatment, each respecting the specialization of the other and generally not seeking to treat illnesses which may fall outside their respective expertise. To paraphase Julius Caesar's opening to his Gallic War Commentaries, "All man is divided into many parts."

However, with the explosion of medical knowledge and discoveries, in addition to the availability and design of technologically-advanced equipment to treat patients in physicians' offices, the demise of the house call and the development of medical specialization was inevitable. But people still remember the days when their family doctor perhaps treated the wholeness of the human being. Today the patient may enter well-decorated offices, remembering a time when the doctor used to enter his home, knowing that his physician may have no conception of his personal economic or social circumstances nor the time to find out, and be prescribed a treatment that he may not be able financially to follow. Yesterday's former trust and respect for the American physician has been replaced by suspicion and doubt. Today patients have begun to realize that many illnesses such as colds, headaches, or backaches will disappear quickly on their own without a physician's examination. It is becoming evident to the public that a cure is more often the work of nature and the person afflicted than it is of the physician. The patient is beginning to realize that he is even more responsible for his personal health than the physician, because his personal well-being is greatly determined by what he eats and drinks, by the exercise he takes or does not take, and by his smoking and non-smoking habits. The patient is beginning to observe that medicine is relatively unable to prevent most illness or disease. It is medicine's enormous potential for good that makes these disappointments so glaring, yet still gives society hope that discoveries will be made which will lead to a more healthful future. Despite such medical miracles as heart transplants, coronary artery bypass operations and CAT scanners, there are illnesses which are chronic or irreversible or part of the aging process, for which cures have yet to be developed. For example, radical surgery for cancer of the breast has been found not to extend life. Cures have so far eluded such diseases as psoriasis, arthritis, or stroke. While the doctors can provide some symptomatic relief, not all lives will be saved or lengthened by what he does. In many instances, scientific medicine is still in its infancy of understanding the basic nature of biological man. This was aptly illustrated when Dr. Richard Selzer commented in his book *So They Say:* "The surgeon knows the landscape of the brain, yet does not know how a thought is made."

So where does organized medicine proceed from here? The demand for health services is not likely to abate in the future and the public's demand on the physician's time, skills and knowledge will only increase. It will take a great deal of individual and collective discipline to return to the ethical ideals which the public once attributed to organized medicine in order to erase many of the negative images and accusations which today confront the American physician. As long as public monies are being expended, society will demand a public accounting of the ways these monies are being spent. With the expectation of a national health insurance program in the not-too-distant future, the present characterizations of the American doctor can either become worse or improve—that decision is up to organized medicine. But one point is for certain: if organized medicine does not take a good hard look at its own behavior and does not try to correct it on its own initiative, then government will certainly take steps to do it. Once government moves into a problem-solving role, it is very difficult and almost impossible for government to relinquish voluntarily its newly found responsibility. There is still time for organized medicine to act so as not to come under the aegis of government bureaucracy. But it will have to act quickly and decisively to bring about those conditions of medical practice which will not penalize the good in organized medicine because of the errant behaviour of a minority within it. Just because society through its government has deemed medical care as a right and not a privilege, organized medicine does not and should not have the privilege to abuse the rights given to it by government. In regard to such abuses, AMA President Richard E. Palmer, MD has stated, "Given the necessary powers and authority, we of the medical profession will make every effort to put an end to the fraud and abuse in the Medicare and Medicaid programs which result from physician activity" . . . The problems of Medicare and Medicaid have been 10 years in the making. They are not going to be cleaned up in 10 days, in 10 weeks or even 10 months.[28] Only the future will be the ultimate judge of medicine disciplining its own house. Whether it be in regard to public medical care programs or other areas of errant medical practice, will the profession have spoken in time and will it be self-policing? Or has the die already been cast as to the manner in which medicine will be treated in the years to come? Will the physician survive?

Figure 5

GENERIC DRUG SUBSTITUTION STATUTE BY STATE AS OF MAY 1978

State	Year Enacted	Formulary Limitations	Two-Line Rx Form Required	Substitution Is Mandatory	Pharmacy Record Keeping Required	Cost Savings Pass-On Required	M.D. Exempt From Liability	Patient/Customer Consent Required
ALASKA	1976	None	✓				✓		✓
ARIZONA	1978	Positive	✓		✓	✓		✓
ARKANSAS	1975	Negative				✓		
CALIFORNIA	1975	Negative				✓	✓	
COLORADO	1976	None				✓		
CONNECTICUT	1976	None			✓	✓		
DELAWARE	1976	Negative	✓		✓	✓		
DIST. OF COL.	1976	Positive			✓		✓	
FLORIDA	1976	Negative		✓	✓	✓	✓	
GEORGIA	1977	None	✓		✓			
IDAHO	1978	None			✓	✓		✓
ILLINOIS	1977	Positive	✓		✓		✓	✓
IOWA	1976	Negative				✓		
KANSAS	1978	None	Optional					
KENTUCKY	1976	Positive		✓	✓		✓	
MAINE	1975	None						
MARYLAND	1977	Negative			✓	✓		
MASSACHUSETTS	1976	Positive	✓	✓				
MICHIGAN	1978	None				✓		
MINNESOTA	1974	None				✓		✓
MISSOURI	1978	Negative	✓		✓	✓	✓	
MONTANA	1977	None				✓	✓	
NEBRASKA	1977	Negative				✓	✓	
NEW HAMPSHIRE	1973	Positive		[2]				✓
NEW JERSEY	1977	Positive	✓	✓		✓		✓
NEW MEXICO	1976	Fed. MAC list				✓		
NEW YORK	1977	Positive	✓	✓	✓			
OHIO	1977	Community Pharmacy NDA-ANDA			✓	✓	✓	
OREGON	1975	None			✓			
PENNSYLVANIA	1976	Positive	✓	✓	✓	✓	✓	
RHODE ISLAND	1976	Positive	✓		✓	✓	✓	
SOUTH DAKOTA	1978	None	✓		✓			
TENNESSEE	1977	Positive	✓		✓	✓		
UTAH	1977	Negative[1]			✓	✓	✓	✓
VERMONT	1978	Positive		✓	✓	✓		✓
VIRGINIA	1977	Positive	✓		✓	✓		
WASHINGTON	1977	Negative[1]	✓		✓	✓	✓	
WEST VIRGINIA	1978	Negative	✓	✓[3]	✓	✓	✓	✓
WISCONSIN	1976	Positive		✓		✓		

[1] The Board of Pharmacy may, but is not required to, adopt a negative formulary.
[2] Substitution is permitted only if M.D. states orally or in writing "or its generic equivalent drug listed in the New Hampshire Drug Formulary."
[3] Pharmacist shall substitute less expensive brand unless in his professional judgment it "is not in the best interest."

NOTES: A *positive formulary* is a list of drugs which may be substituted for certain prescribed drugs.

A *negative formulary* is a list of drugs which may not be substituted for certain prescribed drugs.

A signature on one line of two line prescription permits substitution, while a signature on another line prevents it.

✓ — requirement of a generic drug substitution statute.
☐ — blank space means non-requirement of generic drug substitution statute.

Source: Reproduced with permission of and adapted from chart prepared by National Pharmaceutical Council, Washington, D.C., May 25, 1978.

Professional Standards Review Organizations: Am I My Brother's Keeper?

CONTROVERSY SWIRLS AROUND PSRO'S! Professional Standards Review Organizations seem to stir up or create debate. They will bring more and more of a physician's practice under the scrutiny of organizations sponsored by *government*. To some, this hints of socialized medicine, to others it breaths of George Orwell's world of 1984.

In contrast to today's illumination, invisibility was the watchword when the PSRO amendment meandered its way to law by legislative enactment. On October 30, 1972, President Nixon signed into law the Social Security Amendments of 1972 (P. L. 92-603). Among the provisions of the 989-page bill was an unobtrusive amendment, number 249f. When the amendment became law, it created a new program for monitoring the quality of health care services. The program is called the Professional Standards Review Organization or PSRO. Although the organization has been operating for several years, the changes which it may bring about in patient care are not yet clearly discernable. Proponents view the program as evolutionary for medical practice while critics regard it as revolutionary.

There are many reasons for these divergent views but, essentially, they focus on the purposes of the program. For example, the PSRO is supposed to determine whether the hospitalization of Medicare, Medicaid and Maternal and Child Health Program recipients is necessary, of appropriate duration, and meets professionally recognized standards of quality. If the PSRO achieves its purposes, the concept may be extended to other public medical care programs as well.

While portions of the Social Security Amendments of 1972 attracted a great deal of public attention, the PSRO provision moved quietly through the Senate, with the support of the powerful Senate Finance Committee and without a single amendment offered from the floor. In fact, the House never considered or passed a PSRO provision when it voted on the original Social Security bill, H. R. 1. The Senate's PSRO proposal was adopted by a House/Senate Conference Committee with a few minor changes. It went to the House on the final day and in the last few minutes of the 92nd Congress with a closed rule, (no amendment allowed), and passed 305 to 1.[1]

Thus, almost unnoticed by the public, the federal government took another step designed to reduce or control the costs of medical care while improving its quality. The importance of the obscure PSRO amendment is evident from the comments which attended its enactment. Thus, a staff member of the Senate Finance Committee stated:

"PSROs are the last and best chance for medicine, on an organized basis, to assume responsibility for quality care before the public is overwhelmed by other programs such as national health insurance ... Congress is going to be watching very closely the implementation of this program by the medical profession and HEW."[2]

On the other hand, the conservative commentator, M. Stanton Evans, wrote:

"We are rapidly approaching the point at which American medicine will be conducted bureaucratically with government agents making the key decisions about proper care, regimented procedures and endless involvement by physicians and patients in federal red tape ... PSROs have become possible and allegedly desirable because of the federal government itself ... It is because the government is engaged in subsidizing medical care that the costs for physician's services and hospital care have risen in recent years—a text book case of one sort of intervention by government becoming the pretext for another."[3]

What is the truth about the PSRO? Is it really the messiah for managing the costs of medical care and at the same time upgrading its quality? Or is it the parriah for destroying American medicine? This chapter will consider these questions, examine the facts and fictions attributed to the program, and go behind the rhetoric to see what the debate is really all about.

Although PSROs presently review only the care received by those of our population who qualify for specific public programs, some day they may be responsible for reviewing the care which everyone receives. Although the public cannot participate in the proceedings of the PSRO on the local level, four public representatives can serve on the Statewide Professional Standards Review Council. This Council is established when a state has three or more PSROs within its jurisdiction. These Statewide Councils coordinate PSRO activity within the state and assist the PSROs and the Secretary of HEW in carrying the program forward. Therefore, it is of importance to consider what PSROs are, how they operate, what problems they face and what they hope to accomplish.

Definition of PSROs

According to the U. S. Department of Health, Education, and Welfare (HEW), a PSRO, as seen in figure 6, is organized, administered and controlled by local physicians. Its original purpose, was to evaluate the necessity and quality of medical care delivered in such institutions as hospitals. However, the enactment of the Medicare and Medicaid Anti-Fraud and Abuse Amendments (P. L. 95-142) in October 1977 broadened the mandate of the program. One of the provisions of this law directs HEW to require capable PSROs to undertake ambulatory care review within two years after designation as a PSRO.

Membership in a PSRO is open only to doctors of medicine and osteopathy who are licensed to practice in the geographical area. The program cannot use, as a criterion of participation, physician membership in any organized medical society or association. Any member of a

PSRO is eligible to serve as an officer of the organization and to participate in its activities. The PSRO law requires that the services which a
physician provides to Medicare, Medicaid and child health program recipients be subject to the review of his fellow physicians, otherwise
known as peer review. If a physician's pattern of practice indicates he is
delivering insufficient health care or otherwise is treating his patients
improperly, his physician peers in the PSRO will so advise him and recommend appropriate remedies such as consultation with other doctors.
Also, the PSRO will consult with other health practitioners, such as
dentists, for assistance in reviewing the services they provide. As long as
the physician's pattern of practice falls within the norms and criteria he
helped establish for his PSRO, HEW does not expect the physician's
practice to be significantly altered.

The PSRO is not concerned with the service fees charged by
institutions or physicians. If a physician's colleagues in the PSRO
disapprove of a proposed procedure, or service, or the length of stay
in an institution, then the government does not pay for those
services. However, the physician remains free to provide the care and
services he chooses. Also, he can appeal the decision of his local
PSRO to the Statewide Professional Standards Review Council and
to HEW. Under this program the confidentiality of patient records is
protected. The law imposes severe penalties upon any reviewer or
employee of the program who discloses confidential information.

HEW expects that the standards and criteria used by the PSRO
will be modified as experience is gained and developments in
medicine warrant their modification. Norms, standards and criteria
will take into account professional personnel, facilities and equipment. A National Professional Standards Review Council must
approve those PSRO norms which are significantly different from
professionally developed regional norms. This National Council
consists of eleven physicians of recognized standing who are
appointed by the Secretary of HEW.

As noted in figure 7, HEW designated 203 PSRO geographical
areas throughout the country between January 1974 and January 1,
1976.

The Need for PSROs

In order to understand the reasons for the PSRO concept, it is necessary to travel back several years in order to place, into their proper context, the social and economic conditions which existed at the time the idea of PSRO was conceived. Until recently, the federal government was not involved to any substantial degree as a third-party payor of medical and hospital bills. With the advent of Medicare and Medicaid in 1965 this changed. Overnight, the federal government became the largest health insurer or third-party payor in the nation. The government was now paying hospital and medical bills for millions of aged or poor persons.

Medicare and Medicaid, have been good programs (although Medicaid has been the less effective of the two). Both have enabled millions of persons to meet their own health needs. However, the cost of Medicare and Medicaid have skyrocketed beyond their early estimates. In 1972 alone, the year the PSRO amendment was enacted into law, the Medicaid and Medicare programs were estimated to have cost the federal government $19 billion. In fiscal year 1974, Medicare spent $10.7 billion on the health care needs of the elderly and disabled while Medicaid spent about $10.6 billion on behalf of the poor and the medically indigent, including outlays for premium payments and services not covered by Medicare.[6] In addition, estimates made in 1972 showed that the cost of the Medicare hospital insurance program would overrun the estimates made in 1967 by some $240 billion over a 25 year period. Obviously, the costs of these programs have and continue to be a national problem that requires resolution. Also, up until 1972, Congressional hearings revealed that a significant proportion of the health services provided under Medicare and Medicaid were not medically necessary and some that were necessary did not meet quality standards.

These were the problems—cost and quality—which the Senate Finance Committee had to face in reviewing Medicare and Medicaid. Part of the answer was readily available when the House Ways and Means Committee and the Senate Finance Committee both developed a number of provisions to control allowable unit charges for physician services and hospital per diem costs. But the Committees still were concerned as to whether the services were actually necessary and met proper quality standards. This is where utilization and peer review enter the picture. It was thought that an effective comprehensive professional review mechanism could materially ease the problems of utilization and quality control. A bridge was needed between government and medicine. It had to be a structure in which practicing physicians could, in an organized and publicly accountable fashion, professionally evaluate the quality and necessity of the medical treatment being delivered rather than have an army of government and insurance company employees checking on each medical service. Thus, in 1970, former Senator Wallace F. Bennett introduced an amendment to the Social Security Act designed to establish Professional Standards Review Organizations throughout the country. When reintroducing this amendment in 1972, Senator Bennett noted:

"The relationship between the patient, the physician and the government is at the crossroads in America today. The pressures for increased governmental involvement in the day-to-day practice of medicine are increasing continually as we move toward expanded government financing of health care. Economics, commonsense and morality each demand that the government take an increasingly active role in dealing with the cost and quality of medical care.

The PSRO amendment represents the best, and perhaps the last, opportunity to fully safeguard the public concern with respect to the cost and quality of medical care while, at the same time, leaving the actual control of medical practice in the hands of those best qualified-America's physicians."[7]

Charges and Countercharges

Reactions by the American Medical Association (AMA) to Senator Bennett's comments on the PSRO program were immediate and to the point. The following were some of the AMA allegations:

● "A law of such consequence should have been written with a proportionate amount of forethought. But the forethought was meager. It is the law itself that was creature of impulse—as its background makes clear."

● "The law requires the development and application of 'norms of care' which would lead to cookbook medicine."

● "The PSRO program would violate the confidentiality of patient records."

● "The costs of PSRO review will outweigh any savings."

● "Under the law, fines may be imposed upon a physician and these fines will have a stultifying effect on medical practice."[8]

But the government did not take these charges passively. Issuing his own rejoinder, Senator Bennett stated:

● "The professional standards review legislation was years of effort representing the input and testimony of many individuals and organizations. Its genesis was the American Medical Association's own PRO proposal which they asked me to consider in early 1970.

● "The PSRO legislation seeks to substitute professionally developed norms and parameters of care which are the product of the work of practicing physicians in the area. It seems a far more acceptable approach to have the community of physicians in the area determine these factors than for them to be the province of an anonymous insurance company or government bureaucracy ... The statute doesn't speak to a single norm or way of treatment as the definitive and only type for which payment will be made.

● "The PSRO legislation ... has specific statutory safeguards designed to safeguard patient identity and confidentiality.

● "Considering the $25 billion now spent on Medicare and Medicaid, the costs of PSRO review efforts will be relatively small.

● "In actuality, the law does not contain any provision calling for fines."[9]

Supporting the views of Senator Bennett, HEW issued its own document responding to the charges and allegations raised by the American Medical Association. With respect to the charge of government encroachment on the practice of medicine through the PSRO program, HEW commented:

"PSROs are composed exclusively of local, practicing physicians. Those physicians form, administer and operate the PSRO in their area, hiring and supervising those non-physicians necessary to assist in the operation of the PSRO. The physicians develop, select and modify norms, criteria and standards of care. Only physicians can make final review determinations on care provided by physicians.

The federal government has no desire or authority to perform review of medical care. HEW agrees with physicians that local practitioners are those best qualified to review care provided by their peers."[10]

As far as PSROs violating patient confidentiality, the federal government stated:

"The privacy of patients and physicians is a basic civil right and must be respected. Medical records contain a great deal of privileged information but the data collected for PSRO purposes will be limited to that required for review purposes. While the law requires the development of patient and physician profiles, the identity of these individuals is to be protected from disclosure not only to guarantee privacy but also to assure objectivity . . . Maintaining confidentiality assumes that all personnel involved in the PSRO process are aware of and respect the right of privacy of *all* individuals."[11]

In addressing itself to the costs of the PSRO program, HEW acknowledged that:

There is no question that the PSRO involves administrative costs. There have been expenditures for utilization review activities for a number of years. PSRO brings these activities together and adds important quality assurance components. Taken in proper perspective, the cost of this necessary quality assurance program represents a small proportion of the total cost of the health care programs which PSRO covers. . . . As a result of having PSROs, those health dollars spent will be spent better and patients whose health care is financed by the federal government will be getting better quality care.[12]

With respect to the AMA's charge that the PSRO law requires the development and application of "norms of care" which would lead to cookbook medicine, HEW responded:

"The clear intent is to use norms, criteria, and standards developed by physicians in the PSRO area to aid in selecting cases requiring in-depth review by peers. It is on this more detailed assessment that a peer physician can review a patient's medical and social situation and consider the judgment of the patient's attending physician. Only through such *peer* review—a process repeatedly supported by the AMA—will ultimate decisions regarding the medical necessity, appropriateness and quality of care be made."[13]

Finally, in regard to the AMA charge that the PSRO program will lead to strangulation by paper and the data which physicians must prepare for PSRO ... and acknowledge from it ... will add new mountains to those geology has created and will cut into the time which physicians give their patients, HEW responded:

"The PSRO review system has been designed to minimize physician paperwork. . . . The physician's time will be concentrated on matters requiring professional medical judgment. Other health personnel can be used to do the preliminary screening and handle administrative detail. Paperwork will be kept to a minimum through greater uniformity and standardization in the collection and recording of medical care data. Performing review is on a voluntary basis, as is membership in a PSRO. No physician will be forced to engage in PSRO review activities.

Most physicians already spend time performing peer review and related activities in hospitals. When hospital review is performed satisfactorily, and meets PSRO objectives, the PSRO will not duplicate it. Thus, PSRO review, in most cases, will not require additional time and, therefore, will not decrease the amount of time physicians can spend with their patients."[14]

As can be observed from HEW's responses, the federal agency considers the PSRO to be a well thought-out program with built-in safeguards. These, in turn, should lead to the development of appropriate criteria which will make the program a success on the operational level.

The Bureaucracy Speaks

When the HEW agency responsible for PSRO activities became operational, Dr. Henry E. Simmons, the first director of the program, noted that physician interest in the program, from the viewpoint of applications initially submitted for establishing a PSRO, exceeded the government's most optimistic expectations. This situation existed, according to Dr. Simmons, despite the fact that in 1974 thirteen medical societies were actively seeking repeal of the law. Twenty nine other societies wanted to amend the legislation while several filed court cases challenging the law's validity. In addition, several bills were introduced into Congress attempting to revoke the law. Despite this opposition, Dr. Simmons claimed that there were specialty societies and many independent physicians within organized medicine who disagreed with those opposing the program.[15]

However, not all federal officials involved in the program agreed with Dr. Simmon's views. "No matter what Simmons says, I'm pessimistic about PSROs," one official stated, [16] "I look upon the program as nothing more than an excuse for $1 billion worth of revenue sharing for continuing medical education[17] —or whatever else the medical establishment chooses to use the money for." Another planner asked, "How can PSROs measure up to Henry's expectations as long as Congress insists on giving the regulatory power to those being regulated? It's like letting the oilmen run the Federal Energy Administration."[18]

The members of the PSRO bureaucracy thus raised a very basic question. What will be the ultimate purpose of this program? Will it evaluate the quality and necessity of medical care or will it oversee its costs? According to Dr. Simmons, PSROs have no authority under the law even to examine costs. However, the law does ask physicians to decide on the most appropriate setting in which care should be rendered. Thus, Dr. Simmons concluded, "It's not a cost control program. It's a waste control program."[19] Not all of Dr. Simmons's fellow bureaucrats agreed with his analysis. One stated, "Sure the law says PSRO is a quality assurance program. But you have to remember that the law originated with the Senate Finance Committee and the members of the Committee were frightened by the soaring costs of Medicare and Medicaid. I think that the Committee's emphasis on quality was mostly cosmetic—a gimmick to sell the PSRO concept to physicians."[20] Another bureaucrat stated, "Even 15 or 20 years from now we'll be asking ourselves the $64 question : Have PSROs been worth all the effort? The question may never be answered," he added, "since the law provides for no non-PSRO areas. Lacking any control areas, we'll never know what might have happened without PSROs."[21]

The View From Organized Medicine

Despite HEW's assurances that PSROs will have a positive effect on the quality of patient care, the program has brought no joy to many groups within organized medicine. These factions are still deeply concerned about the program's possible impact on a variety of medical areas. Their concerns include worries about the standards of medical practice which the government might impose, despite federal disclaimers on the subject, as well as worry over increasing malpractice liabilities, breaches of patient confidentiality and possible government fee controls. To anguished opponents, the PSRO stands for "Physicians Should Roll Over."[22] Even the highly respected Council on Medical Services, a standing committee of the AMA's House of Delegates, judged the Professional Standards Review Organization as being more divisive than anything else in the history of medicine! Contradictory characterizations of PSROs at the AMA's annual meeting in 1974 included "virulent, schizophrenic, discordant, PSRO is a malignancy," and, "repeal will be a calamity for health care."[23]

Despite these strident voices, the Association's policy statement on PSROs was stripped to a bare minimum. The new policy, adopted despite pleas for a "clearcut, definitive position," did not urge either PSRO repeal or PSRO sponsorship. Instead the adjusted AMA policy steered a narrow middle course, directing the Association to exert its influence on behalf of "constructive PSRO amendments and sound regulation." While the policy gave tacit blessing to state medical groups which chose to shun participation in the PSRO program, it also urged such groups to develop constructive peer review alternatives. As approved by the AMA's House of Delegates, the

PSRO policy mandated continued efforts to "achieve legislation which allows the profession to perform peer review in accordance with the profession's philosophy." In addition, it specifically reserved the AMA's right to launch a 'legal and legislative attack' on the PSRO if the controversial federal program does, in fact, adversely affect the quality of patient care."[24]

The Positive Aspects of PSROs

The middle course adopted by the AMA was, perhaps, influenced to some degree by those who insist that PSROs hold great positive potential for the practice of medicine. These advocates predict that PSRO review groups will sharply reduce unnecessary surgery and X-rays, decrease the undue length of hospitalization for many conditions such as heart attacks, discourage the unnecessary prescribing of drugs, and generally elevate the quality of care. They also claim that PSRO activities will lead to an increase in the delivery of medical services for those needs which now go unattended.[25] Proponents believe that the PSRO law is written with a complete understanding of what is helpful and fair to competent physicians. They state that the program's emphasis is educational, not punitive; more quality than cost-oriented; and that local medical autonomy is preserved. A physician will be judged by his peers in the geographic area in which he practices not by geographically distant specialists who might not understand the local situation. State and local councils also will be physician controlled. Thus, according to the program's advocates, if medicine accepts the responsibility of establishing viable physician review bodies on the local, state and national levels, there is little danger that the current health care system will be destroyed by bureaucratic red tape or standardization of poor practices.[26]

Proponents also state that education is the cornerstone of the PSRO law—a factor which is the key to higher quality medicine. Both sides of the coin—participation on the PSRO review board and being reviewed by the physician board—provide a means for continuing education in the broadest sense of the term. On a larger scale, these physician-patient profiles will be used to determine the level at which a hospital is delivering over-all care. Thus, the law provides an educational framework not only for the individual physician but also for the entire hospital staff.[27]

In addition, PSRO advocates consider the program to be good insurance for the practicing physician. In their view, malpractice lawsuits would have little chance of success against physicians who follow accepted practices.[28] Those who favor PSROs also suggest that as long as the program's guidelines remain in the hands of the physicians, the doctors will control the paperwork. Doctors will make the decisions concerning procedures, the reasons for reviews and the documentation necessary for review. The proponents also believe that physicians serving on review boards will work continually to minimize and simplify the paperwork, since they will be responsive to the needs of the practitioner.[29]

As far as the quality of physician care is concerned, PSRO advocates suggest that the guidelines for establishing quality standards in the local program are flexible, avoiding the hasty adoption of arbitrary standards for the treatment of disease. First, criteria can be developed in cooperation with the utilization review committees of local hospitals. These standards will improve the quality of care delivered, rather than freezing it at whatever level the physicians may be practicing when the Professional Standards Review Organization is established. Second, the setting of these criteria will be done at the pace set by the local PSRO with appropriate modifications based on experience. Finally, PSRO advocates state there is no reason to fear that the program's criteria might eliminate the exercise of a physician's own medical judgement because panels of local physicians will not only develop the criteria but also continually re-evaluate them.[30]

Finally, those who favor PSROs claim that the program offers organized medicine a chance to improve its performance and efficiency, in addition to providing individual practitioners with an opportunity for improving their medical practice. The PSRO criteria will be addressed to common medical problems which regularly are encountered. These criteria will incorporate the most current information available from medical literature and from local surveys in order to place quality-oriented, definitive guidelines within every physician's reach. Of course, while these guidelines will not relieve the physician of the responsibility of independent study they may aid him in his day-to-day patient encounters.

The state of Utah serves as an excellent example of how PSRO and continuing medical education activities can merge to improve upon the quality of a physician's medical practice. By pinpointing some of the inappropriate therapies physicians had been giving and then correcting these by letters or slide programs, the Utah PSRO has managed to reduce errors and gaps in physicians' performances. For example, the Utah PSRO pointed out 16 physicians who were prescribing tetracycline incorrectly for children. Four months after the Academy of Continuing Education of the state medical society published in its newsletter an item on the use of tetracycline for children's infectious diseases, all the doctors but one had modified their prescription practices. In another situation, 70 percent of expectant mothers in two metropolitan hospitals and 24 percent in another hospital had been getting electronic fetal monitoring during induced labor. After slide shows stressing the importance of monitoring were shown to the hospitals' obstetrics staffs, the rates increased to 90 percent and 70 percent respectively.[31] Utah, thus, serves as an example that PSROs continuing medical education and evaluations of physician competence can be integrated with each other to improve upon the quality of health care services and modify unnecessary costs.

What Does the Physician Think?

In view of the arguments for and against PSROs within and outside organized medicine, it may be interesting at this point to examine the views of the individual physician toward this federally sponsored program. Although few surveys have been published, in 1976 *Medical Economics* did examine and publish the physicians' attitude. When asked if they believed that peer review would improve patient care, a nationwide survey of a cross section of 435 physicians was split right down the middle. Forty-five percent of the doctors said yes; 50 percent said no; and 5 percent were undecided. Moreover, a number of yes and no answers were qualified. Although skepticism was widespread as to the effectiveness of any peer review program, there was hardly any outright opposition of a variety such as of the "no government is going to tell me how to practice medicine." Assuming that outside pressure for tougher quality controls will continue, the slightly skeptical majority has yet to answer the real question: If peer review won't work, what will?[32]

Among the responses and opinions given by the surveyed physicians were the following:

"Problems that any peer review program will have to overcome to be successful include defining such basics as "peers" and "quality care".

"Who knows what good care is? Is poor care worse than no care? Is nonstandard care substandard care? Will standards freeze therapy and not allow new things to be tried?"

"If a specialist must review each case, eventually the workload may become so unbearable that either a rubber-stamp process or random selection of cases for review will result."

"Peer review will probably make patient care more uniform but the average standard of care will undoubtedly be lower."

"It won't change the way physicians practice; it will only make them write the kind of progress notes that they think the reviewers want to see."

"Circumventing rules isn't too difficult . . . The charlatans will just find another way to screw the public, while the good guys will be swamped with yet another batch of paperwork."

"It's going to be like kids in high school grading each other's papers, but perhaps that's better than having an armchair sociologist doing it."

"Peer review is ineffectual because it has no teeth in it . . . One possible solution: Give reviewers the power to revoke or suspend licenses."[33]

Objections to the PSRO program center on cost and bureaucratization rather than on the concept itself. Many physicians wonder if the quality of patient care is the real issue in government-legislated peer review. It is also interesting to note that the practicing physician does not as yet completely believe in the beneficial effects which PSROs are supposed to bring about. Rather, PSROs are still perceived in some quarters as just another mechanism for bringing organized medicine under the watchful eye of the federal government.

The Quality of Medical Care

Who is right—the government or organized medicine? Whose views are correct as to the impact PSROs will have on the practice of medicine and the quality of health care delivery in the years ahead? Are both parties partially right and partially wrong? In any attempt to discuss, and evaluate the quality of medical care, these and many other questions arise. Most are unanswerable in concrete terms. How good is the physician? How good was his medical school and his hospital training? Has he kept up with medical progress? Each year in the United States there are patients who die too soon and needlessly or else have the quality of their remaining life irreparably damaged because of incompetent medical treatment. Although malpractice suits jam the courts, a malpractice award still cannot restore lost health or life or limb.[34]

Will PSROs improve the quality of medical care? A former past president of the American Medical Association, Dr. Russell B. Roth, takes issue with the usefulness of PSROs in this respect. He has stated that the PSRO issue has been written about, argued about, represented and misrepresented, politicized and emotionalized, to the point where any firm meetings of the minds seems beyond accomplishment.[33] Dr. Roth asserts that there will be lengthy professional disagreements as to whether diseased tonsils should be removed in one-day hospital episodes or whether recurrent attacks of tonsillitis should be treated with antimicrobial medications. Is it better medical care to support hernias with trusses or to repair them surgically? What is and what is not unnecessary surgery? When there are choices to be made between operative and nonoperative management of patients, how shall the decision be made? Dr. Roth asks, surely it will not be made by a committee which will not have even examined the patient?[36]

On the other hand, Dr. Charles C. Edwards, a former assistant secretary for health and scientific affairs at HEW, believes that PSROs can improve the quality of care as well as improve the way health care services are organized and delivered. Dr. Edwards states that given the opportunity PSROs can provide a long-needed mechanism for bringing about an improvement in health care services much more rapidly and effectively than in the past. For example, he notes that if cataract patients can be properly and effectively treated without hospitalization then the PSRO movement ought to be able to bring about this major change in the care of such patients. This advance would not only result in the savings of hundreds of millions of dollars, but it would free up valuable and expensive resources which could be used more effectively in other ways.[37]

When we speak of the quality of medical care we are talking about returning the patient to as close to his previous state of health as possible, in the light of present medical knowledge and techniques. In a medically sound review system the following questions must be considered: Did the patient get as well as he should have, compared with other patients having similar problems? Were unavoidable complications managed correctly? Is the mortality rate for a group of patients with similar problems acceptable? With these considerations in mind, it is clear that questions about the patient's recovery cannot be determined until the outcome is known. We must look back on the patient's care with his completed chart in hand. PSROs include such retrospective reviews by insisting on evaluations studies of the quality of medical care given. According to one authority, this activity will help improve the quality of treatment patients will receive in future years.[38] In fact, the PSRO law has already had a positive influence in this respect. Hospitals have intensified their own patient review systems to such a degree that the mechanisms are not only useful for the purposes of the PSRO but also for the hospital itself.

However, when the theorizing on the merits and demerits of PSROs ends and the physician must make medical decisions in accordance with PSRO guidelines, not all doctors consider the development of PSROs as a useful step forward. One such physician is a Mississippi internist who related his own experience:

". . . Again, it was the E. R. (emergency room) doctor who called me—a lot of our troubles start in E. R. these days. An 86 year old man who had suffered an episode of loss of consciousness was admitted to my service. The next day he was mildly addled, but there were no localizing neurological signs. The E. R. doctor had admitted him in self-defense and for the protection of the hospital. He didn't want to send the old man home to die that night of a stroke. There might have been a big hassle. If he died in the hospital, no sweat. Dutifully, acting in accordance with the PSRO cookbook, I ordered the appropriate studies. Three or four days and a thousand or so dollars in Medicare charges later, I sent him home. Twenty-five years ago, I'd have made a $5 dollar house call, explained to the family that Grandpa had hardening of the arteries of the brain, for which there was no effective treatment, and gone my way. The outcome would have been the same. Such is medical progress.[39]

But the problem is not solely PSROs but what PSROs and other watchdog programs represent to this physician and probably to many others—namely, a frustration. Doctors today must spend a large amount of nonproductive time on paperwork and committeework to meet the requirements of insurance companies, certifying agencies, and governmental authorities. The same Missouri internist complained:

". . . What's troubling me is not that I just have *less* time to practice medicine but, more seriously, that outside influences are changing the way I practice—for the worse. Part of the problem is that I find myself doing things my best clinical judgment tells me are completely unnecessary—just to satisfy the watchdogs ... But the pressure to do too much is just one side of the story. There are other times when I don't do things I ought to do and want to do ... Mostly, I believe I still practice a high quality of medicine in my office. I control what's done there. I can hold the volume to what I have time to do well. Not so in the hospital. So there's a paradox: the healthiest patients (the ambulatory ones) get my best efforts, and the sickest (the inpatients) my poorest efforts ... I've said in the past that doctors should exhibit a bit of courage and practice the best medicine they can, in spite of proliferating malpractice suits, government red tape, and everything else. It's obvious that I'm not heeding my own counsel. I'm bending with some evil winds. I think what's happened to me has happened to most doctors in this country. I grew up in medicine when the practitioner trusted his patients and they trusted him. I like being friends with my patients. I don't think medicine is much fun when it's largely an adversary relationship between doctor and patient, or among doctor and patient and insurance company, doctor and patient and plaintiff's attorney, doctor and patient and government bureaucrat, doctor and patient and consumer advocate. And I don't think we can practice good medicine that way, either.[40]

These sentiments and experiences are probably being echoed across this nation as physicians seek to practice medicine within the guidelines established by government sponsored organizations. To many physicians these government actions are more harmful than helpful for maintaining their patient's health and well-being.

How are the PSROs Doing?

The PSRO operational experience is too recent for meaningful data to establish whether they are upgrading the quality of medical care while, at the same time, reducing its costs. But there is tentative evidence available that the program is having some impact on the cost of medical care delivery. In 1976, the U. S. Department of Health Education, and Welfare told a subcommittee of the House Ways and Means Committee that PSRO organizations in Maryland,

Minnesota, Montana and Colorado had saved the taxpayers $22.5 million by reducing the hospitalization stays of Medicare and Medicaid patients. The average decrease in length of stay was approximately 6 percent or one-half day of hospitalization.[41]

However, these initial cost findings are only tentative. In the fall of 1977, HEW reported on a study carried out during the year ending October 1976. The survey compared 18 areas of the country with active PSROs to 26 areas with nonactive organizations. On the whole, HEW could not find any difference in the use of or admission rates to hospitals by Medicare patients in the two areas. In fact, only seven out of 18 closely studied PSROs had achieved reductions in hospital stays. Also, there was no evidence that PSROs had saved any money in most cities during their two years of existence from 1974 to 1976. Even where they had reduced hospital stays, it had cost the PSROs $16 on an average to review each patient's stay, with these federally paid administrative costs adding up to the millions of dollars. On the other hand, when a PSRO allowed hospitals to review themselves the costs were even higher—$18 per patient review—the reverse of what HEW had expected.

The study estimated that the PSRO program, when fully implemented, would have an annual cost of $268.5 million. But this is for only monitoring acute care hospitalizations. The amount does not consider the cost of nursing home or outpatient care. Also, it should be noted the study did not examine the quality of care—only the cost. Thus, it is possible that PSROs are upgrading hospital care even though they are not curbing expenses. Responding to an earlier question as to whether the PSROs are worth all the effort (since we might never know what would have happened without PSROs), HEW has no certain answer. HEW's feelings was reflected by Hale Champion, the Undersecretary of HEW. He warned doctors before a Congressional hearing that they had better help PSROs work—or HEW would have to devise an alternative mechanism which would be less to the physicians' liking.[42] Obviously, HEW is becoming very impatient for results—a sentiment shared by the federal government's Office of Management and Budget.

This budget agency initially ceased funding the PSRO program for fiscal year 1979 until HEW convinced the White House to give the program a little more time to prove its capability and promise. Regardless of the future fate of the PSRO program, one implication is becoming quite clear. While the program's goals may continue to shift from decreased hospital utilization to improved quality care to cost containment, the PSRO program cannot be considered as the sole strategy for reducing health care costs. By concentrating on the utilization of health facilities, PSROs have little potential for offsetting inflation, increases in third-party reimbursement rates, the introduction of expensive new technology into institutions or the increasing charges of the institution themselves.

What About the Future

At what price will the PSRO achieve savings and improve the quality of care? According to the Congressional testimony of a California PSRO medical director, the state health department, in order to curb costs, compels hospitals to discharge Medicaid patients according to a prescribed number of days. Continually, the prematurely released patients who are discharged while still ill end up being readmitted to the hospital a few days later, sicker than ever.[43] If these charges are true, than the allegations that PSROs will lead to cookbook medicine may be more valid than people wish to admit. If reducing costs is the name of the game at the expense of providing medical care of highest quality, then such procedures are inimical to the very purpose of establishing the PSRO program in the first place. Costs should be reduced not by forcing patients out of the hospital but rather by reducing unnecessary hospitalization due to misdiagnoses, thus freeing up hospital beds for those really in need. Reducing costs for improper reasons is an element within the PSRO program which must be carefully watched. In the end the patients for whom the program was created may be the ultimate victims, in the name of cost saving. This type of situation reflects that the program can work but under false premises.

Hopefully, the basic guidelines built into the law will avoid the abuses of achieving cost savings at the expense of patient's health. One such guideline is concurrent review which usually includes reviewing the necessity of a patient's hospital admission and the necessity of his continuing to remain in the hospital. A second mechanism is medical care evaluation studies, as noted earlier, which are designed to improve the quality of care by identifying deficiencies in the treatment given and in the organization and administration of its delivery; correcting such deficiencies through education and administrative change; and periodically reassessing health delivery performance to ensure that the improvements have been maintained. The third mechanism is the development of physician-patient profiles through data collection. Of prime concern in this respect is maintaining the confidentiality of the patient, the practitioner and the institution.

The issue of medical confidentiality became of paramount importance as a result of a court decision on April 25, 1978. On that date a federal court judge for the District of Columbia ruled that the PSRO for Washington, D.C. is an agency of the federal government, subject to the Freedom of Information Act. The judge based his ruling on the argument that the PSRO holds final decision-making authority on the appropriateness and quality of the services under the Medicare and Medicaid programs, making it an agency subject to the provisions of the Freedom of Information Act. The court ruling is not binding on other courts. Moreover, the judge did not decide the question whether any of the exemptions provided in the Freedom of Information Act apply to PSROs.[44] The judge stated:

"The court is well aware that the . . . attitudes of the medical profession strongly suggest that the peer review mechanism, which Congress wisely established in enacting the PSRO program will experience a severe setback, if not a fatal blow, should PSRO records become generally available . . . the remedy for alleviating these justifiable concerns lies with the Congress, not the courts."[45]

The plaintiff had requested the names not of patients but of physicians whose patients were most hospitalized, for what procedures,

procedures, and what if anything was disallowed by the defendant District of Columbia PSRO. The consumer group was seeking information so it could prepare comparative surveys to allow the public to make choices among physicians and hospitals—"a kind of rating system on the quality of care."[46] It is expected that the judicial decision will be appealed and that additional legislation will be sought in Congress to provide PSROs with clear statutory exemption from the disclosure requirements under the Freedom of Information Act. As matters now stand, the PSRO in the District of Columbia must now decide whether its data are exempt from the Freedom of Information Act. If the PSRO makes such a determination, a challenge could be filed in the courts.[47] As has been noted, that issue was not determined by the prior ruling.

But the whole case—the reasons for its initiation and the potential consequences which may flow from its determination— underlines a major concern in health care today. How can the ordinary lay consumer find and assess the quality and skill of a physician and how can his personal medical treatment remain as confidential as it had been prior to the creation of such public programs? If other mechanisms were available to enable the public to judge and choose a physician based upon his professional competence, perhaps the initiation of such a lawsuit would never have been necessary. But such mechanisms are not yet commonplace. On the other hand, physicians also were not without grounds in their charge that the confidentiality of patient treatment might be breached through the creation of such a public program. However, this situation does not appear to be an imminent reality unless the case is finally settled in favor of the plaintiff and Congress fails to pass remedial legislation to prevent such disclosures. But should the unthinkable happen, and our personal medical records be allowed to become available for public scrutiny, then government through the creation of another program will have taken away one more precious element from our right of personal privacy. Who is to say how long patient names will be kept confidential. If PSRO activities were to continue and expand beyond public programs geared to specific groups within our society to embrace the needs of our entire population, then the presently confidential medical records of all of us would be affected. At that moment we will know whether medical practice will have arrived in George Orwell's world where "Big Brother Is Watching You," and how this situation will affect our personal health and well-being during our lifetime.

Figure 6

TYPICAL PSRO ORGANIZATIONAL CHART

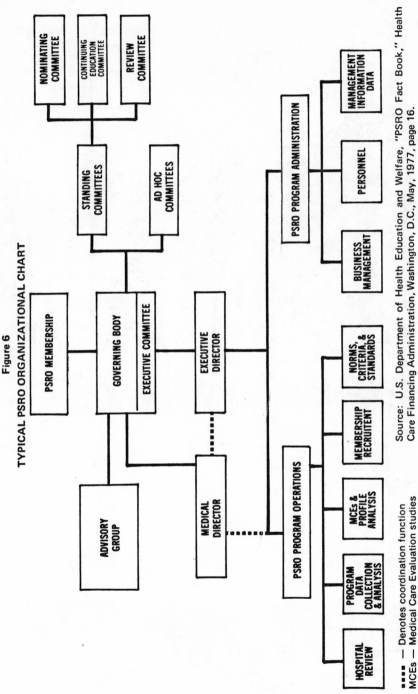

Source: U.S. Department of Health Education and Welfare, "PSRO Fact Book," Health Care Financing Administration, Washington, D.C., May, 1977, page 16.

■■■ — Denotes coordination function
MCEs — Medical Care Evaluation studies

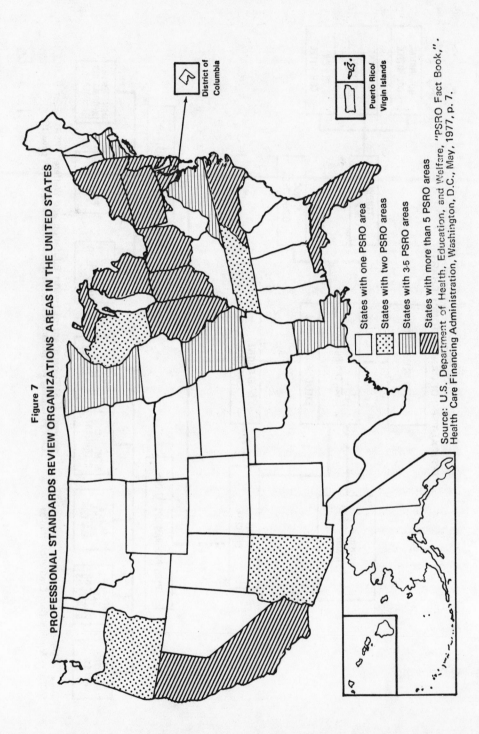

Figure 7

PROFESSIONAL STANDARDS REVIEW ORGANIZATIONS AREAS IN THE UNITED STATES

District of Columbia

Puerto Rico/ Virgin Islands

States with one PSRO area

States with two PSRO areas

States with 3-5 PSRO areas

States with more than 5 PSRO areas

Source: U.S. Department of Health, Education, and Welfare, "PSRO Fact Book,". Health Care Financing Administration, Washington, D.C., May, 1977, p. 7.

CHAPTER 4

Health Maintenance Organizations: The Supermarkets of American Medicine

IT IS AN IDEA whose time has come! It is revolutionary! It will bring order out of the chaos known as the American health care system! It will reduce the costs and alter the delivery of health services in this country! All these exclamations might have been proclaimed back in 1973. At that time the U. S. Congress established a new program to function as an alternative to the private health insurance industry. The law was the Health Maintenance Organization Act of 1973 (P. L. 93-222). Only two years before, the Nixon Administration, in advocating its passage proclaimed that by the mid-1970s more than 1000 of these new delivery systems would blanket the United States, serving 45 million Americans. Moreover, the Administration asserted that by 1980 about 1700 health maintenance organizations (HMOs) would be operating throughout the country, covering 90 percent of the population.

The predictions certainly have not matched reality. By 1975, in the opinion of some health experts, the HMO program was beginning to falter. Federal funds for HMO planning and development were going begging in Washington. HMO advocates began to state that the program had so many deficiencies that it was almost impossible for health maintenance organizations to successfully compete with the private health insurance industry. Instead of 1500 HMOs blanketing the country by the late 1970s, there were only 175 HMO-like organizations operating in the United States, serving slightly more than 6 million people. Even the enthusiasm of Dr. Paul M. Ellwood, one of the fathers of the HMO movement, seemed to be waning as he talked about altering the approach of the HMO concept:

"We're not abandoning it but broadening it (the approach). The key to lowering costs is to reduce hospital use and established HMOs like Kaiser have proven their ability to do this. However, we have been seeing more and more evidence that group practice doesn't necessarily have to be on a capitation basis to hold down hospitalization ... Individuals enrolled in the HMO program were found ... to be experiencing greater hospital use than their fee-for-service counterparts. But both groups showed outstanding low rates of hospitalization."[1]

What has happened? How did a concept which was being heralded as one of the saviors of the health care delivery system begin to evoke so much doubt and negativism in so short a time? Is it really too early to arrive at such judgements? Why were HMOs so ardently championed by the Nixon Administration and others?

In view of these and other questions let us examine the HMO movement in this country. These new delivery systems have great significance for the American consumer. Although HMO premiums in some instances may be higher than those of private health insurance plans, membership in an HMO may reduce the costs of medical bills over the long term. Unlike the usual arrangements between the patient and physician (or the insurance company) under which a doctor is reimbursed for each service he provides, the HMO receives a flat fee for all medical and hospital services. The health maintenance organization's fee does not increase—no matter how much care or how many tests, including hospitalization, a patient requires. In addition, HMOs, as multispecialty medical groups, provide a broad range of benefits. Some services, like preventive care, are not covered by private health insurance to any significant degree. Preventive care tends to identify illness early, treats it efficiently as possible, and hopefully avoids the need for more expensive treatment later, such as hospitalization. Again, such a process results in financial savings.

Health maintenance organizations as a concept have been in operation for half a century. They were known as prepaid group practice plans. These latter organizations are now redefined as operational entities by Congressional law. It is of interest to know what these HMO organizations are, how they have evolved, what services they can offer and how they will effect your personal physician and his private practice of medicine. Although only 61 organizations, serving more than 4 million people, were federally qualified as HMOs by the spring of 1978, their growth may become more rapid in the ensuing years. You may even have an opportunity at some future date to join an HMO through your place of employment. Early in March 1978, Secretary of HEW, Joseph A. Califano Jr, convened a meeting of representatives of the nation's 500 leading corporations to discuss how to foster the growth of HMOs in order to lower their company's and employee's health care costs. It may be that you are the employee and your company the employer which HEW has in mind. It is the purpose of this chapter to discuss one of the newest innovations in the delivery of health care services. You, as a patient-consumer, can benefit from this knowledge and join an HMO, should one be available in your community.

Definition of an HMO

However, before examining these and other issues, it is first necessary to define the concept of an HMO. Prior to the enactment of the Health Maintenance Organization Act of 1973, group practice plans such as Kaiser Foundation Health Plan on the West Coast functioned in this country for many years. In terms of definition, prepayment plans are those to which payments (premiums) are made beforehand or in advance into a fund used to pay for an individual's health services when the need arises.[2] Such services may be provided, for example, by a medical group practice. Group practice, on the other hand, is more difficult to define. The term has a variety of meanings to different people, depending upon the aims which they believe the group should seek. To some individuals group practice means non-medically controlled, closed panel and prepaid medical care by physicians on salary.[3] To others, group practice has other meanings. The difference in meaning centers around the concept of who controls and administers the multi-speciality groups. However, in its most basic form, group practice is a systematic relationship between physicians or dentists who are organized for the conduct of their practice. A variety of group practices exist, depending upon the scope and content of the relationships. The U. S. Public Health Service has defined group practice as:

"any group of three or more physicians (full-time or part-time) formally organized to provide medical services, with income from medical practice distributed according to some prearranged plan. Comprehensive group practice may include the provision of preventive, diagnostic and curative services by family or personal practitioners, specialists and other professional and subprofessional technical staff working as a team in a center, pooling their knowledge, experience and equipment as well as their income."[4]

This previous description covers what is meant by a closed panel group of physicians. The doctors are working together as group, pooling their income, sharing common facilities, support staff, and medical records. Such an arrangement is the more traditional type of prepaid group practice in this country. However, with the passage of the Health Maintenance Organization Act of 1973, the concept of prepaid group practice was refined even further. An HMO was now defined as a legal entity which provides a prescribed range of services, known as basic health services, in return for a prepaid, fixed and uniform payment. An HMO also had to provide its members with an equal opportunity, on a prepaid basis, to contract for certain prescribed optional health services, known as supplemental services, if the HMO found it feasible to make such services available.[5] HMOs have three variations—the staff model, the individual practice association, and the group practice:

- A staff HMO provides services through physicians who receive salaries from the HMO. In some cases physicians may receive incentive payments in addition to salary. Services are provided in a clinic setting with the number of service outlets depending on the number of enrollees and their area of disbursement.

- The individual practice association is usually sponsored by the state or county medical association. Enrollees pay monthly premiums to the HMO, which contracts with physicians to provide services on a fee-for-service basis.

● A group practice is an HMO which contracts with a medical group, partnership or corporation composed of health professionals to provide health services. All physicians are usually located in one facility and are paid a salary or on the basis of the number of persons for whom they are responsible.[6]

In the previous description, the individual practice association (IPA) would be considered an open panel of physicians engaged in group practice. The physicians maintain their own existing fee-for-service practices and individual private offices. They agree to provide prepaid health care to HMO members in much the same way they provide services to their other patients who are covered by Blue Cross-Blue Shield or commercial health insurance. Such is the conceptual nature of the health maintenance organization.

Evolution of HMOs

In terms of history, the development of prepaid group practice plans in this country during the past half century has been marked by great controversy. Opposition from medical societies at the local and national levels often led to bitter litigation. These lawsuits involved the rights-of-membership in medical societies and the right-of-hospital privileges for physicians with closed panel groups. Yet, despite these obstacles, a number of plans have survived and the concept of prepaid group practice has received renewed stimulation with the passage of the Health Maintenance Organization Act of 1973.

For purposes of this discussion, two kinds of group practices must be distinguished. Some groups consist primarily of specialists and act as referral centers. Examples of such groups include the Mayo Clinic of Rochester, Minnesota, the Lahey Clinic of Boston and the Ochsner Clinic of New Orleans. In the other category, groups consist of a substantial number of personal physicians and provide not only referral service but also comprehensive care for the patient or for the patient and his family. In addition, such group practices also may be prepayment plans to which the patient and/or his family is a subscribing member. Examples of the latter organizations include the Group Health Association of America in Washington, D.C. and the Group Health Cooperative of Puget Sound in the state of Washington.

The expansion of prepaid group practice has been the result of many pressures. As stated by W. P. Dearing, former director of the Group Health Association of America, Washington, D. C., the educated desire for more health services, together with the economic capability of purchasing more has been accompanied by a demand for efficiency and quality control of the more costly product. Not only are consumers—as individuals and as groups in labor unions, cooperatives, and the like—demanding more and more comprehensive care with quality controls but also business management increasingly is insisting upon efficiency, quality and cost controls.[7] Prepaid group practice is becoming widely recognized as an effective method for achieving these ends.

These attitudes have taken a long time to develop for the very early era of group practice pre-dates the large scale expansion of voluntary health insurance. Most of the early attempts at group practice emanated from the labor unions and industrial organizations as the only viable means of bringing a minimum of health services to workers. Typical industrial developments included the early health service programs of the railroad, lumbering and mining industries, while medical centers of the International Ladies Garment Workers were large scale union prototypes in this field. But these programs had poor financing. They never really succeeded in developing the king of popularity and appeal which voluntary health insurance has had since the end of World War II.[8] Yet these organizations, despite their lack of universal appeal, did establish excellent reputations as being providers of high quality care through an organized system. They emphasized ambulatory care and preventive services in an effort to maintain the health of their members and to minimize inpatient care.

There are various reasons for the failure of many prepaid group practice plans since their initial establishment in the 1920s. Some people have perceived these organizations as being impersonal, inconvenient and involving long waiting periods prior to their delivery of health services. Others felt that there was a clinic or charity atmosphere in the health care facilities. In addition, it was difficult to attract doctors to these plans. Many did not wish to practice medicine in a prepaid group practice setting. Even today these problems remain and continue to hamper the development of HMOs in this country. Yet, various studies have shown that the operation of a prepaid group practice system reduces the number of days of inpatient hospital care by as much as 50 percent, while its members receive more outpatient and preventive care services than in the traditional-fee-for-service system.[9] Thus, despite some negative impressions the evidence has pointed to the fact that HMO type systems significantly reduce the cost of care without lowering its quality.

Consequently, when health care costs began to rise dramatically in the period following the implementation of Medicare and Medicaid, a re-examination of the health care system seemed urgent. The Nixon Administration undertook such a study. In the course of analyzing the system, the Administration considered health maintenance organizations as one means to contain the runaway costs of health care. After a thorough study of the concept, the government decided to promote HMOs as a major federal initiative.[10] Former President Nixon announced this undertaking in his 1971 health message to the Congress. The Administration noted in a White Paper on health care that HMOs emphasize prevention and early care; provide incentives for holding down costs and for increasing the productivity of resources; offer opportunities for improving the quality and distribution of care; and by mobilizing private capital and managerial talent HMOs reduce the need for federal funds and direct control.[11]

But despite this Administration prognosis, there were various reasons why prepaid group practice required federal assistance at this point in its history. First, the movement was growing at a slow rate.

While the older plans were well established, there was not enough pressure or incentive for their expansion or for the development of new plans in other locations. Second, health care providers were not readily convinced that HMOs should grow in great number. Hospitals had little to gain from a system which stressed outpatient care; and many medical professionals viewed any form of organization, even if privately controlled, as a step toward socialized medicine. Furthermore, the American Medical Association, in strong opposition, had raised serious questions about the ability of HMOs to deliver high quality care. Even without opposition from the health care establishment, HMO growth still faced an uphill battle. Financial requirements for organizing even a modest HMO system and covering its early operational deficits were prohibitive to all but the wealthiest of potential sponsors. Consumers were expected to support the HMO movement once they understood its long range promise of financial savings and better care, but consumer education is an expensive effort. Finally, the laws in many states were unfavorable to the operation and formation of HMOs. The existence of all these impediments made it clear that the federal government had to give some kind of assistance if a substantial number of HMOs were to develop.[12] Consequently, a series of bills were introduced in Congress in the early 1970s. One was introduced by the Nixon Administration, another by Senator Edward M. Kennedy and still another by Congressman William R. Roy. Public hearings were held on these bills and discussions took place with representatives of various elements of the health care industry. Legislative language was revised, compromises achieved and, finally, in the late Fall of 1973, the Health Maintenance Organization Act was passed by Congress, and former President Nixon signed the bill into law in December of that year.

During this same time period of 1971 to 1973, HEW's Health Services and Mental Health Administration (HSMHA) had undertaken an experimental program to determine how effectively HMOs could operate in a variety of managerial formats and environmental settings. Of the 79 organizations awarded developmental funds in this experimental HMO program, 29 were operational by 1975, serving more than 150,000 people. In 35 instances the decision was reached that HMO activity was not feasible and the remaining 15 organizations were completing the process of becoming operational units.[13]

But the federal government was not the only resource developing HMOs during this period. The private sector also began to examine these prototype organizations as another way to lower the costs of deliverying health care. Physician and consumer groups, Blue Cross-Blue Shield and commercial insurance carriers, to name but a few sponsors, began to establish HMOs. From February 1971 to December 1975 the number of HMO-like delivery systems had increased from 33 to 178 organizations, serving almost 6 million persons compared to 3.6 million in 1971.[14] In fact by the mid-1970s thirty Blue Cross plans were involved in 98 HMO-like organizations. During 1975 enrollment in Blue Cross affiliated HMOs increased by 14 percent to 1,168,900 people compared with an estimated 8 percent increase nationally for all HMOs. Blue Cross plans presently have another 30 HMOs in the developmental planning stage. By 1980 Blue Cross estimates that it will have invested $57 million in an effort to offer subscribers HMO programs as an alternative to traditional health care coverage.[15] When the Blue Cross effort is coupled with that of other insurance carriers and groups, it would appear that the HMO movement will grow more rapidly than in the past if certain problems can be resolved. Before discussing these obstacles to HMO development. I will briefly describe the original law which has given impetus to the movement.

Health Maintenance Organization Act of 1973

The HMO law of 1973 contains several sections which enable the American public to have a serious alternative to the way they may wish to receive their health care services in future years. One section stipulates that every employer subject to section 6 of the Fair

Labor Standards Act, who employs 25 or more persons to whom a health benefit plan if offered, must, under certain specified circumstances, offer those employers the option of membership in a qualified HMO. Another section supersedes certain restrictive provisions in state laws which would have prevented the operation of otherwise qualified HMOs. A third section offered a five year $325 million federal assistance program to organizations wishing to develop HMOs. The financial support was designated for feasibility studies, planning, initial development and initial operations. Another section of the Act defines an HMO in terms of the services which it must provide and the manner in which an HMO must be organized and operated.[16] Since the passage of HMO Act of 1973, another bill, the HMO Amendments of 1976, was signed also into law on October 8, 1976. The new legislation (P. L. 94-460) corrected several aspects of the 1973 law which made the certification of HMOs a difficult problem. However, in order to understand the necessity for the 1976 amendments a brief description of the organization and operation of an HMO, as specified by the 1973 law, is relevent. In order to qualify as a health maintenance organization under the 1973 Act, an organization had to provide its members with the following set of basic benefits without any limitation as to time and cost:

- Physician services, including consultation and referral;
- outpatient services;
- inpatient hospital services;
- medically necessary emergency services;
- short-term outpatient evaluative and crisis intervention mental health care services;
- diagnostic laboratory and diagnostic and therapeutic radiological services;
- home health services and preventive health services including voluntary family planning services, infertility services, preventive dental care for children, and eye refractions for children;
- medical treatment and referral services for abuse of or addiction to alcohol and drugs.[17]

The 1973 law required that an HMO provide in addition to the offering of basic benefits, certain supplemental benefits if the HMO had the manpower to do so and if its members wished to purchase such services. The supplemental benefits included the services of intermediate and long-term care facilities: vision, dental and mental health care; long-term rehabilitative services; and prescription drugs. The payment for basic health benefits is on a community-rated basis, that is, everyone, regardless of individual health status, pays the same premium rate. The cost of the premium payments varies in one respect. A single person pays a specified amount, while a family, regardless of size, pays a higher but uniform rate. In this fashion community rating spreads the cost of illness evenly over all HMO members rather than charging the sick more than the healthy for health insurance coverage. On the other hand, an HMO could provide supplemental services both on a community-rated and fee-for-service basis. In addition, the 1973 law allows an HMO member to make a co-payment as long as this cost sharing does not prevent an individual from receiving health services. A co-payment means that the insured patient pays a fixed amount for a unit of service such as $2 for a doctor's visit or for a unit of time such as $10 per day in a hospital and the insurer pays the remaining amount.

As far as HMO organization and operations are concerned, the HMO must:

- show fiscal soundness and provide safeguards against insolvency;
- take full financial risk with only limited reinsurance;
- enroll persons broadly representative of the service area;
- provide for open enrollment periods;
- not expel any member because of health status;
- have a policy making body, of which at least one-third consists of members of the HMO;
- provide meaningful hearings and grievance procedures;
- show that it has satisfactory quality assurance arrangements;
- provide medical social services and health education to its members;

- provide continuing education for its health professionals;
- report to the Secretary of HEW, to the public and to its members data relative to the cost and utilization of its services.[18]

While some harbor negative feelings for the HMO as a conceptual and operational entity, many do not find its services inferior to the traditional fee-for-service system of medicine. Certain aspects of the HMO still have appeal for potential enrollees including:

- one stop medical care where services are available for all family members and for all conditions;
- 24 hour service;
- convenient location;
- more benefits including preventive services for the same money;
- a physician who is the total health care manager;
- a physician who is backed up by a range of specialists.[19]

Prospective members view the HMO as the kind of organization where it is easy to receive the care they need, when and where they need it. Patients enrolled in HMOs know their entry point into the health system—they do not have to seek out a specialist or worry about where to go after hours or on weekends. The HMO provides full-time coverage and arranges necessary referrals. From the HMO's viewpoint this situation makes its planning more efficient. At the beginning of the year the HMO can estimate the number of patients it will be serving and, accordingly, can arrange for hospital beds and specialists. At the other end, the consumer knows in advance the total cost of the HMO's services. Yet, despite the appeal of the HMO to some members of the public, there are additional reasons, besides a mixed public image, why the HMO has not lived up to its predicted expectations in the past few years.

Federal Impediments to HMO Growth

One of the causes for the HMO's slow development is the federal government itself. The General Accounting Office

(GAO)–the official watchdog agency of the U. S. Congress–recently studied HMOs. In its findings of 1975 the GAO concluded that the program had administrative weaknesses. The U.S. Department of Health, Education, and Welfare did not have a single unit which was responsible for HMO operations; ten governmental regional offices administered the program; and the program lacked coordination. The ability of the regional offices to handle and counsel HMO-aid applicants ranged from nil to expert. Overall, HEW lacked the right number and kind of personnel who were needed to evaluate and process grant applications as well as to give legal opinions. The GAO noted "a significant staff turnover" since the program's inception, a euphemism for the heated controversy taking place between career civil servants and former President Nixon's political appointees over the priorities of HMO development.

In addition, the law itself seemed to hinder HMO growth. When the HMO bill was originally considered, some Congressmen viewed the proposed HMO as being inferior to the care being delivered by such veteran prepaid group practice plans as the Kaiser Foundation Health Plan. Thus, the Congress stipulated a wide range of benefits in the HMO law as a condition for federal recognition and aid. But the law also included organizational and financing restrictions as well. The net result of all these diverse legal provisions was summarized by the Institute of Medicine of the National Academy of Sciences. The Institute noted that the various legal requirements made it very difficult for HMOs to become competitive in a market dominated by the fractionated fee-for-service traditions. In fact, the Institute of Medicine thought that the legal restrictions were preventing the HMOs from receiving a fair market test in deliverying health care services.

The HMO benefit package is an excellent example of how government actually can create the obstacles rather than foster the solutions for bringing high quality health services to the nation. As already noted, Congress mandated a very broad benefit package. In fact, it was so expansive that HMOs had to charge high premiums.

As a result, especially during the recession of the mid-1970s, HMOs could not compete financially with other health insuring organizations. It seems that provision was not made for people who might not want HMO coverage either because of its cost or because they might want to purchase part of the HMO benefit package from other sources. But under the 1973 law, the HMO had to provide all the mandated services to all of its members whether they wanted the benefits or not. Unlike most insurance companies and Blue Cross, the HMO could not offer its members a low benefit package. Thus, if a federally qualified health maintenance organization found that its basic benefits were too high priced and thus unmarketable in its service area, there was no way for the HMO to seek relief. Similar regulatory conditions were not being imposed upon the HMO's competitors whether they were health insurers or other kinds of organizations.

HMOs also confronted another problem. The 1973 law required HMOs to open their enrollment at least once a year for 30 days. In addition, HMOs had to provide health care services at a single community rate regardless of the health status of those who applied for membership. These requirements, like the broad benefit package, are desirable features in a health care delivery system. However, many health experts argued that to require both an open enrollment and community rating for an HMO but not for its competitors placed the HMO at a very serious disadvantage. Some suggested that insurance companies, which use experience rating, simply could leave the chronically ill and disabled to the HMOs which would be legally obligated to provide these groups with benefit coverage at ordinary rates.[20] Since it costs more to treat those in poor health than those in better health, the HMOs therefore would have to increase their premium costs and thereby become financially unattractive.

The Aetna Life and Casualty Company is an excellent example of how the 1973 HMO law actually deterred an organization from successfully establishing an HMO. Aetna had planned to start an ambulatory HMO in Tampa, Florida, with an ultimate projected enrollment of 20,000 to 25,000 members. The HMO, called the Hillsborough Health Plan, would have used existing hospital beds. But preparation for the HMO ended in November 1974. A market survey indicated that the Plan would have to charge approximately $70 per month for a family of four or about $840 per year for membership in the Plan. The price exceeded the ability of both employers and employees to pay for such care. Inflation only made the problem worse.[21] However, this situation should not have been too surprising. The benefits mandated by Congress have been estimated to have made HMO payments 5 or 10 percent higher than standard health insurance premiums. According to one corporate official who is involved with HMOs, "the law designed a cadillac".[22] Even Dr. Paul M. Ellwood, Jr. has been critical of the HMO benefit package and its impact of the HMO movement:

"If the federal government persists in applying a standard quantity of benefits that HMOs must provide . . . more than anyone else has to provide, then HMOs are not going to make it."[23]

In view of these cost issues, do HMOs really achieve the kind of savings which served as the rationale for the 1973 law? On a month by month examination, HMO premium costs, when compared to other programs such as Blue Cross, are higher in some instances. In fact, during 1976 the average national family cost for HMO membership was $89 per month or almost $1100 per year. But the higher HMO premium costs, compared to other insuring organizations, has been changing lately. For example, while the monthly family premium for the Harvard Community Health Plan (an HMO) was $7 per month higher than that of Massachusetts Blue Cross-Blue Shield seven years ago, the premiums of the Harvard Plan increased by 93 percent and the competition's by 199 percent in the ensuing seven years. As a result, the family premium of the Harvard Plan was $28 a month less than that for Massachusetts Blue Cross-Blue Shield in 1976.[24] One of the reasons for this change is the lower hospitalization rates of HMO members compared to individuals covered by other health insuring organizations. In fact, during 1976 Blue Cross and Blue Shield plans in some areas of the country increased their premium rates about 35 percent, while the average federally qualified HMO held its premium increase to 19 percent.[25] Thus, we are finally reaching a point in terms of hospital costs where programs such as HMOs, which de-emphasize hospitalization, are beginning to achieve a distinct price advantage over their competitors. Even Medicaid experiments involving HMOs in the District of Columbia and Washington state have demonstrated cost savings of 20 to 30 percent to HMO members compared to individuals receiving fee-for-service medicine. Seven HMOs involved in experimental Medicare programs sponsored by the Social Security Administration also have shown that their total costs average about 15 percent below the costs of the traditional fee-for-service system. The Group Health Cooperative of Puget Sound in Washington state has demonstrated that its costs are about 30 percent below the average for the same services offered under other health delivery systems.[26] As a result of these cost saving demonstrations, the Carter Administration has become an ardent advocate of HMO development. In the words of Hale Champion, Undersecretary of HEW:

"How much more proof does one need than the studies that show HMOs' ability to provide care for at five to 35 percent less than the fee-for-service sector? What is there left to demonstrate when over 25 HMO-type organizations have been providing good quality care to four million enrollees for the last 10 years, and Kaiser and others have been going strong for over 30 years?"[27]

But, despite such support, HMO development must overcome additional obstacles besides those caused by the law itself or the federal agency responsible for the program's operation.

State Government Problems

Another hinderance to HMO growth is state government. One of its legislative tools, the state enabling act, thus far has hampered the establishment and economic viability of HMOs. By 1974 seventeen jurisdictions had enacted such laws. On the positive side, most state enabling acts require that the jurisdiction monitor the quality of the care which the HMO delivers, that HMOs have an established mechanism for processing the grievances of their membership, and that HMO members participate in establishing organizational policy. In addition, almost all enabling acts release the HMOs from various restrictions and the corporate practice of medicine. On the other hand, the enabling laws also impose requirements which may be burdensome to the HMO and not in the consumer's interests. For example, several states impose financial reserve requirements which are similar to those which are applied to insurance companies. While these financial reserve regulations may be appropriate for insurers, these requirements are not beneficial for HMOs which contract to provide medical services and not dollar benefits. Some states also require the approval of HMO premium rates and most fail to exclude HMOs from certificate-of-need laws. Several states require HMOs to have various open enrollment provisions, which can be expected to increase significantly an HMO's cost and decrease its ability to compete. Few states impose similar requirements on insurance companies or traditional providers. Few state enabling laws have dual choice provisions which would increase an HMO's access to the market. As of 1975 only one state (Michigan) required that the dual choice provision apply to more than state employees. In the view of some health experts, an HMO enabling act may not adequately protect consumers in many states from HMOs of poor quality or encourage fair competiton between HMOs and other modes of health care delivery.

In addition to enabling legislation, certificate-of-need laws also hinder the development of HMOs on the state level. These laws presently require hospitals and certain other health facilities to obtain approval or a certificate-of-need from a regulatory authority prior to undertaking new construction or certain modifications of their health services. These laws originally were enacted as a legislative response to the continuing increases in the costs of hospital care. These rising costs are due, in part, to such factors as an oversupply of beds, third party reimbursement incentives for overutilizing hospital services and the excessive zeal of nonprofit hospitals for undertaking new capital expenditures for elaborate and, at times, economically inefficient facilities. But as of January 1974 most of the 23 states with certificate-of-need legislation applied these laws to HMOs as well. Unlike other health care institutions, the central characteristic of HMOs is their incentive to minimize the costs of needed medical care. Because the HMO receives a flat fee for all medical and hospital services, it has an incentive not to engage in excess hospitalization, not to run duplicative or unnecessary tests, and not to refer a patient to an unnecessary specialist. The HMO not the patient pays for wasteful and unnecessary procedures. Thus, when controls are imposed upon the HMO the outcome is likely to be a reduction in effective competition between HMOs and the other health care delivery approaches. The controls only add needless costs to the HMO's operation which must be passed along to its membership in the form of higher premiums. In a 1973 survey of HMOs where certificate-of-need laws were in effect or pending, 48 percent of the responding HMOs cited these laws as being moderate or severe barriers to their growth.[28]

Thus, it is clear how state and federal regulations affect the formation of health maintenance organizations whose length of time in becoming operational during the 1970-1973 period was estimated to be 2½ years.[29] This time span can be appreciated by examining the various procedures outlined in figure 8 for establishing an HMO. Also, when all these laws are translated into the responsibilities which an HMO administrator must assume to make his organization a successful entity, their effect become even more clear. In a survey of HMO administrators, three-fourths felt that gaining access to employers and other potential member groups was their most serious organizational and growth problem. At this juncture it can be seen how important the dual choice provisions of state and federal law become for gaining HMO membership. The second most serious obstacle was the opposition of other health providers to the health maintenance organization. The third was problems of financial support. The fourth most serious barrier to an HMO's formation and growth was expanding its staff of physicians, while legal barriers were generally considered to be the fifth most serious issue which they faced.[30] Other managerial problems with which the administrator must deal include the following operational requirements. Each federally qualified HMO must have one-third of its policy making board composed of its members, one-half of its revenues must come from HMO activities after three years, the HMO's purchase of reinsurance, which is insurance coverage for its insurance losses, is limited, and the HMO also must meet reporting, quality assurance and continuing education requirements according to federal law. Neither state nor federal law imposes these requirements upon other insurers or other health providers. As a result, the HMO again is placed at a competitive disadvantage in the market place.

In comparison to states without HMOs, states with such organizations tend to have higher incomes, larger and more urbanized populations, more physicians per capita, higher per capita and per diem hospital costs as well as greater public and private expenditures.[31] HMOs seem to locate where they can be most competitive with conventional delivery systems and where consumers spend considerable amounts of money on medical care. These sums may be out-of-pocket expenses, health insurance or public program payments. It also appears that HMOs tend to form in those urban areas where another HMO has already appeared and has broken the ice. Three-fourths of the HMOs established in the 1972-1973 period located in metropolitan areas which already had one or more HMOs by the end of 1971.[32] In fact, a 1977 Federal Trade Commission study analyzed HMO-Blue Cross competition and reported some interested findings. When an HMO came to town and captured a significant part of the market, the rate of hospitalization in that community decreased. There were also indications that when an HMO became established, Blue Cross formed its own HMO or increased its range of benefits and concentrated on more effective cost controls. In addition, the arrival of an HMO often seemed to be followed by the formation of an individual practice association (IPA)—which is an HMO established by physicians. As already noted, the principal objective of such an association is to maintain the traditional payment system—a fee for each service performed for the patient. IPA generally attempts to institute cost controls while preserving the patient's free choice of physician. The FTC study showed that HMOs preceded the formation of IPAs in 11 of 13 states and in 10 of 17 metropolitan areas. However, the data was not conclusive that HMOs cause the formation of IPAs and that IPAs actually control health care costs.[33]

HMO Operational Problems

Despite the seemingly advantageous areas in which HMOs tend to locate, it has already been noted that their failure rate is high and their rate of formation is slow. So slow, in fact, that the General Accounting Office reported that by June 30, 1976—2½ years after the passage of the HMO law—only seventeen health maintenance organizations were certified by the federal government as complying with the Act's requirements. By the Spring of 1978 the number had increased to 61 HMOs. However, during this 2½ period up to June 30, 1976, 168 projects received grants for feasibility studies, planning and early development activities. HEW anticipated that only 80 HMOs might be certified under the Act by the end of the demonstration program. Examples abound of HMOs which began and subsequently failed because of government overregulation or the profit-motive which sponsors see in this new health care delivery system. For example, in 1975 forty or more HMO-like organizations known as Prepaid Health Plans (P.H.P.) held contracts with the state of California to provide services to Medi-Cal (Medicaid) patients who comprised all or most of their enrollments. But the State Attorney General filed cease and desist orders against many of the plans for a variety of reasons. These included financial instability, failure to meet the registration deadline and non-compliance with parts of the state law. By the winter of 1978, only thirteen Prepaid Health Plans were in operation, serving 125,000 Medicaid patients out of a total of more than 2 million eligibles.[34] Make no mistake, HMOs are viewed as a business and not as an idealistic way of improving the health care delivery system. As one consultant has remarked:

"An HMO is a business. Unlike a clinic or hospital, you have to market your product aggressively. If you've got an attractive well-priced product, somebody is going to buy it."[35]

But, as of the fall of 1977, not too many people were buying the HMO product. In fact, of the 3.8 million persons enrolled in HMOs as of November 1977, about 3.2 million were enrolled in four Kaiser Foundation Health Plan HMOs and the remainder were members of 43 other HMOs.[36] In addition, more than two-thirds of all HMOs serve fewer than 10,000 members.

When an HMO becomes operational, experts say that to break even the prepaid health plan should enroll about 30,000 persons and spend more than $2 million on marketing, staff and facilities over a three year period. This knowledge did not prevent Healthcare, a Brooklyn New York HMO, sponsored by the Connecticut General Life Insurance Company, from going out of business in 1975. The HMO's total enrollment numbered 500 people after 15 months of operation. Its premium of $69.75 a month for a family of three or more exceeded some New York Blue Cross plans by as much as $30 per month.[37] This price differential constituted part of its marketing difficulties. The HMO was established initially to provide ambulatory care for about 4,000 patients and 35,000 members, when fully staffed.[38] As a result of the HMO debacle in Brooklyn, New York it is easy to theorize that HMO managers should price their services low enough to attract patients, yet high enough to avoid financial losses. But what is easy to theorize is much more difficult to carry out in practice.

Established HMOs have shown that the best hope for achieving economic viability over a period of time is shortening the length of a patient's hospital stay. However, HMOs presently have within their managerial arsenal another weapon for realizing economic soundness—one which has the endorsement of the federal government. In October 1975, HEW published the HMO "dual option" regulations which are mandated by the 1973 HMO law. The regulations require companies which offer their employees a health insurance benefit plan to give these employees the option of joining a federally qualified HMO, if such a program exists in their area. This dual option was modified slightly by the HMO Amendments of 1976, of which more will be said later. This dual option is so important that prepaid health plans which are not as yet federally certified as HMOs fear that they might suffer unfair competition when federally certified HMOs are offered as an alternative to their own programs.[39] Consequently, we have a situation where federally qualified HMOs must compete with prepaid group practice plans which are not federally certified as HMOs. Both of which, in turn, must compete with other health insuring organizations in order to survive as operational entities.

HMO Amendments of 1976

The difficulties raised by the HMO law of 1973 did not escape the attention of Congress. Vexed by the program's lack of progress and recognizing those aspects of the original Act which may have contributed to the HMO's slow growth, Congress re-examined the law. As a result of its review, Congress enacted the HMO Amendments of 1976. President Gerald R. Ford signed the Amendments into law (P. L. 94-460) on October 8, 1976. The 1976 Amendments made major alterations in seeking to correct the deficiencies of the 1973 law. The first important modification relates to the dual option regulation. As already noted, the original law required any employer with more than 25 employees to offer membership in a federally qualified HMO, if one were available, as a health benefits option. Now the employer must offer that benefit only if 25 employees reside in an HMO service area. Also, if the employees are represented by a union, the union may turn down the HMO option for its members.

Another important alteration relates to open enrollment and community rating. Existing HMOs will not have to enroll members under the community rating system, but new HMOs seeking federal qualification will have to do so. In addition, open enrollment is now required only for those HMOs which have been operating for five years or those with 50,000 members and no financial deficit in the previous year. These HMOs must enroll a number of individuals equal to three percent of the total enrollment increase for the previous year. Also, open enrollment does not have to include people who are institutionalized with a chronic illness or a permanent injury if these conditions would economically impair the HMO. A 90 day waiting period is allowed before new benefits apply to new members. Open enrollment can be waived entirely if it would jeopardize the HMO's economic viability.

In addition, the benefit package which HMOs were required to offer under the 1973 law was somewhat modified. Preventive dental services for children were eliminated from the list of basic services. Also, HMOs will no longer be required to make all supplemental benefits available to members. The HMO will have the option of choosing from among the supplemental benefits and may offer all, some or none of these. Also, the category of preventive services was modified to include: periodic health examinations for adults, immunizations, well-child care from birth, voluntary family planning services, children's eye and ear examinations and infertility services.

Finally, the 1976 Amendments stipulate that Medicare and Medicaid beneficiaries cannot constitute more than half of an HMO's membership, but this requirement can be waived by the Secretary of HEW for three years.[40]

Hopefully, these modifications of the Health Maintenance Organization Act of 1973 will help overcome the developmental problems which have plagued HMOs the past few years. However, much still may have to be done in order to make this program a nationwide success. From the viewpoint of federal administration alone, there is a need of additional staff, especially in the HEW regional offices, who are experts in marketing, actuarial analysis and financial management. But the 1976 Amendments, at least, may begin to spur the growth of HMOs. Only time will determine what other measures are necessary to make this new delivery system economically viable as an alternative to our other modes of health delivery.

HMO Impact on Physicians

The establishment of an HMO in a community has various implications for the physician in private medical practice. First, he may lose part of his private patient population to the HMO. This may happen if private corporations follow the 1976 experience of the R.J. Reynolds Industries of North Carolina and establish their own HMOs to reduce their corporate health costs. Also, in early 1976 HEW issued regulations which required all prepaid group health plans to provide a 30 day open enrollment period for Medicare beneficiaries. Officials in the Social Security Administration believe that up to 10 percent of all Medicare beneficiaries will decide to enroll in an HMO. The health maintenance organization, however, can discontinue a Medicare enrollment if the patient loses his eligibility for Part B of Medicare, moves outside the HMO service area or use fraud to obtain treatment.[41] As of the winter of 1978 only 1.5 percent or under 700,000, of the Medicare and Medicaid recipients (which total almost 50 million) were enrolled in HMOs.[42]

Second, there is a mixed impact for the physician who wishes to choose between practicing medicine in an HMO versus the traditional fee-for-service practice. A physician who is working for a federally certified HMO must devote a substantial amount of his time to the HMO. Under the 1976 HMO Amendments this is interpreted to mean about 35 percent of his professional time compared to 50 percent as interpreted under the 1973 regulations. Although allowed three years in which to work up to that division of time in a new HMO, many highly qualified solo and group practitioners have been turned off by the 1973 provisions. How can they be sure, they ask, that in three short years their—as yet—faceless HMO patients will outnumber their familiar fee-for-service clients?[42] But, it is possible for the physician to remain on a fee-for-service arrangement, even in a health maintenance organization, while still practicing in his own office. As already noted, this HMO arrangement is known as an individual practice association (IPA). The individual practice association operates, however, at risks; if the total capitation money disappears before all the fee claims have been made, the doctors are out of luck. But there is still another alternative. Even if all the HMOs become subject to federal standards—including the requirement that doctors give the HMOs a certain percentage of their time—the physician will still be free part of the time to see patients on a fee-for-service basis. And if the physician does join an established HMO on salary, he will have all the advantages of any large multispecialty group practice such as less paperwork, ready consultation, and regular hours plus a secure comfortable income.

On the other hand, despite security, an HMO also could mean less professional independence for the physician. Under the current federal program, peer review and other quality controls are mandatory. So is continuing education. It is also possible that an HMO might have its own drug formulary and might require the physician to prescribe generically. Finally, federal standards require consumer participation. One third of the positions on the policy-making board of a federally qualified HMO—but not an individual practice association—must be allocated to laymen enrolled in the HMO. This requirement gives consumers, along with doctors, a management voice in such matters as grievance hearings, quality assurance programs, continuing education courses for staff members, costs, utilization patterns and availability and accessibility of services.[43] It will be up to the individual physician to decide whether he feels comfortable with lay consumers contributing to decisions which are of importance to his practice of medicine. That seems more negative than positive in view of the tradition of independent thought and action which the physician develops in his medical training.

The Future

At one time HMOs projected an image of becoming a network of integrated delivery systems blanketing the nation in numbers of more than a thousand, sweeping into their institutional framework thousands of physicians as well as other health professionals and bringing efficiency as well as organization to the delivery of health services. The fear that socialized or bureaucratically-run systems were at hand, spelling the demise and the disappearance of the traditional private practice of medicine, loomed large. Yet, in the latter part of the 1970s the projected explosion of the HMOs has, thus far, turned out to be a dull thud. Only a handful of HMOs can even meet federal standards for becoming organized and operational. If that network ever develops, it looks like it may be many years away. Yet, it is still a threat to those physicians who prefer the private practice of medicine—not at the moment—but as another concept which is being tried and pushed with the full backing of the federal government. The issue at hand is not whether HMOs will become operational throughout the nation. Rather, the concept of prepaid group practice which had been lying relatively dormant for almost half a century suddenly has become a very viable idea for government to support as it seeks another solution to contain the runaway costs of health care. Of course one solution is available—but an answer which everyone wants to avoid if possible—a brake of last resort. A solution in which the government assumes total control of the entire health care industry through the nationalization and ownership of hospitals, nursing homes, drug companies, and private medical practices whereby it sets the fees, the prices and the profit margins. However, in trying to preserve the free enterprise system of the health care system, nothing seems really to work. But every time a new concept is adopted such as a Professional Standards Review Organization or revived or modified such as a health maintenance organization, another part of the health care system has been, perhaps, forever altered. The inability of health care institutions and professionals to discipline their own house creates the problem.

When they cannot do it for themselves, government fills the vacuum and performs the task for them. This is the significance of HMOs. Some time in the future—and when that day will be is indeterminable—the physician and other health professionals may very well be swept into this nationwide system and will ponder how and why it came about. They will only have to look back to a time when the costs of health care became so burdensome for society that the federal government became an activist in the health care field to find the answers. One of its solutions was the creation and fostering of an HMO—three letters which undoubtedly will be an integral part of the medical alphabet for many years to come.

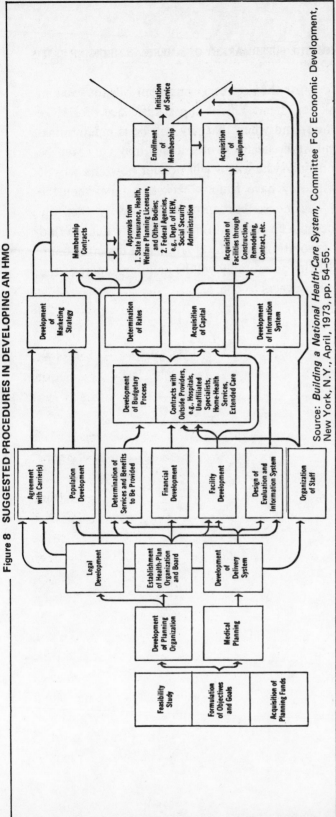

Figure 8   SUGGESTED PROCEDURES IN DEVELOPING AN HMO

Source: *Building a National Health-Care System*, Committee For Economic Development, New York, N.Y., April, 1973, pp. 54-55.

Figure 9

BASIC BENEFIT SERVICES PROVIDED BY A FEDERALLY-QUALIFIED HEALTH MAINTENANCE ORGANIZATION AS OF JANUARY 1976

- Physician services (including consultant and referral services by a physician)
- Inpatient and outpatient hospital services
- Medically necessary emergency health services
- Short-term (not to exceed twenty visits), outpatient evaluative and crisis intervention mental health services
- Medical treatment and referral services (including referral services to appropriate ancillary services) for the abuse of or addiction to alcohol and drugs
- Diagnostic laboratory and diagnostic and therapeutic radiologic services
- Home health services
- Preventive health services (including immunizations, well-child care from birth, periodic health evaluations for adults, voluntary family planning services, infertility services, and children's eye and ear examinations that are conducted to determine the need for vision and hearing correction.)

Note: Ancillary services mean hospital services or other inpatient health program, other than room and board, and professional services.

Source: U.S. Department of Health, Education, and Welfare, Health Services Administration, Division of Health Maintenance Organizations, Washington, D.C., January, 1978.

CHAPTER 5

Health Care Planning: Who Speaks for the Patient's Well-Being?

"It is the single most dangerous piece of legislation ever enacted by a United States Congress . . . it will totally restructure the practice of medicine, make the HEW Secretary an absolute czar of the delivery of health care and give nonmedical people the power to decide whether or not a service to be rendered in a hospital is the appropriate one."[1]

WITH THIS STRONG DENUNCIATION, Dr. James H. Sammons, the executive vice president of the American Medical Association, succinctly gave his view of the National Health Planning and Resources Development Act of 1974 (P. L. 93-641).

A decade earlier the Comprehensive Health Planning and Public Health Service Amendments of 1966 were enacted into law. At that time, Dr. William H. Stewart, then Surgeon General of the U. S. Public Health Service, stated that "the people shall be served and new social instruments, institutions and patterns of operation shall be developed to serve them".[2] That statement has proven to be prophetic. In the intervening decade organized medicine has seen enacted into law such programs as the Professional Standards Review Organization, the health maintenance organization and the new health planning law which it has so emphatically condemned. What happened to the health care field during this period of time to necessitate all these changes, especially the enactment of still another health planning law? What *is* health planning? Why do we need it? What implications does it have for the future practice of medicine? What do these divergent views, between the representatives of organized medicine and the federal government expressed nearly a decade apart, mean to you both as a patient and consumer? When we hear about present health care we listen to figures that boggle the human mind. We hear about the hundreds of millions of dollars spent for this social service each year and about health professionals who themselves number in the several millions. We hear about scientific advances in health fields whose technology and subject matter have become so complex that, as laymen, we have little everyday understanding as to their nature. Under these circumstances, some basic questions arise. How can I, just an ordinary consumer and patient, have influence over such a complex system which keeps absorbing more and more of my personal income? How can I exert some control over the prices which I must pay for health care services? How can I make any kind of input which will ensure that I will receive quality health care at reasonable cost and not inferior care at expensive prices? After all, it is my out-of-pocket expenses, it is my personal income taxes and it is my insurance premiums which are supporting the health care system. How can I be assured that the decisions which the health professionals are making are for my best interests as a patient rather than for their personal self-interests? Where is the entrance into the health care system which everyone keeps talking about? How can my voice be heard and my rights and interests, as a patient and consumer, protected and respected? These are some of the legitimate questions which the people have begun to ask as they realize that it is getting terribly expensive to become sick in this nation.

From a practical viewpoint, as a single individual you cannot affect the billions of dollars which are being spent nationally on health care services. Nor can you specifically affect the national costs of hospital care or physician services, nor the costs of the other health care services and problems which you hear or read about daily. But as an individual you can have a significant influence on the cost and quality of health care in the area where you live. For wherever you dwell—in urban or rural areas, North or South, East or West—there now exists an organization called a Health Systems Agency (HSA) which represents your geographic area. This agency, along with others at higher levels of government, was established in accordance with the requirements of the health planning act of 1974. As a consumer you can sit on this agency's governing board as part of the majority representation while the providers of health care services, such as physicians, constitute the minority representation. You now can have your voice heard as to how you think health care services should be delivered in your locality. By participating in the proceedings of this agency you can create a dialogue with the members of your community upon whom your health care depends—your doctor, your pharmacist, your hospital administrator and your health insurer, to name but a few. You can now help decide whether your hospital should build a new wing or purchase various kinds of expensive equipment. It is not only your judgement which is involved but also your money. Your decisions will be reflected in your hospital's daily charges, your physician's fees and your health insurer's premiums.

You can now contribute directly to the planning of your community's health care services because the 1974 planning law was designed, in part, with you, the consumer, in mind. Whether or not you participate in the deliberations of your local Health Systems Agency is, of course, your own decision. But the opportunity does exist for you to do something to control the cost of health care in your locality. And when all the communities collectively attempt to control their health care expenditires, then national health care costs also will be affected. But health care planning not only involves consideration of costs but also of the quality of care which you will receive from those who provide the services. There are many who negatively view the role which Health Systems Agencies will assume in the health care delivery system. These opponents consider HSAs to be a potential evil rather than a positive good. These detractors of the planning process have many reasons for their beliefs. In view of this dichotomy of opinions, let us examine the issue of health care planning—what it is, how it has evolved, the conflicts it has created within the health care field and what it may mean for the future of those who deliver, as well as those who receive, health care services.

Definition of Health Planning

Health planning is part of an evolving process called creative federalism—a term which is used to described a pluralistic approach to solving the problems of urban society. Creative federalism engenders an environment which Nelson Rockefeller described as "the free play of individual initiative, private enterprise, social institutions, political organizations and voluntary association . . ."[3]

As a concept, there are many varieties of planning. But they have the common basis, that planning is the opposite of improvisation. Planning is a process of developing alternative courses of action and predicting foreseeable results. Planning is not just a decision-making process. It is also a process of projecting and documenting choices of action. The selections are to be made through the political and social decision-making system of society. Dr. William H. Stewart, former Surgeon General of the U. S. Public Health Service, gave a good explanation of the planning process when he stated:

". . . there are at least two kinds of planning, interrelated but distinct from each other, that need to go simultaneously if we are to fulfill the expectations of the society we serve. One type is largely operational—it is directed toward day-to-day and year-to-year decisions on specific activity directed toward a specific objective. It is the kind of planning done by a program manager to carry out his program mission. The other type of planning is truly comprehensive. It is less concerned with targets and more concerned with directions. Ultimately, it must be tuned to values—the changing aspirations of society that require translation into changing goals for health and changing patterns of relationship among target-oriented activities.[4]

In a further refinement of this working planning concept, certain questions may be asked when attempting to accomplish the objectives of comprehensive health planning. They include:

● What is the problem for which you are developing a plan?
● What information do you need for developing a comprehensive plan?

- Who has the information—including the experience and judgement—required as an input into the development of the plan?
- What groups and agencies do you expect to act on your plan?[5]

In seeking the answers to these questions, planning essentially involves four basic steps—the survey, its analysis, the plan and its implementation. These steps are the basis upon which the principles of health planning are carried out. Although these principles seem quite simple and direct in their approach, the process of health care planning has evolved slowly and has been characterized as much by failure as it has by success.

The Historical Development of Health Planning

The evolution of health planning in the United States has several phases, the first of which evolved during the early 1920s. During this period the public became aware that hospitals throughout the country required some kind of planning effort. In 1921, the New York Academy of Medicine issued a report which found there was one hospital bed for every 200 persons in New York and concluded this ratio was sufficient. At the time, under the prevailing standard of the U. S. Public Health Service, it was estimated that about 2 percent of the population would be sufficiently sick at any given moment to require hospital care. However, during the ensuing decade, the realization developed that the method for determining a community's need for hospital beds had to be refined. Separate criteria had to be established for beds in a general hospital, beds for contagious diseases, maternity beds and beds for mental and tubercular patients. By the 1930s, local socio-economic conditions were the primary criteria for making these hospital bed determinations. These criteria included the economic status of the community, the character of housing and industry, education, morbidity levels and the caliber of the local medical profession[6]. In addition to the U. S. Public Health Service, other estimates of ideal bed size were made at this time. In the late 1920s, both the Duke Endowment and the American Hospital Association's

Committee on County Hospitals agreed upon a ratio of five general hospital beds per 1000 population. In addition, the Duke Endowment established bed ratio standards for contagious, children's and tubercular disease.[7] In 1945, the U. S. Public Health Service sanctioned a ratio of 4.5 beds per 1000 population which, with slight refinement, because the national standard for the Hill-Burton law of 1946.

As planning agencies increased in number during the 1930s, there was a general belief that the quality of health services would be greatly improved if working arrangements among hospitals became closer. Thus, planning agencies became interested not only in hospital beds but also in the organization of health facilities. However, by the 1940s a general shortage of hospital beds, their uneven distribution throughout the nation, and a lack of coordinating operations among hospitals was observed. Rural areas especially faced a crisis not only in terms of bed supply but also in regard to the availability of medical personnel. The way was paved for the second period of health planning which began when the U.S. Congress passed the Hospital Survey and Construction Act of 1946 (Hill-Burton). This law offered federal funds to states for the construction of hospitals and related facilities, pending a survey by each state of its existing institutions and the submission of a state plan to meet its bed needs.

Although the Hill-Burton Act did not make any reference to the coordination of facilities on a regional basis, the Act did give limited recognition to planning and regionalization by means of area-wide planning councils.[8] As a result of Hill-Burton, all states between 1946 and 1961 developed plans and established priorities. A total of $1.6 billion in federal monies and $3.4 billion in state funds was expended in the construction of 239,000 general hospital beds. One-third of these beds were in communities of less than 50,000 population. Although hospital design and construction were improved during this period of time, no real progress in terms of the coordination or integration of facilities on either a regional or local level was achieved.[9]

However, interest in the subject did not wane. It was rekindled by a series of meetings which were held in 1958, under the co-sponsorship of American Hospital Association and the U.S. Public Health Service. These meetings developed a joint report which assisted in the organization and operation of planning agencies. In 1961 the planning process was bolstered further by the passage of the Community Health Service and Facilities Act which authorized grants for area-wide planning and the development of hospitals and related facilities. This act became part of the Hill-Burton program and, together with the 1964 amendments to the Hill-Burton Act, provided financial impetus for health planning agencies. With these changes came a resurgence of interest in planning for other health services as well. For example, the enactment of the Community Mental Health Centers Act (P.L. 88-164) in 1963 encouraged the planning of mental health services.

By 1966, there were about 60 voluntary health planning agencies operating in the country. The focus of these agencies was on the supply and geographic distribution of hospital beds; on controlling duplication of services and facilities; and on encouraging activities and programs of coordination between institutions. Thus, the agencies were involved with institutional planning such as with hospitals. Physicians were not the subject of the planning process at this time. Consequently, they were not directly affected by the decision of the agencies. Agency planning was more technologically oriented than systems oriented.[10]

As the concept of health planning evolved during this period together with the establishment of planning agencies and the funding of such programs with federal monies, Congress became increasingly aware that the changing character of American health care demanded new governmental initiatives. These included comprehensive health planning for health services, health manpower and health facilities at every level of government; revitalized administration of health agencies at the state level and broader and more flexible support of health services at the community level as well. This perception led, in part, to enactment of the Regional Medical Program (RMP) in 1965 (P.L.89-239). This program originally was intended to encourage regional planning and the transfer of medical technology for the categorical illness of heart disease, cancer and stroke from university medical centers to the community providers of health services. Over the years the program shifted its focus toward regionalizing health-care delivery, facilitating co-operative action among health care providers and designing as well as testing innovative ways to improve health care services.

Despite the passage of the Regional Medical Program in 1965, health planning activities were still considered too narrow and not sufficiently oriented toward the problems of upgrading the health status of the public, improving the environmental and raising the quality of life of the American people. Therefore, the Partnership for Health Act (P.L. 89-749) was enacted in November 1966 and then amended in 1967. It was passed to correct the earlier flaws of health planning and to undertake once again the rationalization of our health delivery system. The Comprehensive Health Planning Program (CHP) established gradations of agencies within state and local government including the 314 (b) agencies which were named after the authorizing section of the Act. The CHP (b) agencies were charged with the responsibility of planning the total needs of their region. They were expected to build on the activities of the area-wide Hill-Burton agencies, whose federal support was phased out with the passage of P.L. 89-749. However, in some states, Hill-Burton continued to exist with local funding.

The legislative intent of the Regional Medical and the Comprehensive Health Planning Programs was to improve the health care system without interfering with existing patterns of medical practice.[11] However, the concerns and focus of the new agencies were at times so broad that the planners went from problem to problem, never quite solving one before another became pressing. Too often more time was spent debating what should be done rather than doing anyting. But, by the late 1960s, despite these problems,

CHP agencies were given some powers to influence health activities through their review and comment role in statewide certificate-of-need (CON) programs, where they existed, and in the award process of federal grants for some Public Health Service programs. One of the important ways in which CHP had an impact on the health system was through its participation in Section 1122 of the Social Security Amendments of 1972 (P.L. 92-603).[12] Under Section 1122, a hospital or other health care institution cannot recoup a major financial capital investment by adding charges to the bills of Medicare or Medicaid patients unless the improvements were first allowed by an authorized state agency. However, despite having the authority to make these reviews, both the Regional Medical and the Comprehensive Health Planning Programs remained still dependent on whatever powers of persuasion they could marshal to encourage the development of health-resources among their regional constituencies.

Also, by the late 1960s, emphasis on deliverying health services began to shift to organizations other than just hospitals, such as neighborhood health centers, community mental health centers and health maintenance organizations. By the early 1970s, the rise in the cost of medical care, growing concern with the quality of care which was being delivered and the re-emergence of national health insurance as a major policy issue added impetus for designing a more effective health planning system. By about 1972, there was general agreement that comprehensive health planning had been a failure. After a brief flirtation with substitute experimental health service delivery systems, the U.S. Department of Health, Education, and Welfare began to look for a wholly new approach to health planning. This search ultimately led to the passage of the National Health Planning and Resources Development Act of 1974. The Act was signed into law on January 4, 1975.

The 1974 legislation combined aspects of the Hill-Burton, Regional Medical and Comprehensive Health Planning Programs into a new generation of agencies. These organizations take over the health planning and resource development functions previously performed by the Comprehensive Health Planning and Regional Medical Programs which were phased out of existence under the 1974 health planning law. Also, the experimental health service delivery systems which HEW was testing for purposes of public demonstration were also terminated upon enactment of the 1974 legislation.

Health Planning Act of 1974

The National Health Planning and Development Act of 1974 not only establishes a new program of comprehensive health planning but also empowers a system of local planning agencies to oversee the use of some federal funds, including funds for new hospital construction. The goals and purposes of the new law are increased accessibility, acceptability, continuity and quality of health services; restraint of the rising costs of health care services; and the prevention of unnecessary duplication of health resources. The law thus establishes a prospective national framework for reviewing the funds which will be expended under any future national health insurance plan.

At the core of the new program is a network of local health planning agencies called the Health Systems Agency (HSA). A total of 205 geographic areas throughout the country have been designated for these agencies. To the maximum extent possible their area boundries are "approximately coordinated" with Professional Standards Review Organizations, existing regional planning areas as well as state planning and administrative areas. Each of these agencies will serve, except in special cases, a defined population of between 500,000 to 3,000,000 people. These local agencies can be either a nonprofit private corporation or a public agency operating under the auspices of a unit of general-purpose local government or a public regional planning body. The Secretary of HEW must certify these agencies according to the criteria laid out in. the law. In addition to the Health Systems Agency, there are planning bodies on the state and national level which form policy and supervise the work of these local agencies. These include the National Council on Health Planning and Development, which assists the Secretary of HEW in developing national health planning guidelines; the Statewide Health Coordinating Council, which draws up the state health plan, which in turn, can supersede the plan developed by the local HSA, and monitors activities of the HSA, reporting to Washington on its importance, and the State Health Planning and Development Agency, which can enforce the HSA's decisions on major equipment purchases and new construction since the state agency administers the state's certificate-of-need laws.[13]

On the local level, the Health Systems Agency is required to:

- gather and analyze data;
- establish area-wide long-range health systems plans and annual implementation plans;
- provide planning assistance to organizations seeking to develop plans;
- review and approve or disapprove applications for federal grant funds for health programs in the health service area;
- assist states in reviewing capital expenditures under Section 1122 of the Medicare Act;
- assist states in their mandated certificate-of-need programs;
- recommend to states projects for modernizing, constructing and converting medical facilities;[14]

The Health Systems Agency develops a health systems plan for its geographic service area. This plan, in turn, is approved at the state level. Eventually, the HSAs may control who may be reimbursed with federal funds under national health insurance or Medicare/Medicaid, including possibly physicians! For the more immediate future, they directly control only federal grant monies which are spent for health projects in their areas under the Public Health Service Act, the Community Mental Health Centers Act, and the Comprehensive Alcohol Abuse and Alcoholism Prevention, Treatment and Rehabilitation Act of 1970. Even though HSAs receive their guidance from HEW regulations out of Washington, they are very important to organized medicine and the rest of the health care field. Some day their plans and recommendations may determine which new hospital, nursing home or, perhaps even which physician's office, receives the all important building permit—the certificate-of-need from the state agency.[15]

In addition to the aforementioned responsibilities, the new health planning law creates a national set of health care guidelines which local communities, through the activities of HSAs, will try to incorporate into their health systems. They include the following:

● provide primary care for medically underserved populations;
● develop "multi-institutional systems" to coordinate obstetrics, pediatrics, emergency medicine, intensive and coronary care, radiation therapy and other services;
● develop group practices, especially those linked to institutional health services, as well as HMOs and other organized systems for the provision of health care;
● train and use more physicians' assistants, especially more nurse clinicians;
● develop multi-institutional sharing of support services;
● promote improvements in the quality of health services, including those identified by PSROs;
● provide various levels of institutional care on a "geographically integrated basis", including intensive, acute general and extended care;
● promote "prevention" of disease, including studies of nutritional and environmental factors;
● get health service institutions to adopt a more uniform and simplified form of cost accounting, better management procedures, reimbursement arrangements and utilization reporting in order to improve the management of health care programs;
● develop effective methods of personal health education for the general public.[16]

Before the passage of the 1974 planning law, very few constraints existed for controlling the costs of health care. Until this law required that all states enact certificate-of-need laws, only slightly more than one-half had done so of their own volition. Also, only a small number of states have attempted to regulate health care costs through the establishment of state rate setting commissions. But the new law provides monies for up to six states who wish to do so in the future. Before this law, if a group of doctors in a hospital wished to add a service or increase their rates, they only needed the approval of the hospital board of directors—bodies which are not known for contradicting the wishes of their physician staff. But under the 1974 law, both the local HSA and the state planning agency will conduct at least every five years elaborate reviews of existing facilities, services and of any proposed construction to determine the need or lack of need for these addition. While no sanctions exist at present in regard to an HSA's findings, it is obvious that the law creates a mechanism which may be equipped with enforcement powers at a later date. Even the Hill-Burton hospital construction program was affected by the 1974 law. Rather than concentrating on the building of new inpatient facilities, as in years past, the Hill-Burton program received new directives under the 1974 planning law. These included concentrating on the construction of ambulatory care facilities, improving and converting existing facilities to new uses and constructing new inpatient facilities, but only in areas of rapid population growth.

A final example of the new planning law's orientation is the emphasis it places on the consumer movement within the health care field as well as the greater voice it gives to planning professionals in directing the future course of health delivery. At the state and local levels, governing boards oversee health planning activities. These boards will be carefully consti-tuted so that a majority of its members will be consumers, professionals and government officials. The providers of health care—the doctors, hospital administrators and others who have a vested interest at stake—are legislated to form a minority on these boards.[17]

The AMA Fights Back

By making the physician take a back seat to the majority representation of the consumers and other non-health providers on local and state planning boards, government appears to have given American medicine another indication of lack of confidence in the ability of the physician to plan our present and future health care services. Rather, government is turning to the consumer whose vested interest in the system is not personal economic gain but receipt of the highest quality service at reasonable cost. Is it any wonder that executive vice president of the American Medical Association lashed out at the 1974 planning law by stating that it sets up the Secretary of HEW as a medical czar? According to Dr. James H. Sammons:

"It is the secretary who's going to issue guidelines on national health policy that will continue standards for the appropriate supply, distribution and organization of all health resources. It's the secretary who's going to approve or disapprove the annual budgets of the local planning agencies. It's the secretary who's going to establish procedures and criteria to be used by the planning agencies in performing reviews of state medical facility plans, appropriateness of existing institutional health services, proposed new institutional health services, and use of federal grant funds. It's the secretary who's going to decide how the state health plan, the local health system plan, and the annual implementation plan are going to be developed. It's the secretary who's going to make grants available to states to demonstrate the effectiveness of rate regulation.

"And that's just the start. The secretary has so many other responsibilities that it takes too long to list them. For trivia-minded people like me, I should point out that the secretary is identified 281 times in a 59 page act. Now that ought to give you some idea of the incredible amount of power over health care and its delivery that has been massed and placed in the hands of a single individual—an individual who is not elected."[18]

Although many may dispute this characterization of the law's intent, it expresses organized medicine's exceeding displeasure with the new planning Act and its implications for the future practice of medicine. It has seemingly placed the profession on a direct collision course with the federal government. Early in 1976, Dr. James H. Sammons stated:

"We at the AMA are concerned with maintaining the quality of care. The government has taken the position that quality can go to hell in a basket as long as costs are contained.

"This law would put medical decision-making in the hands of consumers. It scares me to death.

"Well, we will communicate and co-operate with government if they are reasonable. And you people in the states should do the same if government is reasonable. But this type of regulation is an abridgment of freedom, and if government is to be unreasonable, then we will fight. And if we end up standing alone, then we will stand alone."[19]

Not long after this statement was made, HEW issued, in March 1976, some proposed regulations governing the activities of state government under the planning law. The massive set of regulations spelled out in detail the organization and functions of the State Health Planning and Development Agencies (SHPDA) and the Statewide Health Coordinating Councils (SHCC) which were to be established under the planning law. In addition, the proposed regulations covered such items as review of the need for certain health expenditures, the minimum requirements for state certificate-of-need programs, the review of proposed institutional health services by local Health Systems Agencies (HSA) and statewide bodies, and the program of capital expenditures review as authorized by Section 1122 of the Social Security Act. Although retaining the terminology "ambulatory surgical facility," the regulations dropped the term "organized ambulatory health care facility" from the definition of a health care facility. Thus, for the moment, at least, the operations of a physician's office in the private practice of medicine were assured of not being placed under the review authority of the planning law. But in October 1976, three weeks before the Presidential election, a curious event took place in Washington. Draft guidelines for a national planning policy, which had been scheduled for publication in the *Federal Register* of October 13, 1976, were withdrawn at the last minute by HEW.

A departmental spokesman stated that the hold-up was purely procedural and not substantive. According to the assistant secretary of health and scientific affairs, the draft guidelines were not to be considered regulations nor even a formal notice of proposed rulemaking. The guidelines emphasized consumer participation and sometimes were specific to the point of setting goals for a patient in a doctor's office. Among the guidelines were such goals as suggesting that the appointment waiting time for primary care service be no longer than one week and in-office waiting time be no more than 30 minutes.[20] Three weeks before a Presidential election the federal government was getting close to suggesting how the private physician should conduct at least one small aspect of his office operations—a prerogative organized medicine is fighting fiercely to protect. This group within our society had contributed heavily to the upcoming federal elections about to take place at the time the proposal was, perhaps, coincidentally withdrawn. But only time will be the ultimate judge as to whether or not these guidelines become federal regulations under the planning law in the future. However, they do serve as an excellent indication of how government may someday attempt to regulate the practice of medicine. Waiting a maximum of thirty minutes to see a physician is appealing for the patient who now must remain much longer in the waiting room after scheduling his appointment in advance. But it is not very appealing for the patient being treated when the physician may say "I'm sorry your thirty minutes are up, won't you please come back again so that I can finish the treatment". Although this situation is a highly unlikely scenario for an ethical physician, its possibility is not as unseemly as it may appear. On October 5, 1977, the Columbia Broadcasting System aired on national television a film entitled "Mary Jane Harper Cried Last Night"—a movie dealing with the battered child syndrome. In one sequence of the film, the abusing mother began to tell her psychiatrist about some childhood experiences which may have subconsciously contributed to her adult behavior. Although the mother was anxious to complete her narrative to the psychiatrist on a particular childhood episode, the psychiatrist forced the mother to end her discourse because her session time was completed. Because of the literal minutes on the clock, the patient's emotional cry for help went unheeded as the psychiatrist told her to come back the following week and continue her dialogue from its point of interruption. Eventually, with no one listening to her problems, including her parents and her psychiatrist, the mother, in a state of emotional trauma, killed her child. A movie and fiction—yes; but how often have we observed life imitating art? Although this case—whether fiction or reality—may be considered an extreme case, the guidelines can create all kinds of problems for the delivery of health services because of the manner in which they are expressed. And the guidelines are required to be published in accordance with the 1974 health planning law as part of the development of a national health policy which local Health Systems Agencies can implement.

Thus, it is not surprising to find the American Medical Association opposing those health planning regulations which already have been published and which may be published in the future. For example, on May 3, 1976, the American Medical Association wrote to the Secretary of HEW objecting to the previously mentioned regulations proposed by HEW in March of that year. The AMA said that the proposed rules are contrary to Section 1122 of the Social Security Act and the planning law; exceed and misinterpret statutory authority and Congressional intent; contravene the Privacy Act; and would have an "adverse impact on the availability and quality of health services." The AMA noted that the regulations "would usurp local and state responsibility proclaimed by the advocates of the Act as the hallmark of the legislation."[21] The AMA contends that the planning law itself violates the Constitution because it transfers to the federal government authority that it constitutionally reserved to the states. According to the AMA's general counsel:

"It places the control of health facilities and, thus, ultimately the control of medical practice, in the hands of the federal bureaucrats. It's an unwise law—restrictive, oppressive and impractical"[22]

The aforementioned rationale served as the basis of a lawsuit which the American Medical Association filed on May 13, 1976 against the federal government seeking judicial relief from the law. But in September 1977, the U.S. District Court Judges in Raleigh, North Carolina unanimously ruled the health planning act does not invade the sovereign rights of the states nor interfere in the private practice of medicine. On April 17, 1978, the U.S. Supreme Court affirmed without opinion the ruling of the U.S. District Court upholding the constitutionality of the 1974 health planning law. But in addition to seeking judicial relief, there appears to be a need for some alphabetic relief from the law as well. As one of the law's inner workings noted:

"The HSA will develop a Health System Plan (HSP) and an Annual Implementation Plan (AIP). In most states, the various HSPs and AIPs developed by local HSAs will be forwarded to the State Health Planning and Development Agency (SHPDA), which will presumably integrate the HSPs into a State Health Plan (SHP) and a State Medical Facilities Plan (SMFP), both to be coordinated through a Statewide Health Coordinating Council (SHCC). All according to HEW guidelines."[23]

To some authorities the mix of HEW, HSA, HSP, AIP, SHPDA, SHP, SMFP and SHCC add up to bureaucratic confusion.

Implication of Law to Physicians

While the American Medical Association wages a national fight against the 1974 health planning law, the significance of the law can also be examined in terms of its effect on the individual physician and his everyday practice of medicine. One important impact of the 1974 law stems from the certificate-of-need legislation (CON) which all states must enact by October 1, 1980 if they hope to obtain federal funding for new health facilities. The certificate-of-need laws will limit the building of excess hospital beds. Under-utilized wards and wings may be shut-down and entire hospitals eventually may be closed through the review-of-need provisions which the law contains.

Since the establishment of state and local planning units does not occur quickly, it could be as long as five or six years before a physician's medical practice begins to feel the effect of the new health planning system. Facilities are now generally felt to be overbuilt in many parts of the nation and further regulations will be issued to identify and close those facilities which can be eliminated without impairing the delivery of health-care services.

Another provision of the law calls for the Secretary of HEW to develop a classification system for primary, secondary and tertiary health-care facilities with progressively sophisticated resources. Although the law does not specify that such a system must be put into effect, it is possible that it could be done. Thus, if and when it is used, some of the services a physician may like to use at his hospital may be eliminated. Coronary-care, cobalt therapy, renal dialysis and other highly specialized units may be centralized within many communities. That could result in inconvenience for the patient and his physician, though such consolidations and centralization also could result in reducing health care costs. According to former Congressman William R. Roy, a doctor who helped shape the 1974 planning law:

"The day is past when a physician on a hospital staff can assume his requirements will not be met without challenge. From now on his needs will be weighed against the community's financial resources."[24]

Dr. Roy's statement is a true reflection of the times. In March 1978, the U. S. Department of Health, Education, and Welfare issued final planning guidelines which local Health Systems Agencies can use in determining the future of hospitals and health services in their geographic areas. According to HEW officials, one major goal of the federal guidelines is to cut back about 100,000 unneeded hospital beds by 1984—about 10 percent of the total bed capacity of community hospitals throughout the country—in order to boost occupancy rates and reduce health care costs. The federal guidelines call for no more than 4 community hospital beds per 1000 population in a given health service area and an average occupancy rate of at least 80 percent for all hospitals combined in such an area. There are also proposed restrictions on costly medical services the intent of which, according to HEW, is to improve the quality of care by limiting the use of these services to those facilities which perform them on a regular basis. Thus, the guidelines, like other governmental activity whose basis emanates from the 1974 health planning law, will have a great impact on a physician's private practice of medicine. Among the remaining guidelines issued by HEW are the following:

- Obstetrical services should be planned on a regional basis. Hospitals providing care for complicated obstetrical problems should have at least 1,500 births annually. Average occupancy rates for units of more than 1,500 births per year should be at least 75 percent.

- Neonatal services should be planned on a regional basis. An area should have no more than four neonatal intensive and intermediate care beds per 1,000 live births per year. A neonatal special care unit should contain at least 15 beds.

- There should be a minimum of 20 beds in a pediatric unit in urbanized areas.

- Average annual occupancy rates for pediatric units should range from a minimum of 65 percent for 20-39 bed units to at least 75 percent for units with 80 or more beds.

- Institutions performing open heart surgery for adults should do at least 200 open heart procedures per year, and there should be no additional units established in an area unless all existing units are handling at least 350 adult open heart surgery cases per year. For pediatric heart operations, a minimum of 100 operations is required, at least 75 of which should be open heart surgery, and no new units should be established unless existing units are handling 130 pediatric open heart cases.

- There should be a minimum of 300 cardiac catheterizations annually in an adult catheterization unit, and at least 150 cardiac catheterizations annually in any pediatric catheterization unit.

- A megavoltage radion therapy unit should serve a population of at least 150,000 persons and treat at least 300 cancer cases a year.

- A computed tomographic scanner should perform at least 2,500 "medically necessary" patient procedures per year.
- Local health plans should be consistent with HEW regulations regarding end-stage renal disease services.[25]

In issuing the guidelines, HEW Secretary Joseph A. Califano, Jr. stated that "these standards provide a solid basis for controlling excess capacity in the health care industry—an excess which has needlessly added billions of dollars to hospital costs".[26] The Secretary also pointed out that the standards are subject to adjustment at the local or state levels to meet special circumstances and requirements. However, the American Medical Association had a far different reaction to the standards issued. In commenting upon the preliminary guidelines upon which the final standards were based and issued without any significant alterations, the AMA stated:

"We still believe that the mandatory nature of the department's actions distorts the Congressional intent behind health planning and ignores the realities of medical care and the education of health professionals . . . We continue to believe that the present approach HEW is taking is contrary to the needs and interests, of the patients"[27]

Needless to say, HEW does not agree with the views of the American Medical Association as to the purpose or the intent of the standards. But what we have in this confrontation is a very serious question. Who speaks for and represents the patient's well-being in these matters—the government or organized medicine?

Upon publication of the standards, local planning agencies have a year to incorporate them into their plans and have five additional years to carry out the stated objectives. It should be noted that up until the announcement of the previous standards, a number of states were already "rationing" facilities and equipment under certificate-of-need regulations. For example, in northern New Jersey two hospitals and two groups of physicians all applied to buy $400,000 brain scanners. But the local health planning board could authorize only two in its region. It chose as the location for one scanner the larger hospital which has a university medical center affiliation. The two physician groups merged and installed the second scanner in a free-standing diagnostic center. Instead of four under-utilized units, there were two scanners operating at near capacity.[28] If hospitals in other communities throughout the nation begin to centralize their services, it would undoubtedly impact upon thousands of physicians. Centralization could harm medical practice unless the physician is able and willing to make adjustments if the hospital reduces its services, transfers its services to a more centralized location or even shuts down. Although the 1974 health planning law does not yet call for mandatory closings of beds or whole institutions, it does require each unit of the Health Systems Agencies to review all facilities in its area at least once every five years for continuing appropriateness, as already noted. So far the law dictates nothing more than a public release of agency findings about duplicative services and excess beds. But the publicity attracted by such reports alone will generate more pressure to eliminate waste.

On the other hand, a physician's practice can actually get a boost from hospital or service consolidation, especially if his institution is chosen to serve as the area's hospital center and if its facilities and services are augmented to meet this new responsibility. But should a particular service such as a radiation center be denied to a hospital because such a center already exists a few miles away, then the physician is likely to receive courtesy accreditation at the other institution. If he does not mind travelling or is willing to relocate his office, it is likely that he will be able to obtain privileges there as well. Otherwise, the physician may find himself referring more patients than at present to other practitioners.

Another major concern to physicians is the possibility that planning councils in states with strong certificate-of-need laws would try to dictate the location, equipping and expansion of private medical offices. Thus far, private physician offices are not subject to certificate-of-need controls under the federal health planning law. However, this situation does not mean that one day a physician's desire to spend monies for his private office—whether it be for equipment or construction above a certain monetary level would not be subject to the decision of area health planners who are seeking to reduce health expenditures in their community. Under the circumstances. Max H. Parrott, MD, who served as President of the American Medical Association, stated that the 1974 health planning law represented a giant step toward making American medicine a public utility rather than an independent profession:

"Why are the AMA and most physicians fighting so hard against the health planning act? We are doing so because our whole medical philosophy is at stake, a philosophy that will determine what the future of health care in America is to be. We doctors simply cannot be doctors unless we approach care from the standpoint of human beings, of patients. Government tends to see the people as abstract, statistical building blocks, and to fancy that the better it plays with these blocks, the more it does for people. This kind of all-too-serious play has led to disaster in public housing, urban renewal, highway development, welfare and other areas . . . Let us ask ourselves where is man in the planning act. Will it do him any good, or will it do him harm?[29]

In November 1977, many people in Northern Virginia also were asking themselves as to whether the 1974 planning law was going to do any good or any harm. At that time, the Northern Virginia Health Systems Agency (HSA) released its plan for public comments. The plan outlined how health care services should be provided to the residents of Northern Virginia for the ensuing five years. If the reaction of the doctors, nurses and hospital administrators to the Northern Virginia health systems plan is any indication of what will happen in the rest of the country when other agencies release their plans, then the health care provider and the American consumer-patient may be about to go to war. In general, the Northern Virginia plan emphasized the problems of escalating health-care costs. It called for a moratorium on the building of more hospitals, emergency rooms, obstetrical units, operating rooms, and X-ray units until existing facilities were used more heavily. The physicians argued at public hearings on the plan that the agency's standards were not realistic. They stated that heavier use of these facilities would lead to longer waiting lines, poorer care and eventually higher costs. And all the underlying friction between the health provider and the consumer-patient over the whole philosophy of health planning came to the surface. Their antagonism toward each other centered on the key health planning question—who has the ability to plan most effectively for the public's health and well-being—the health provider or the layman? Their opinions are most likely to be echoed many times across this nation before health planning becomes an effective instrument for solving the many health problems which ail the nation. The comments are also indicative of the frustrations which today bedevil the health providers as they observe the government encroaching more and more on their freedom of professional decision-making as government attempts to contain health care costs while improving its quality. Similarly, the consumers also are frustrated over their personal inability to control the rising costs of health care with which they must deal with in their everyday lives.

The following comments, indicative of the frictions and frustrations, were made at the hearings:

". . . the vehement testimony from doctors and hospital administrators is understandable for a group that really has grown under its own rules, and all of a sudden is confronted with consumers trying to take a role. There's a natural human reaction to protect their own turf."—HSA Board Chairman.

"Regulations are written by people who don't understand the problem, to the distress of the enforcer and to the ultimate detriment of the supposed beneficiary."—a doctor.

"HEW's new national planning guidelines are a giant step in the wrong direction . . . We must be allowed leeway. We must be allowed to learn from experience."—a doctor.

"Congress has been stampeded into passing a law which has effectively excluded health providers from participating in the planning process . . . The total law has to be changed. The total philosophy and intent of Congress is inappropriate but this HSA took it to the nth degree."–a doctor.

"Planners have no constituency in our community and no expertise in the delivery of health . . . I have a constituency. If a patient is displeased, who does she call up and complain to, whether it's the cost of the bill or the quality of her care? If doctors don't represent her in her health needs, then who does?"–a doctor.

"I go to most of the (HSA) meetings, and I do not see many from the provider side there."–a consumer.

". . . the HSA had done a good job of addressing the concerns that worry me–higher costs, too much dependence on doctors to treat minor ills, too much use of emergency rooms for routine care . . . These guys (in the medical profession) have blown it . . . They haven't given us a reasonable system and Congress reacted . . . The HSA (board members) are my neighbors and they listen to me, which is more than some of the providers can say. The overall impression I got (at the hearings) was, 'we don't want the status quo changed'."– a consumer.[30]

Upon receiving the public comments, the agency's board of directors then reviews the plan to determine what changes, if any, should be made prior to sending the plan to the state and then to HEW for final approval. But the public hearings and the comments which they elicited answer, in part, a question posed earlier in our discussions–what do the divergent views between organized medicine and the government mean to the patient-consumer in terms of who should plan for his health care services? On the local level it means everything. This community dialogue with health providers will determine the quality and the cost of the health care services which the patient will receive in years to come. His most valuable possession–namely, his personal health and well-being–will be affected by the outcome of the community's debate. His life literally will depend upon the final answer.

Conclusion

"We are now very definitely intervening in the private practice of medicine and in the organization and operation of health care institutions and the primary reason is dollars. More and more of the federal budget is going toward health expenditures. As inflation has eaten up all of the benefits of Medicare, there has been an overwhelming need to say that government can no longer play the passive role of simply paying the bills."[31] This statement, by a former director of HEW's Bureau of Health Planning and Resources Development, can well summarize the whole thrust of government activity into the health care field. Health care planning is here to stay and the penetration of the federal government into the health care delivery system with each succeeding law becomes deeper and deeper. As yet, no one can foresee what impact the mixture of conflicting and overwhelming political interests will have on the final shape of the planning systems. But one point is for certain − the private physician and the way he practices medicine will be materially affected by the 1974 law, another example of government intervention. This health planning law is far more ambitious and far more complex to understand than other health programs which have preceded it. Once again, another alteration has been made to the way medicine will be practiced in this country, although the magnitude of the change is difficult to perceive at the moment. How wise and reasonable will be the individuals who run the new system is not known. However, the quality and cost of health care which the American public will receive and pay for in future years will well depend upon their future decisions and actions. A decade after the enactment of Medicare and Medicaid, when the government began to finance health care services on a massive scale, the continuing creation of a health care system of labyrinthean complexity may well make the former cottage industry, as health care has often times been called, look well-organized indeed.

Figure 10

———— THE NEW HEALTH PLANNING ALPHABET ————

NHPRDA
National Health Planning and Resources Development Act of 1974– the new law.

NCHPD
National Council on Health Planning and Development– a new HEW advisory council which sets national health policies and guides health development.

SHPDA
State Health Planning and Development Agency– the state planning agency which replaces the old CHP(a) agency.

SHCC
Statewide Health Coordinating Commission– advisory council for SHPDA, containing representatives from all HSAs in the state.

SHP
State Health Plan– the policies, goals and objectives the state will follow in developing health care.

SAP
State Administrative Program– the plan the state agency will follow to achieve its goals and objectives within a given year.

MFP
Medical Facilities Plan– equivalent of the old Hill-Burton state plan.

DPA
Designated Planning Agency– a familiar acronym for the state agencies which conduct both Section 1122 of P.L. 92-603 and certificate-of-need review.

HSA.
Health Systems Agency– the area-wide planning agency which replaces the old CHP (b) agency; usually serves multicounty area.

HSP
Health Systems Plan– the statement of over-all policies, goals, and objectives for the area served by the HSA

AIP
Annual Implementation Plan– the work program the HSA will follow to achieve its goals and objectives.

AHSDF
Area Health Services Development Fund– the money available to HSAs for promoting local health care development.

HPD
Health Planning and Development– refers to the combined activities of comprehensive health planning (CHP), regional medical programs (RMP) and Hill-Burton.

Source: Adapted from Robin E. MacStravic, "Provisions of the National Health Planning and Resources Development Act,", *Hospital Progress,* April, 1975, p. 49. Reproduced with permission from *Hospital Progress.* Copyright, 1975 by the Catholic Hospital Association.

CHAPTER 6

Medical Malpractice Insurance: To Sue or Not Sue — That is the Question

DOCTORS' STRIKES, WORK SLOWDOWNS, formation of physician-owned and operated insurance companies, the ordering of extensive and possibly unneeded medical tests—is the revolt finally taking place? Is the American physician finally striking back at an over-regulated government health program which is oppressing his freedom to practice the kind of medicine he deems best? No! Instead, this is the American physician's response to another and more immediate crucial situation affecting the way he conducts his medical practice—namely, *the medical malpractice suit.*

Professional journals, and other communication media announced initially that a new crisis had hit American medicine. Warnings proclaimed that, unless solutions for the problem were found and found quickly, the American public would face additional staggering increases in the high costs of medical care. But was it really a new crisis? Why does it still persist? Why is it a matter of grave concern to those within and outside the medical profession? What precipitated its sudden transformation from discussion in the back pages of professional journals to the front pages of our daily newspapers and prominence on our evening television news?

Whether or not you know the answers to these questions, you are not fully insulated from the medical malpractice dilemma. For even if you, as a consumer-patient, never file a malpractice lawsuit against your physician, you are still involved in the malpractice quandry. Every time your physician sends you his bill, part of his charge reflects the cost of purchasing medical malpractice insurance to protect himself against the lawsuits which other patients may file against him. As an innocent bystander, you are paying for that insurance. And when your doctor's insurance rates rise so do the charges in your medical bill. Certainly, this is a situation that urgently requires a resolution which is equitable to the insurance carriers who provide the malpractice coverage and to the physicians who purchase it and fair as well to the public who ultimately must pay the bill.

A very basic question arises. Why are so many lawsuits now being filed against the American physician? There are many explanations offered for this problem. One of the principal ones is that the system in which you, as a patient, receive your medical care and the climate in which it is delivered has changed greatly from the recent past.

As more and more people obtain the means to finance health care, whether it be through public programs which are established for this purpose or through the expansion of private health insurance plans, a larger number of people are able to pay for their physician's treatment. The more they are able to pay for their medical care, the more they can afford to visit their physician. In fact, HEW has noted that about one billion patients visits were made in 1976. The more patients visit their doctor, the greater is the number of physician-patient contacts. The greater the number of patient contacts, the more hurried and more impersonal may be the physician's attention to each patient. The more hurried the doctor's attention, the greater is the risk that he may make mistakes in his diagnosis or treatment, particularly given the complexity of medical technologies and the nature of the new miracle drugs. The greater these risks, the greater the chances of a malpractice suit. With increased chances of a malpractice suit, the premium rates will be higher, or those rates will rise which the carrier will charge the physician to cover the costs of his insurance. And the higher the premiums, the more the physician has to charge the patient to cover the cost of his insurance. The higher the medical bills, (of which malpractice insurance is but one of many cost items,) the more the public complains that health care has become a service which it no longer can afford. With increased public complaint there is more of a cry for additional government intervention into the health care field. And the more the government intervenes, the more it undertakes such measures as expanding existing programs, creating new plans for those who have difficulty in purchasing medical care, or increasing public regulations over health care providers in an attempt to reduce their service costs. The more the government undertakes such measures, the more health costs increase as health care providers comply with additional government regulations and as more people are able to pay for their medical care because of the expansion or establishment of public programs. And the larger the number of people able to pay for their medical care, the more often they can visit their doctor to receive treatment and we are back to the very first step of the dilemma relating to malpractice suits.

On the other hand, if a physician tries to reduce the cost of his medical practice by dropping his malpractice insurance, he may administer medical tests for his own legal protection which a patient does not need. This kind of practice is known as "defensive medicine." In this fashion, the physician drives up the cost of his medical bill in particular, and health care in general. On the other hand, the physician may become more cautious in treating his patient and cut back on ordering procedures which may result in a malpractice suit being filed against him if such procedures are improperly administered. And even if public or private programs did not exist to help an individual purchase medical care or did not cover a wide variety of health services, a patient still might need a particular medical service. If a patient has to be in a nursing home, that need exists regardless of the availability of nursing home coverage which may pay for all or part of his care through either public or private programs. And if a patient has to pay for his medical service with his own funds, he may not be able to afford such care. So again, we have a situation where the public demands that some kind of mechamisn be created to help it pay for health care. Thus, public and private programs are established to provide financial protection against the costs of ill health. And, again, the public can pay for its medical care and visit the doctor more often than when this assistance did not exist. So once again we are back to the very first steps of the scenario where the increasing demand for doctor's services could lead to hurried attention which could result in misdiagnoses or mistreatment which, in turn, could result in the patient's filing of a medical malpractice suit.

What does all this mean? Simply stated, the rising costs of health care services, of which malpractice suits are but one of many contributing factors, is an issue whose many components defy an easy singular solution. However, there are health authorities who believe that reorganizing and restructuring the health care system into an integrated, rationale and coordinated whole, developing new health delivery systems such as health maintenance organizations or developing a comprehensive national health insurance plan will accomplish these goals. But the medical malpractice dilemma, like the issue of health care costs, may be likened to the late Winston Churchill's description of the Soviet Union. It is "a riddle wrapped in a mystery inside an enigma." Thus, because the medical malpractice issue is important to the cost and the quality of medical care today and in the future, this chapter will examine the medical liability insurance problem—its background, the reason for its emergence as a national dilemma, the physician's reaction to it and the remedies which are proposed.

Definition of the Problem

In order to understand the significance of medical malpractice litigation, it is first necessary to define malpractice. The 1971-appointed HEW Secretary's Commission on Medical Malpractice has offered one definition. This body stated that medical malpractice is an injury to a patient which is caused by the negligence of the health care provider. The malpractice "claim" itself is an allegation, with or without foundation, that an injury was caused by negligence. "Injury" implies either physical or mental harm which occurs in the course of medical care whether or not it is caused by negligence.

Consequently, compensation to patients for malpractice claims requires proof of both injury and professional negligence.

The issue of compensation, as reflected by the enormous awards given by some juries, is one of the problems which makes medical malpractice litigation a knotty dilemma to solve.[1] The difficulty of resolving the problem becomes readily apparent when we realize that the financial reserves of the medical liability companies could be exhausted if large malpractice awards become epidemic in scope. In order to balance their costs the insurance companies must increase the premium rates of their medical liability insurance. This increase, in turn, has resulted in the inability of some physicians to afford the higher premium. Therefore, they either practice medicine without malpractice insurance coverage, (otherwise known as "going bare"), or cut back on the kind of medicine they practice by becoming more cautious in the way they prescribe their treatments. Indeed, the costs of malpractice have been soaring. In 1960, total malpractice premiums in this country were $60 million and in 1975, insurance industry estimates were well over $1 billion.[2] In terms of actual claims filed and awards made, it was estimated in 1970 that 39 percent of the incidents reported to the companies did not reach the claims stage. About 65 percent of the claims filed were disposed of before they came to trial. Less than 10 percent of the cases went to final judgment after trial, as was true for the year ending June 30, 1976. Eighty million dollars were paid out in 1970 for the 12,000 incidents for which claims were made; the median judgment was $2,000 and only 3 percent of the litigants received awards of $100,000 or more.[3]

According to a survey carried out by the National Association of Insurance Commissioners (NAIC), the claims picture began to change by late 1975 or early 1976. In a study of 44 companies in which 9,471 claims were examined, about two-thirds of the reports (6,160) showed that the physician defendant did not make any payments. But the remaining reports listed payments totalling more than $57 million. The average payment per claim was $14,369.

However, the average payment per claim for cases settled through arbitration was only $6,291.[4]

The NAIC survey found that deaths accounted for 29 percent of the awards; while emotional damage represented only one percent of the funds paid out. Temporary injuries accounted for 49 percent of the reported incidents but only represented 15 percent of the monies awarded. Permanent injuries (other than death), on the other hand, accounted for only 27 percent of the payments made. The kind of procedures which caused the injuries for which awards were sought ran the gamut, with operations on the musculoskeletal system costing the insurance companies the largest proportion of payments (15 percent), followed by the digestive systems (13 percent), miscellaneous diagnostic and theraupeutic procedures (11 percent), gynecologic surgery (10 percent) and drug treatments (10 percent).[5]

In terms of the kind of doctors who were sued, the survey showed that board-certified physicians outnumbered noncertified physicians, 796 to 758. The percentage of defendants who were board-certified was larger for surgical specialties than for others. Comparing the types of specialists who were sued, the NAIC survey found that anesthesiologists, heart surgeons, neurosurgeons, obsteticians and gynecologists, orthopedists, plastic surgeons and thoracic surgeons generated a relatively high volume of claims.[6]

The question arises—why such large awards? Perhaps because of sympathy for the plaintiff who is filing the suit; or because huge sums in other settlements are often quoted in the communication media; or a jury or judge looks at the poor plaintiff and then at the wealthy doctor or insurance company and considers large awards just payment for the agonies which the patient has suffered. The physician, on the other hand, places the blame on a combination of circumstances—a litigation conscious public, aggressive trial lawyers and liberal juries, inflation and the breakdown of the insurance system. The legal profession, in turn, stresses the faults of the physician, that the public expects too much, and that there is poor communication between the physician and his patient. In addition, lawyers say that the physicians may neglect the necessity of obtaining consent of the patient, may have inadequate training and in some cases may abandon a patient or clearly may be guilty of negligence.

However, regardless of the reasons for the size of the awards, there are a number of legal doctrines which bear upon the outcome of any malpractice litigation. They include the following according to HEW Secretary's Commission on Medical Malpractice:

- *Burden of proof.* This rests upon the plaintiff.
- *Expert testimony.* In general terms, such testimony is required to establish negligence.
- *Standards of care.* The usual standards of care must be maintained. Formerly, the locality rule was employed in which doctors were judged on the basis of standards of care maintained in similar communities. This rule . . . is rapidly disappearing in the country because it is assumed that all doctors now have access to medical information wherever it may originate.
- *Proximate cause.* It must be determined whether the injury was due to the underlying disease or due to the physician.
- *Res ipsa loquitar–* "the thing speaks for itself." As an example of this doctrine, a patient who has lost a leg after treatment for a fractured knee could be shown to the jury. The surgeon will have the burden of proof, and unless he could in some way establish his innocence, would be judged guilty. (This doctrine is not recognized in Canada.)
- *Procedural issues.* For example, instructions to juries by judges may include statements to which one of the lawyers had raised objections; this lapse could be considered a cause to initiate an appeal.
- *Statute of limitations.* They may be influenced by the date of injury, the discovery rule, and fraudulent concealment. Suits may be brought, depending upon state laws, either during a specified period after commission of the injury or after discovery of the injury. ("Discovery" usually relates to retained foreign bodies after surgery.) Statutes of limitations regularly specify longer periods for infants or children than for adults. Statutes of limitations vary in different states.
- *Erroneous instructions to juries by judges.*

- *Respondeat superior.* By this doctrine an employer is held responsible for the acts of his employees. Hospitals are affected by this consideration.

- *Informed consent.* "Informed consent" requires more than the blanket approval for anything that might transpire during a hospital admission. Without belaboring the point, it is obvious that this consent could be made so detailed that it might become an actual danger for a patient. Any unauthorized procedure, even for a patient's good, could legally be construed as battery. Furthermore, oral assurance of good results by doctors has been made the basis for suits.

- *Charitable and governmental immunity.* Charitable immunity is not applicable in Massachusetts since by statute charitable institutions can be held liable for injuries. The federal government may be sued for injuries caused by individuals; if negligence is proved, as in the case of a medical office, the government pays the award.

- *Breach of contract.* If a physician has guaranteed a complete cure, which is not attained, suit may be brought for this purpose.[7]

Given the aforementioned list, it should be noted that many states are presently reviewing and examining their law of tort to determine which doctrine should be eliminated or modified in order to alleviate and ameliorate the current crisis. For example, it has been estimated that the cost of medical malpractice is nearly $6 billion a year, at least half of which is attributable to defensive medical practice.[8]

Medical Malpractice Situation In 1976

Just as the year 1975 saw the medical malpractice liability issue became a national crisis, the outlook for 1976 was even more grim than that of the year before. The list of states with problems of insurance availability or exorbitant rates (anything less than $10,000 for the highest risk categories is now viewed by doctors as being inexpensive) had grown to include all but a few states. Even in these states—specifically, Colorado, Georgia, Nebraska and Oklahoma—physicians were deeply concerned about their futures. The crisis was so bad in Alaska that 30 percent of its 270 physicians were practicing without malpractice insurance by the beginning of 1976. A fifty state survey by *Medical World News* revealed deterioration in every state during 1975, even among those which passed comprehensive malpractice legislation in that year. A company writing malpractice insurance, the St. Paul Minnesota Fire and Marine Insurance Company had pulled out of 17 states and another company, the Argonaut, pulled out or attempted to leave all of the states where it was a major carrier. Several other insurers, such as the Employers Insurance of Wausau and Lloyds of London, had either voluntarily dropped out of the malpractice insurance business or, like Signal Imperial of Los Angeles, California, had been forced out of business through insolvency even though malpractice premium rates had been rising during this period of time. Rates filed by the Insurance Services Organization (ISO) for its member companies raised the costs of malpractice insurance for orthopedists and other high-risk specialists purchasing million dollar policies, where they can find them, to as much as $10,000 or more in such previously low costs states as Alaska, Hawaii, Kansas and Montana. In expensive states such as California and Michigan, many of the same high-risk specialists pay more than $36,000 for the same policies–again where they can find them. There are only a few states like Colorado where physicians have not had much trouble either in terms of the availability or the price of the medical malpractice insurance.[9]

However, *Medical World News,* in another 50 state survey, found that at the end of 1976 malpractice insurance costs, though still high in some states, had begun to level off in other jurisdictions. In addition, medical society officials reported that virtually in every state basic coverage–if not umbrella coverage–was readily available to all licensed physicians.[10]

But physicians are not the only ones suffering from high malpractice insurance rates. Hospitals also are finding themselves under the same intense financial pressure. J. Alexander McMahon, president of the American Hospital Association, stated in 1976 that "the situation is bad and will be getting worse. There is no end in sight to the premium increase. I know of some hikes exceeding 1400 percent."[11] Adding to Mr. McMahon's comments was George B. Allen, President of the New York Hospital Association, whose member hospitals during 1976 were being hit with 200 to 600 percent rate hikes. According to Mr. Allen, there are two main reasons for this situation. One is that liability insurance companies fear that the incidence and the size of the malpractice award will continue to rise. Thus, they have to be prepared to pay out large financial judgements four or five years from now. Another is the fact that the insurance companies did not have adequate reserves and are only now beginning to catch up. The effect of the insurer's increase is dramatic to say the least. The Louis A. Weiss Memorial Hospital in Chicago, Illinois, unable to find an American insurance carrier which would sell it more than one million dollars in liability coverage, was forced to buy from Lloyds of London. By 1976, the hospital had $10 million of insurance coverage, but its total premium of $1.7 million exceeded the size of almost every malpractice award in the history of Illinois. Another example is the Cornwall (N.Y.) Hospital which paid $24,000 for $11 million in coverage in 1974 and then had to spend $486,000 in 1975 for only a $6 million policy. The premium amounted to 10 percent of the institution's operating budget and because of the state's freeze on Medicaid and Blue Cross reimbursement at that time, only part of the cost could be recouped by raising patient charges.[12] In trying to solve these financial pressures, hospitals, by the spring of 1977, had set up their own captive insurance companies in about 13 states. This solves the availability problem but not the problem of cost. The premiums of these captive insurance companies usually are on a par with private carriers. But as time passes, the captive insurance companies expect to be able to keep their rate increases lower than the private carriers since they do not seek a profit. Only time will determine whether the hospitals have found a solution to their dilemma.

Part of the hospital's dilemma involves an individual's perception and adjustment to an environment with which he may have little personal familiarity and understanding as a patient. This situation can lead to much misunderstanding and miscommunication between hospital personnel and the patient, which, in turn, can create an atmosphere for potential malpractice liability and litigation. The general director of the Beth Israel Hospital in Boston, Massachusetts best described this hospital atmosphere when he illustrated a patient's view of hospital care:

"He enters somewhat anxious, if not outright scared, about the illness. He is then stripped of his clothes and given a restrictive set of rules: where he may go, what he may eat, and what he must *not* do. In a typical day, he might have contact with admitting personnel, several shifts of floor nurses, the attending physician, radiology and laboratory technicians, operating room nurses, house staff, aides, and volunteers. All the highly developed clinical procedures of modern medicine are focused on the patient. It is not surprising that this array of hospital rules, tests, instructions, and contacts holds a large potential for miscommunication.

The patient may become angry because no one knows when his physician is coming, no one can reach the physician to prescribe a stronger medication, or no one knows when surgery is scheduled. Some staff members are sympathetic about his pain; others don't seem to care. Perhaps one individual was cross when the patient asked a question, and now he is scared to ask anyone anything. Or perhaps the patient is irritated over a nonclinical problem: the television doesn't work, the admitting office can't find his insurance card, or whatever."[13]

In the seemingly foreign environment over which the patient has little control, there is an almost limitless universe of people, procedures and places which may lead to a malpractice suit. The individual sued may be a renowned physician or a student technician. The procedure may be a complicated surgical technique or a simple dosage of medication. The hospital location may be literally anywhere, from the emergency department to the operating room or the patient's bedside. For example,

● A patient is transferred to a new department shortly before evening medication is to be administered, and the floor nurses do not communicate until the next day whether the medication was in fact given.

● The attending physician does not carefully check the nursing notes, which indicate critical changes in the patient's condition of which the patient is unaware.

● A nurse is transferred from her regular floor to a department that is short-staffed, and she misses the briefing meeting on the status of each patient.

● A technician is told to draw blood from the patient in 905, Mrs. A, who is quite groggy and incoherent and, in fact, is not Mrs. A, who was transferred to 906. The technician fails to check with the nurses' station because no one is there when he arrives and he is running late.

● A surgeon left a hemostat in a patient. The hospital had no procedure for counting surgical instruments before and after surgery (although it instituted one after this occurrence). Court found potential liability for both physician, as controller of operating room, and hospital, which is responsible for operating room procedures.[14]

In an effort to reduce these and other preventable injuries and accidents and minimize the severity of claims, some hospitals have begun on an experimental basis to test a systems approach to liability control. A systems approach encompasses every aspect of patient care, from the time the patient enters the admitting office through diagnosis, treatment, recovery, and discharge. It is a program which allows the hospital to act upon the root causes of liability claims. Through various sources such as incident reports and medical audits, the hospital can identify individuals and procedures which are deficient. It can spot communication failures and isolate breakdowns in care immediately before an angry patient files a claim. Whether such a system will work and be able to reduce to any significant degree the kinds of hospital incidents which lead to malpractice litigation is not yet known. But hospitals, as well as individual physicians, are exploring many avenues to reduce the financial burden caused by malpractice litigation, the cost of which is ultimately borne by the patient.

The People Speak

In view of the problems which the malpractice insurance crisis presents throughout the nation, it is interesting to consider how the public views this situation—the same public who must bear the costs of the increasing premium rates in the form of higher medical bills. When a statistically valid sample of the adult American population was asked in a 1975 Louis Harris poll if they sympathized with a physician's refusal to handle any cases except emergencies until insurance rates were lowered, they responded as follows. Fifty-four percent said they sympathized with the physician, another 30 percent did not and 16 percent were not sure. The respondents were much less sympathetic to lawyers, however. Seventy-three percent said that smart lawyers have made a racket out of malpractice suits by encouraging patients to sue their doctors. (The Harris organization stated that the low opinion which Americans hold of lawyers is reflected by many of its polls which showed that only 16 percent of the people surveyed trusted lawyers compared to 44 percent who trusted doctors.) However, when it came to the question of favoring an out and out doctors' strike, 55 percent of those polled said it was *wrong* for a doctor to strike for any reason. Although people apparently empathized with the physician on the insurance problem, they still felt the physician had no right to take any action which might jeapordize the public's health.

When respondents sympathetic to the physician's plight were asked to explain their feelings:

- 19 percent said malpractice premiums were too high and doctors cannot afford them;
- 12 percent said they were satisfied most doctors do their job of helping people and caring for the sick;
- 12 percent said people tend to sue without justification and that malpractice suits have become fashionable today;
- 7 percent said doctors are only human and should be allowed some error;

- 9 percent stated that doctors are in an unfair position and are taking advantage of in lawsuits;
- 6 percent said malpractice claims are too high and should be limited;
- 6 percent said lawyers encourage dubious suits;
- 4 percent said higher insurance costs would be passed on to the patient;
- 5 percent said doctors are victimized by insurance companies.

As far as those who were sampled and were negative to physicians:

- 15 percent said doctors should not strike because of the Hippocratic oath;
- 7 percent said doctors make enough money to cover their premium;
- 5 percent said doctors overcharge;
- 5 percent said some doctors are out for themselves or cheat people;
- 5 percent said doctors can be careless and deserve malpractice suits;
- 1 percent said doctors have a high and mighty attitude and should be checked up on.[15]

Physicians React

How are the physicians responding to the malpractice situation? In seeking to answer this question the American Medical Association conducted a poll of a random sample of 1000 physicians in 1976. Of the 419 respondents to the survey, about one out-of-three doctors was considering letting his malpractice insurance expire, while 13 percent were already practicing medicine without malpractice insurance coverage. The poll indicated that 49 percent of the surgeons surveyed, 44 percent of the obstreticians-gynecologists, 41 percent of the psychiatrists, 35 percent of the general practitioners and family physicians, 31 percent of the anesthesiologists, 26 percent of the internists and 13 percent of the pediatricians were considering their malpractice insurance coverage.[16]

The Countersuit

However, while some physicians are trying to decide whether they should drop their malpractice insurance coverage, others have begun to fight back in various ways. Many physicians become angry when they are sued for malpractice not only because of professional pride but also because they feel the patients have acted unfairly out of malice or greed. Few doctors believe that a malpractice suit is justified. Until now, the majority of physicians, encouraged by their attorneys and by their insurance companies which hesitate to spend large sums of money on court cases, settled their medical liability suits out-of-court by giving some amount of compensation to the plaintiff who filed the lawsuit. Generally speaking, only the most clearly defensible medical malpractice cases reach a courtroom judgement. This is evidenced by statistics which show that physicians win 80 percent of jury-tried cases. The high number of out-of-court settlements does not mean that most physicians sued for malpractice admit to charges of negligence. Rather, the physician and his insurance company preferred not to fight the lawsuit because the plaintiff (the patient) has a better than even chance of receiving some kind of payment and generally has no risk of ever losing money because of the contingency fee system. Under this system, the lawyer agrees to accept as his fee a certain percentage of the malpractice suit award. In such a case, if a lawyer does not win a financial settlement, then it does not cost the client anything. The client does not pay for the lawyer's time, or other costs except, perhaps, some out-of-pocket disbursements such as filing fees for the case. On the other hand, regardless of whether the physician wins or loses, he still has to pay the lawyer's fees and other expenses directly or more usually through his insurance carrier who either will demand higher malpractice insurance premiums or else cancel the physician's coverage. Thus, as the costs of malpractice insurance begin to rise out of sight and as insurance companies cease conducting business in more and more areas, the once passive physician is now taking the offensive. His mechanism of attack in such cases is *the countersuit* in which the physician becomes the plaintiff, countersuing his patients or their attorneys, or both when the physician believes that the malpractice suit against him is totally unfounded. As one physician stated:

"We have to begin realizing that the defendent actually supports this whole system . . . The plaintiff doesn't pay anything, whether he wins or loses. The system really encourages the filing of suits–he can keep going back to court until he eventually wins. In the past we've been willing to pay the blackmail, to settle and end it, but we can't afford to do that anymore; we've got to fight back."[17]

The number of countersuits being filed by physicians has been growing since 1974. A few physicians have met with success despite the lack of supporting legal precedents in this area. For example, on June 1, 1976 a Chicago area physician was awarded $8,000 by a circuit court jury who found that the patient, her husband-attorney and their two attorneys had willfully and wantonly filed a lawsuit without cause against the physician. As yet no final judgement has been rendered on the appeal of this case. In response to this legal decision, a former president of the American Medical Association, Max H. Parrott, MD, stated that:

"The action serves notice that doctors intend to fight back against non-meritorious cases and puts lawyers on notice that they are placing themselves in jeopardy if they do not adequately investigate a case before filing it . . . A major factor in the huge increases that doctors have to pay for insurance has been the vast increases in the number of cases that have been filed. Many of these cases have no merit either in law or medicine and, in fact, the majority are not even brought to trial. Yet, insurance companies estimate that it costs $2,500 to open a claim. These costs are borne by the doctors and ultimately, of course, by the patient. If this case stands up on appeal, it should discourage the filing of frivolous or non-meritorious cases and should have a beneficial effect on the professional liability situation in the long run."[18]

Information is still scarce on the exact number of countersuit actions being filed by physicians. However, research conducted by several state medical societies indicates that the countersuit definitely is gaining momentum. For example, a survey by the California Medical Association in the early part of 1976 indicated that at least ten such cases have been undertaken in that state. In Florida two physicians, one in May 1977 and another in January

1978, were awarded financial damages in successful countersuit actions against the attorneys of their former patients who had initially sued them for malpractice but without success. While in New York in early 1978, the Supreme Court Appellate Division–the second highest state court–upheld the right of the physician to countersue when he has been unjustly sued for malpractice.

Physicians use a variety of charges as the basis of their countersuit actions, the following being the more common:

Malicious Prosecution

This charge requires proof that the original malpractice suit which the patient lost and physician won was brought without cause and for malicious reasons. An action in a malicious prosecution cannot be started until the termination of the first suit. Any type of settlement would preclude such a termination. Most legal experts agree that proving malice on the part of the patient or his attorney is difficult.

Abuse of Process

This charge requires that the physician show an intentional misuse of the legal system on the part of those bringing malpractice charges. Again, malice must be demonstrated but the original suit does not have to be terminated.

Defamation

This charge requires proof that false statements by the patient or his attorney have defamed the physician. Since broad privileges are granted litigants in their statements during court proceed most false statements are not actionable.[19]

However, not everyone is enthralled by the prospect that countersuits may become the vogue for dampening the filing of malpractice lawsuits against the physician. According to Sheila Birnbaum, Professor of Law, Fordham University:

"The trend toward countersuit action has to have a very dampening effect on litigation–it is really bad for everyone concerned. Bringing countersuit action could mean that litigation could go on forever. The people representing the physician could be subject to further suits themselves. You know, it could just go back and forth and on forever–where will it all end?"[20]

Physician-Operated Insurance Companies

In addition to utilizing the countersuit, the physician has begun to adopt another approach for alleviating the malpractice crisis, namely learning the malpractice liability insurance business and entering it himself! As Dr. James H. Sammons, executive vice president of the Medical Association, commented in May 1976:

If someone would have told me a year ago that I would be opening a conference on Physician-Owned Medical Liability Companies, with such a large attendance, I would have told him he was out of his mind."[21]

The physicians who attended the conference, represented almost every medical society, and were mindful of the fact that unless they learned the ins and outs of the complex world of insurance in record time, the delivery of health care services in their state could be seriously jeopardized. By the middle of 1976, only twelve major insurance carriers were still writing medical malpractice insurance coverage and, those who did, were doing so reluctantly. But the physicians must have learned their lessons well. By the fall of 1977, 15 medical-society-sponsored, doctor-owned malpractice carriers were in operation, covering 60,000 physicians in 13 states.

However, the process of establishing a physician-owned insurance company is far from easy. Private insurers which have been in the business for years claim that they cannot make a success of it. The question remains as to whether physicians can be successful. Nevertheless, physician-owned and operated companies are said to have several unique advantages compared to commercial insurance carriers. First, physician-owned companies have peer review committees which can recommend limiting an area of a doctor's coverage if he is not qualified to perform surgery or other procedures. Second, physician-owned programs can serve as a membership strengthening device. The companies will not be subjected to sales and administrative costs, such as high salaries and costly commissions, or the profit objective which necessarily motivates commercial carriers in order to satisfy their stockholders. These differences allow additional premium dollars to be available to physician-owned companies for the payment of claims and for investment purposes which, in turn, affect premium rates. Finally, since physicians are both the owners of the company and its policyholders, they can serve both as underwriters and claims consultants. In this fashion, they can recognize a malpractice lawsuit which is justified and move for a swift settlement or can insist on a legal defense where the claim is groundless.

One insurance authority warns physicians not to succumb to the temptation of trying to save money for doctors through these physician-owned companies. The business must be managed on the basis of statistics. Rates will be high and the members won't like it, but his advice is, "don't knuckle under."[22] For this reason, actuarial soundness is a necessity and insurance companies, when becoming operational, must have sufficient capital, surplus finds, and reinsurance, (which is basically insurance coverage for insurance losses). In addition to having to meet managerial problems to be successful, a physician-owned company may also have to overcome a distrustful public and court system, which may feel that physicians, unlike their commercial insurance competitors, are unwilling to pay "just" claims of patients injured by an alleged malpractice.

Given these social and business conditions, physicians and hospitals are not only forming their own insurance companies within the United States but also they are establishing such organizations in offshore areas which are not subject to American taxes. One example is a group of Boston hospitals and health centers which set up their own insurance company in 1976 on the Caribbean island of Grand Cayman where there are no corporate or other income taxes. Through this venture they hope to save $2 million in malpractice premiums. The institutions hope to pass on these savings to their patients by reducing their hospital room rates. The Boston plan also eliminates a present practice of the malpractice insurance system of charging a single rate to high and low risks alike.[23]

In addition to the problems involved in operating a medical liability insurance company, physicians also have to understand the conceptual environment in which they are working if they are to make their companies a success. According to Alfred Hofflander, Professor of Finance and Insurance at the UCLA Graduate School of Management, poor planning on the part of the insurance companies is partially to blame for the malpractice crisis. Medical malpractice has historically constituted only a small percentage of the total written volume of insurance. As long as medical liability insurance was profitable the companies did not devote a great deal of attention to managing it. Medical malpractice is the kind of business in which a company collects the money as premiums today but does not pay out the money as claims for 5 or 10 years—a situation often referred to as the "long tail." This delay gives the insurance company an opportunity to invest these funds. If the investment yield is profitable, the company can lower the cost of its product as well as increase its financial strength.

On the other hand, the passage of time also can have other effects. It usually takes 7 to 10 years before an insurance company knows whether it has made a profit or loss on the policies which it wrote during a given period. During these same years, however, the company will continue to write new policies at rates which may be either too high or too low. If there is high inflation and increasing jury awards during those years, company payments may be greater than initially anticipated when the firm set the premium rates. Also, insurance companies believe that the frequency with which doctors are being sued is rising.

Thus, in Professor Hofflander's view, companies have decided to leave the medical malpractice insurance field or push the insurance rates out of sight for a variety of reasons. The departing companies fear rising costs, the spectre of more malpractice lawsuits and large settlements, and, without good data or the time for basic research, they cannot estimate what their future costs will be.[24]

Joint Underwriting Associations

Other ideas have been conceived which will hopefully alleviate the problem of supplying malpractice insurance to the physician. One of these concepts is the Joint Underwriting Association (JUA) which sells malpractice insurance to doctors as a last resort when no other seller exists. By the winter of 1978 some 33 states passed legislation creating such entities.[25] But the JUAs have been criticized severely by physicians because their premium rates are higher than those which physicians were accustomed to paying. As a result there has been an attempt to reduce the rates. One approach is being tried by the Joint Underwriting Association in New York state where deductibles were being used in 1976. A New York state physician who elected to be insured by a JUA could select either a $3,000 deductible or a 25 percent co-insurance up to a maximum limit of $3,000. An internist could remove $112 from his annual premium of $2,480, or $76 in return for placing himself at risk for $3,000 if he wished to retain his right of consent to a settlement. Savings rose with medical specialties which are of higher risk. An orthopedic surgeon, for example, could reduce his annual premium of $17,195 by $787 if he chose the deductible and waived consent. In doing so, he was gambling that he would not be sued for malpractice for a sufficient number of years so as to offset his share of an eventual payout. So far, only a few doctors have decided to take this chance. Of the 4,000 doctors who were enrolled in JUAs in early 1976 only a few purchased either option.[26] How much effect the deductibles will have on preventing malpractice incidents is open to debate. There is no clearcut answer to this dilemma.

With his own money on the line, a physician not only may become more conscientious in treating his patient medically but also in relating to his patient personally. This could be helpful in deterring or preventing malpractice suits. Some doctors might begin to think more carefully about performing procedures for which they lack the skills if their own money is at stake and leave those procedures which they have performed only on rare occasion for the experts. On the other hand, it is possible that with his own money on the line, a doctor might be hesitant to treat a difficult case when no other doctor is available to handle it and the patient might suffer accordingly. Either way, it is the patient who pays the penalty—whether he is treated by an unskilled physician or not treated by a physician who may be skilled not sure of a particular procedure.

However, high prices are not the only problems with the Joint Underwriting Association. Most of the organizations now in operation limit their coverage to between $100,000 and $200,000 per claim and from $300,000 to $600,000 in the aggregate per year. As a result, many doctors feel dangerously exposed in terms of the amount of coverage. A third major problem with JUAs is that malpractice insurance carriers, especially those which find operations unprofitable in a given state, sometimes use that fact that a JUA exists as an excuse to leave the state. This was said to have been the case when the St. Paul Fire and Marine Insurance Company decided to leave South Carolina and Massachusetts. This company withdrew knowing that criticism of its departure would be lessened because of the existence of another source of malpractice insurance coverage.[27] Finally, another concern of many state medical society officials is fear the commercial malpractice insurance carriers will not return to states which have actually established JUAs as an exclusive seller of professional liability insurance, even though JUAs formation is usually only for two year periods.

Changes in State Tort Laws

The use of countersuits by physicians, and the establishment of doctor-owned insurance companies or Joint Underwriting Associations are not the only weapons being used to resolve the malpractice suit dilemma. One of today's most popular legislative proposals is reforming the state's tort laws. A tort, according to legal authorities, is a wrongful act which results in injury to another person's property, business, emotional well-being or reputation for which the injured person is entitled to recover damages. Tort action in the U.S. Courts is based upon the demonstration of culpability of the defendant plus a lack of contributory negligence on the part of the plaintiff. A familiar exception is Workmen's Compensation—where legal responsibility for work-connected injuries automatically falls on the employer regardless of fault. In a tort action, on the other hand, the plaintiff must demonstrate that the defendant is at fault.[28]

Some of the tort law reforms being sought in the state legislatures include the elimination of *res ipsa loquitor,* which puts the burden of proof relating to negligence on the doctor; prohibition of *ad damnum pleas,* as these pleas result in publicizing multi-million dollar lawsuits; institution of a collateral source rule to require deduction of health insurance and other reimbursements from any ultimate judgment; adoption of a local-witness rule, which forbids the use of itinerant "experts"; and the establishing of short (usually two year) statutes of limitations which begin running from the date of the injury rather than from the date of its discovery. Another reform which is being sought in legislation would permit a successful defendant in a test case to recover his legal fees from the plaintiff where the lawsuit is found to be frivolous and totally devoid of merit.

In addition to seeking changes in the tort laws, some states, like Indiana, have attempted through legislation to place a "cap" or a ceiling on the total amount which may be awarded in a malpractice case. In this manner it is hoped that insurance companies will be encouraged to reduce their premium rates or at least slow down the level of their rate increases. Indiana passed a law, effective July 1, 1975, which placed a limitation of $500,000 on a recovery in any single case involving one plaintiff, that is, the person filing the lawsuit. The individual physician's liability is limited even further—to $100,000. The other $400,000 would be recovered under a state-operated fund which is established by a surcharge of not more than 10 percent of a physician's insurance premium. As another means of reducing payouts, the Indiana law created a screening panel of three physicians and a nonvoting presiding lawyer to review all claims and decide whether they are justified. The opinion of the panel is not binding on the insurance company or the lawyers who are handling the case, but the opinion is admissible in any court proceeding that involves the claim.[29] By the summer of 1977, the Indiana Medical Association stated that the number of malpractice claims which had been filed since the law was passed had decreased by 90 percent. Also, all the panel resolved cases had been settled out of court. In addition, malpractice insurance premiums had only risen an average of 8 percent annually since 1975, compared to annual increases of 75-100 percent in the two year period prior to 1975. Indiana's Patient Compensation Act has been upheld as constitutional by a U.S. District Court. In addition, the pretrial screening panel which the Indiana law created has also withstood constitutional challenges in the Supreme Courts of Arizona, Massachusetts, and Wisconsin. Hence, the initial data and legal judgement from Indiana's experience makes it appear that appropriate state actions may have a positive effect on alleviating the medical malpractice crisis. Another proposal for changing the tort system involves the use of contingency fees. As already mentioned, under this system the lawyer agrees to take a certain percentage of the award if he wins the case. The lawsuit does not cost the client any money if the lawyer loses, except, some out-of-pocket expenses or, perhaps, some filing fees for the case. The medical profession regards contingency fees as an important culprit in the rise of malpractice insurance premiums. Various authorities believe that contingency fee percentages should decrease as the amount of the award increases. It is said that if the contingency fee system were to be totally eliminated about 90 percent of the new malpractice suits being filed against hospitals and physicians probably would disappear because patients could not or would not otherwise finance the prosecution of their claims.[30] In the United States,the legal profession clings firmly to the contingency fee system on the grounds that this fee system enables a poor person to obtain legal services which he could not otherwise afford. In any event, it can be shown that an American lawyer's contingency fee (which averages about one-third of the amount awarded to a plaintiff in a malpractice suit,) is far greater than the 20 percent average fee taken by Canadian lawyers. It can be argued that such large percentages are not economically justified because the contingency fee system arose at a time when today's large malpractice awards were not contemplated.[31] Thus, applying to the larger award the same percentages as was originally intended for smaller amounts is not appropriate.[32] According to one legal expert, lawyers in Great Britain are forbidden to accept contingency fees in their legal practice. It would constitute a serious disciplinary offense for any lawyer in Great Britian to undertake a case on that basis.[33]

In spite of the current debate over contingency fees, the different philosophies and size of awards in different countries, it seems unlikely that contingency fees will be eliminated as part of the American legal system.

Despite all the criticism of the tort system, it has important good features:

- The tort lawsuit brings redress to patients who have been wronged;
- It is the only weapon which society has with which to enforce and improve standards of care;
- It has uncovered malefactors whom medical societies have not been successful in ousting.[34]

In addition to the aforementioned solutions, other proposals for controlling malpractice insurance rates are also being offered.

Arbitration

Another idea that is gaining popularity for lessening the impact of the medical malpractice crisis is the proposition to establish arbitration panels to settle disputes. These panels might include doctors, lawyers and members of the public. The decisions of the panels could be binding or the losing party could retain the right of appeal.[35] Although such panels might be partially effective in reducing the time and the publicity associated with the processing of claims, arbitration merely changes the format through which the award decision will be made. People other than doctors may be making the decision and the rules governing the admissability of evidence in such a proceeding would even be more liberal than those presently existing in a court of law. Arbitration conceivably could even enhance the frequency of successful claims. It is also suggested that arbitration panels might not be consistent with the Seventh Amendment of our Constitution which guarantees the right of trial by jury. But the report of the HEW Secretary's Commission on Medical Malpractice concluded that a medical malpractice arbitration plan would survive the test of constitutionality under any theory so far devised.[37] In fact, a Maryland law requiring that medical malpractice suits be submitted to a pretrial arbitration board was declared constitutionally sound in every respect on April 5, 1978 by a court of that state. Under the 1976 Maryland law, the findings of the arbitration panel can be admitted in court as evidence; an objection to the findings carries the burden of proof. While the arbitration panel determines liability and recommends awards for damages, its findings are not binding because it has no enforcement power.

At present, most states have laws which specifically authorize the physician to contract with his patient so that any future claims for medical injury made by the patient will go to binding arbitration and not to a court proceeding. However, many doctors do not like the idea of confronting each patient with a piece of paper which, in effect, says that if you think I will commit malpractice we are going to ask an arbitrator, and not a court or jury, what he thinks. Physicians are not so much afraid that the piece of paper will give the patient ideas about suing but rather that the idea already may be there in view of all the malpractice suits which are being aired publicly. So far, the experience of arbitrating medical malpractice suits has been too limited to support any sweeping conclusions about its effect on the incidence of claims. But it does seem probable that arbitration does reduce the severity of claims, without having any significant effect on increasing or decreasing their frequency. A doctor-patient contract does not automatically take a dispute to arbitration; one of the signers must invoke the right. Usually, the doctor takes that step after the patient sues. A court must then decide whether the arbitration takes precedence over the malpractice suit–a ruling that the patient's attorney may seek to forestall. Once a case goes to arbitration, however, the plaintiff must bear the burden of proof as he would in a court of law. Experimentation has shown that the cost of defending a charge of medical malpractice through the process of arbitration is far lower than the cost of going to court. In fact, the most recent full-year statistics–for the period ended in June, 1976–show that the average payout on claims in which a trial-court award was made was $27,000; the average for all other forms of disposition, including settlement and arbitration, was $12,700[38] Hopefully, if arbitration succeeds in lowering defense costs and reducing the size of the awards, then hopefully the insurance carriers would pass on such savings by reducing the amount of the medical malpractice premiums. But, there is no certainty that this will take place. However, one positive contribution of the arbitration process is minimizing the physician's trauma of being sued and of all that is involved in the proceedings of a courtroom trial. Despite its advantages, no one knows for certain how rapidly arbitration will be used by doctors in private practice. Physicians in rural areas, where juries tend to be more sympathetic to the medical profession and where awards are generally lower than in urban areas, may prefer to remain with the status quo. Thus, authorities have concluded that arbitration will probably not become the standard of all private practices or even in the majority of them for some time to come. On the other hand, physicians have little to lose if arbitration does not work and much to gain if it does.[39]

No-Fault Insurance

Another alternative solution for the medical malpractice problem is the proposal that no-fault insurance be adapted to the malpractice insurance area. This kind of insurance might require a payment by every person who enters a hospital or becomes a patient in a physician's office. These contributions would then go into a fund which could be used to pay for medical injuries. This idea has arisen as a result of the introduction and success of the no-fault concept in the automobile liability field. The basic principle of no-fault in the automobile field is that an accident victim is paid by his own insurance company, so that only the fact that he is insured has to be established. The question of fault does not have to be determined. Thus, much of the expensive litigation which raises the costs of automobile insurance can be avoided. However, the application of the no-fault concept to the medical field is much more difficult. If all medical injuries were to be compensated, then the number of claims, including many which may be of a nuisance nature, could indeed be incalculable. This situation might make the system very expensive. Consequently, some authorities have suggested that no-fault medical insurance should restrict its benefits to injuries of major importance and of a permanent nature, such as blindness. Specified amounts then could be established for each kind of injury. Other injuries, minor in character, such as a broken tooth or an infection might be handled by a simple grievance procedure.[40] As with any no-fault system, patients would waive their claims to compensation for pain and suffering in return for the immediate award of medical expenses and loss of salary. Although the no-fault approach might appear to be a bad bargain for the patient, a number of surveys show that most accident victims are more upset about obtaining any financial reimbursement at all rather than getting the big award that might be years away. With today's crowded court agenda, the path to the final award involves years of waiting without any certainty of payment.[41]

The Physician Speaks

Given many diverse proposals for solving or at least alleviating the malpractice issue, how does the physician feel about these various concepts and suggestions for solving or at least moderating the malpractice problem? What does he think should be done in order of priority? In seeking answers to these questions, *Medical Economics* conducted a survey of 417 physicians in 1976 to rate the effectiveness of 10 solutions which are being set forth by activists within and outside the field of medicine. Simply stated, the results indicate that physicians are ready to fight back and attorneys will be their chief target. But the survey also noted that doctors can and should upgrade their own practices to help forestall malpractice claims. The following is the percent of physicians who favor various concepts and propositions:

- 83 percent favored legal limits on plaintiff attorney fees.
- 81 percent endorsed legal limits on awards.
- 76 percent approved shorter statues of limitation.
- 69 percent supported compulsory binding arbitration.
- 61 percent preferred no-fault malpractice insurance.
- 59 percent endorsed stricter peer review.
- 55 percent favored compulsory (non-binding) arbitration.
- 48 percent supported doctor-operated malpractice insurance plans.
- 46 percent preferred a surcharge on patients' bills to help pay malpractice premiums.
- 43 percent approved federal subsidy of malpractice premiums.[42]

As can be noted from the previous figures and proposals, the four measures which physicians favor most for resolving the malpractice dilemma would place restraints on the lawyers. In suggesting alternatives to the ten leading remedies, about one-third of the physicians spoke in terms of striking back at the plaintiffs and their attorneys chiefly through the use of countersuits as noted. There was deep animosity towards lawyers among the physicians surveyed. Another course of action favored by a minority of physicians is for doctors dropping their malpractice insurance and thus reducing the amount of money which may be available to the plaintiffs who are filing the lawsuits. A large number of doctors suggested lobbying for corrective legislation while others called for strikes. But the number of physicians calling for remedial legislation outnumbered those calling for strikes by a ratio of 2 to 1. On the other hand, many doctors believe that patients deserve some sort of compensation, most of the physicians favoring a no-fault system. And some doctors would have patients purchase their own malpractice insurance just as airline travelers buy flight insurance. Finally, another recurrent idea is that doctors should establish better rapport with their patients in order to reduce the number of malpractice suits which are being filed. In other words, physicians should exercise greater vigilance, diligence and attention to the details of patient care, especially in communicating with the patient. But whatever the method being advocated, and physicians are not united by any means on a single course of action, one fact is certainly clear—physicians are not about to accept passively the current malpractice crisis. They will fight back in some manner, shape or form.

Conclusion

The American physician is under attack as never before. The idealistic picture of the kindly family practitioner going out in the darkness or through storms to treat his patients is a long gone memory for many people. The public is expressing its displeasure with the "new" physician and the quality of medical care by filing malpractice suits. The day of the corporate physician (meeting government regulations and lawsuits like any other business) is at hand and seems to be a sign of the future. The omen of increasing litigation against the physician became apparent when the American Bar Association held its mid-winter meeting in 1978. In essence, the Association's policymaking House of Delegates rejected proposals designed to reduce the cost of medical malpractice litigation and insurance, thus giving lawyers additional economic incentive to initiate lawsuits on their client's behalf. More specifically, the group *voted against* the following recommendations of an American Bar Association commission which had studied the medical malpractice problem for several years:

- placing a ceiling on the amount a plaintiff can recover in a malpractice case; either for measurable dollar losses or for reimbursement for pain and suffering resulting from a medical problem;

- limiting the contingent fees charged by lawyers in such cases and placing such a fee arrangement under court jurisdiction;
- permitting judges in malpractice cases to deduct from jury damage awards the amount the plaintiff is due to receive from insurance benefits;
- permitting defendants who lose malpractice suits to pay damages assessed against them in installments;
- requiring suits on behalf of children, usually based on their birth, to be filed before they reach 8 years of age;
- giving doctors and hospitals three to six months' notice of patient's intentions to file malpractice suits in order to provide a cooling-off period during which disputes might be settled out of court.[43]

After the debate a member of the American Bar Association commission, which had drafted the program, warned the House of Delegates: "This is a very serious issue. You'll have the problem back in your hands. You have not faced the issue."[44] Is it any surprise that physicians feel such deep animosity toward the legal profession and consider lawyers the culprits in the malpractice dilemma. Here is an instance where the legal profession, through the American Bar Association, had an opportunity to endorse measures which could have contributed toward ameliorating the malpractice crisis. But when the moment beckoned, the legal profession failed to live up to the challenge at hand. It refused to approve the reforms.

What is the solution to the medical malpractice crisis? Unfortunately, there is no single answer or consensus to this question. If there were, it would have been adopted to the satisfaction of all who are concerned—the patient, the doctor, the lawyer, government and the insurance carrier. But one fact appears certain—unless a solution is devised and devised quickly, the American public will continue to pay the consequences. The situation is aptly illustrated by the following comments of a physician who no longer will exercise one of his medical skills, the loss of which may be felt by those of his patients who might have wished to be treated by this particular doctor:

"When my partners and I got the bill for our malpractice insurance last year, we saw that the premium, which had doubled in 1976, had more than tripled this time—a sixfold increase in two years. We've never had a single suit against us. We're internists, practicing in Mississippi, where the risk of a suit is supposed to be one of the lowest in the nation. We quizzed our agent. He quizzed the company. What is boiled down to was that most of the new increase was levied because we did lumbar punctures and needle biopsies of the liver. So we had a simple problem of economics: our income from those two procedures was less than $1,000 a year, and we were to be charged $3,000 a year for their coverage. We decided to stop. Surgical colleagues, who have to be covered for invasive procedures anyway, agreed to handle them for us.

Well, I've been doing lumbar punctures for 30-plus years. I've never had a significant complication. One of my partners did almost all the needle biopsies of the liver in our hospital for 10 years. He's had more experience with the technique than the rest of the staff put together. Yet our skills in these areas will now atrophy and be denied to our patients because of the vagaries of insurance coverage."[45]

These comments are an excellent example of how the medical malpractice crisis is affecting medical practice today. In fact, the findings of a poll released by the American Medical Association in April 1978 reveal:

- one out of eight physicians (12.9%) had been sued for malpractice since 1975;
- about one of twelve doctors (8.5%) is presently not buying professional liability insurance;
- about three out of five (57.8%) office-based physicians have raised their fees to cope with climbing malpractice insurance premiums. Another 21.5% have limited their practices and no longer do procedures which put them into higher risk more costly insurance categories;
- almost three out of five (56.8%) doctors state that they are ordering more tests and procedures for patients today than previously to protect themselves against possible legal action.[46]

Consequently, no one wins when a physician concludes it is not in his economic interest to have malpractice coverage for performing a particular procedure; or when he hesitates to render medical treatment out of fear of a malpractice suit; or when he overpractices to the extent that he orders procedures necessary for his legal protection and not for the patient's health. In the final analysis, it is the patient who is the ultimate victim—either directly by paying higher medical bills, or indirectly by paying higher insurance premiums to a third party who pays the bill on his behalf, or by not receiving the care he requires because of the actions of a minority of the patient population who file malpractice suits—be they justified or not. It would indeed be a sad day if one of the finest health systems in the world were to be destroyed by one of the finest legal systems in the world—both of which should be operating in tandem to protect the physical and legal well-being of the American public.

CHAPTER 7

Private Health Insurance: The End of the Beginning?

THE HEALTH INSURANCE INDUSTRY has arrived at its moment of truth! Higher costs for the American consumer have resulted in a demand for relief. Americans want the protection that the word insurance implies. But, they find that the more they spend, the less protection they receive!

"I doubt that health insurance as we know it and as you design and sell it will survive the changes that government and consumers are going to bring about. For the past 20 years, the insurance industry and the "Blues" have watched a bad situation get worse and have not developed the machinery to cope with the problems. The health insurance industry has not earned the confidence of the working man. You have a big task ahead of you, which is to demonstrate that in a rapidly changing industry you are socially responsible and economically relevant. I believe you must either find new products and shape them for better informed, more critical consumer markets or face obsolescence as an economic institution."[1]

Eight years after a vice president of the International Brotherhood of Teamsters labor union issued this warning in 1970 to the commercial health insurance industry, the situation for those purchasing private health insurance has not improved in terms of the product which they are buying. For example, in 1976 a *Business Week* survey found that some companies actually had doubled and tripled their employee health insurance outlays during the preceding five years. For many, the higher costs had led directly to lower benefits rather than more improved ones.

While the private health insurance industry claims that its coverage has been greatly broadened in recent years to keep pace with inflation, not everyone agrees with this view. Continental Airlines serves as an excellent example of the problems which private industry faces in this area. In 1970, Continental Airlines paid $2,120,000 to purchase health insurance for 8,329 employees and in 1975 spent $7,000,000 to cover 9,256 employees or only 927 more persons.[2] Officials of various other companies have stressed that the bulk of the extra dollars has gone to pay for the higher cost of the old benefits rather than the purchase of new ones. While companies can pinpoint the exact causes of the increase in health care costs, they express little agreement on how to reduce them. Some try one thing and some try another, and *most* apparently feel helpless. An official of the Halliburton Company, a Dallas oilfield and construction firm, typifies corporate ambivalence on the subject. He opposes national health insurance because, he says, the government messes up whatever it touches. But unless someone takes some action to control health costs, he adds, "Lord knows what's going to happen."[3] The question which immediately arises is 'why'? What has happened to the private health insurance industry in this country? What has made it so incapable of fully protecting the individual against the costs of ill health at prices which are reasonable for the public to afford. Why do many voices, both public and private, declare that a new social mechanism, as exemplified by national health insurance, is needed to afford every individual his right to comprehensive health care. Part of the answer lies in the convergence of a variety of forces at work in our society. They include the facts that the demand for health care is rising along with the cost of providing it; the consumer's voice is becoming more militant as his frustrations and expectations in regard to this service continue to increase; and shortages of manpower and facilities continue to persist. Another part of the answer can be found in the role which health insurance has assumed in our society as a mechanism for helping us pay our medical bills. For example, in 1950 you paid about 70 percent of your personal medical bill out of your own pocket. By 1976, you paid about 32 percent of your medical bill with your own money and health insurance took care of the rest.[4] Thus, health insurance has become an almost indispensable underpinning to the whole structure of financing medical care.

The importance of health insurance to the whole medical industry has been noted in our previous discussions. We have shown, for example, how the American public is becoming increasingly disturbed over the rising costs of medical care. Consumer groups criticize hospitals and physicians for charging too much for their services; for building hospitals in areas where they are not needed; and for allowing the costs of health care to skyrocket because they know they will be reimbursed by health insurance programs. In reply, some hospital administrators and physicians state that the huge sums of money which are available from government programs are among the reasons why health care costs have risen so rapidly. Another cost-inducing factor, they say, is physicians who feel pressured into ordering more and more expensive laboratory tests and other patient services in order to protect themselves against the possibility of malpractice suits.[5] And health insurance—both public and private—underwrites the costs of all these activities. Because of the existence of health insurance our whole philosophy and attitude toward seeking medical treatment and paying for such care has also been changed. By enabling millions of Americans to finance their personal medical expenses, health insurance has severely distorted the sensitivity of both the patient and the health provider toward the costs of medical treatment. As individual patients we now can say that as long as other groups—the third parties such as Blue Cross and commercial insurers—are paying our bills why shouldn't we seek out the best care available, often meaning the most expensive. Why worry about the cost? It is similar to the hobo who when asked why he sought treatment from the most expensive doctor in town, knowing that he could not pay his bill, answered simply, "when it comes to my personal health no one but the best will do." It must be borne in mind that only 17.5 percent of all policies are written for individual policyholders and paid for entirely by them; most people have varying percentages of their premiums picked up by Medicare, their employers or unions.[6] So what happens? By not being responsible individually for a large portion of our medical expenses since someone else is paying the bill, we become responsible collectively as a group of consumers. We have to pay higher insurance premiums to cover the rising costs of health care and, thus, take home less personal income from our work; we have to pay higher taxes under public programs such as Social Security to cover the rising costs of government medical programs in which we might not even be qualified to participate; and we observe government intervening more and more into the health care field in an attempt to control its costs and frequently driving up these costs as a result of its increasing regulation and intervention.

By developing a product called health insurance which enables us to pay our medical bills, thereby performing a social service, the private health insurance industry now ironically finds itself accused of being one of the culprits of our present health care crisis. One of the primary reasons for this accusation concerns the way the insurers reimburse the providers of health care services. For example, the reimbursement to hospitals is usually on a retrospective basis after the costs have been incurred. Debate has been so critical of the ability of private health insurers to control health care costs, notwithstanding the accusations that they are also contributing to these rapidly rising expenses, that drastic measures are being advocated in regard to this industry. Voices in this country have begun calling for the demise of the private health insurance industry and for the establishment of a national health insurance system in its place within which the private health insurers would have little, if any, important role. This feeling is well summed up by Dr. I. S. Falk, one of the architects of the Kennedy-Corman national health insurance plan which advocates this approach. Dr. Falk has stated:

". . . Now, that which has been good should not be the enemy of the better. Private health insurance should no longer stand in the way of insurance that can be designed to meet the public need, not only on the extensiveness of the populations it reaches, but also in the effectiveness of the protection it provides."[7]

But the private health insurance industry is not giving up its role in our society complacently. In appealing for a chance to prove that a public-private partnership can solve the health care crisis through the industry's own sponsored Burleson-McIntyre national health insurance bill, Robert F. Froehlke, President of the Health Insurance Association of American, which represents the commercial health insurance industry, has asked:

"Why not give us the chance to prove it? Let the health insurers backing this plan either put up or shut up. Then if we do not perform, other—more costly and disruptive—solutions can always be attempted."[8]

This struggle among the various special interest groups in our society whether it be labor, private business, professional health providers or others will not be abating in the ensuing years as each attempts to influence the future course which this nation will take in financing and delivering health care services. And because of the political and ideological conflicts involved, the enactment of a national health insurance program is not an imminent reality at the present time. Yet, in the absence of such a national program, you will still have to cope with the cost of your personal health care and private health insurance is one mechanism available to help you. Consequently, it is the purpose of this chapter to explore the issue of private health insurance—what it is, why it has problems protecting you fully against the costs of ill health, what you should look for when purchasing health insurance policies, the economic impact which health insurance has on our society, and what groups such as private business are doing to control their personal health expenses and through such measures the costs of health care to you, their employee. However, before discussing these and other issues, it may be of interest at this point to discuss the historical development of private health insurance in this country.

History of Private Health

Private health insurance originated in the United States in the middle of the nineteenth century when a few insurance companies responded to the public's demand for coverage against rail and steamboat accidents. Then, during the latter half of the 19th century the concept of the mutual aid society which had originated in Europe, notably in Germany, was adopted in the United States. Essentially, this was a movement in which workers banded together into membership organizations. Small contributions were collected from each member in return for the promise to pay a cash benefit in the event of disability through accident or sickness. Early providers of health insurance therefore included fraternal benefit societies. Also, a number of mutual benefit associations, called "establishment funds", began to be formed in 1875 within the United States. Comprising the workers of a single organization, these funds, sometimes financed partially by employers, provided small payments for death and disability. Toward the end of the nineteenth century, with the entry of accident insurance companies into the field, health insurance began to demonstrate substantial growth. At about the same time, life insurance firms first made accident and health insurance available. Thus between two eras—the mid-nineteenth and the late twentieth centuries—the private health insurance system evolved. During this period, the number of people protected by policies steadily increased. By 1976, it was estimated that 183 million Americans were protected by one of more forms of private health insurance.[9]

In general, private health insurance presently encompasses five broad categories, as noted in figure 11: namely, protection against hospital expenses, surgical costs, regular expenses, major medical and wages lost because of illness or accident.

In its initial stages, the primary emphasis of health insurance was not toward hospital and surgical benefits. Rather, the insurance was designed to protect the individual against the loss of earned income which resulted from his contracting any one of a limited number of diseases such as typhus, typhoid, scarlet fever, diphtheria, and diabetes. Although subsequent plans expanded the number of diseases covered, eliminated medical examinations and included surgical fee schedules, this emphasis on the income aspects of insurance continued until the initial stages of the Depression in 1929. As the Depression worsened, the public became increasingly aware of the need for improved methods for sharing the costs of medical care. On the other hand, hospitals were faced with empty beds and declining revenues. These conditions prompted the formation of a mutually advantageous arrangement between a number of teachers and the Baylor Hospital in Dallas, Texas, to provide the teachers with hospital care on a prepayment basis. This was the origin of the Blue Cross service concept for financing hospital care. It had a profound effect on the insurance industry by foreshadowing the development of reimbursement policies for hospital and surgical care. At the same time, another form of prepayment service was developing in Los Angeles, California where a group of health care providers assumed the responsibility for organizing and integrating medical services on a prepaid basis, that is, combining group practice with prepayment. This physician sponsored organization, continuing today as the Ross-Loos Medical Group, served as the forerunner of such eminently known programs as the Kaiser Foundation Health Plan of California, the Health Insurance Plan of Greater New York, the Group Health Association of Washington, D. C. and the prototype for today's emerging medical care foundations and health maintenance organizations.

During World War II, a major change occurred in the health insurance field when the freezing of industrial wages made fringe benefits a significant element of collective bargaining. Eventually, group health insurance became part of this package. In the postwar years, three powerful forces interacted to provide modern health insurance with its strongest momentum for growth. The first of these was a 1948 decision of the United States Supreme Court, which held that fringe benefits, including health insurance, were a legitimate part of the collective bargaining process.[10] The second impetus was the sharply increasing cost of medical care. The third force was the ability of the private health insurers to introduce new kinds of coverage and broaden existing benefits.

Thus, as the nation emerged from the Depression economy to a more affluent status, insuring organizations began to develop more extensive benefits and, in the early 1950s, introduced the most comprehensive insurance program yet devised—major medical expense coverage. This policy has been defined as insurance especially designed to offset the heavy medical expenses resulting from catastrophic or prolonged illness or injury. The policy is often superimposed or provided as a supplement to basic protection; that is, benefits do not begin until regular hospital-surgical or medical insurance programs are exhausted, or the policy can be provided as comprehensive protection where both the basic and extended benefits are a single unit. From its start, major medical has grown rapidly in response to the family's need for protection against swiftly escalating hospital, medical and surgical costs.

In addition to the development of major medical expense coverage, the rapidly developing economy of the post World War II era also led to the reemergence of yet another form of protection. The health insurance industry began to make available long-term disability benefits, reemphasizing the income replacement concept during times of disability and other financial emergencies.[11] Thus, it appears that the health insurance industry has come full circle since its early beginnings when the industry emphasized income replacement rather than health care service benefits in its insurance policies.

Private Health Insurance Industry

Underlying the development of private health insurance programs are three fundamental principles which are used in making the actuarial determinations from which premium rates are derived. They are:

First, the unpredictability of risk for the individual. Simply stated, no one can foretell with certainty which persons will suffer illness or injury. Nor can anyone predict the effect of a disability on a particular individual.

Second, a reasonable predictability of the degree of risk for a group–the larger the group, the more accurate the prediction can be. As an illustration, studies of people with high blood pressure reveal an extra hazard for the group, even though particular individuals in the group have a favorable outlook clinically. Thus, by drawing upon the past experience of groups, risks can be evaluated.

Third, transfer of risk from the individual to the group, through the traditional pooling of resources.[12]

The industry which operates on the previous principles is comprised of three broad categories: Blue Cross and Blue Shield, commercial insurance companies and independent plans. These organizations offer group as well as individual coverage. In 1976, seventy Blue Cross plans covered 83.9 million persons for hospital care and seventy Blue Shield plans insured about 72.6 million persons for medical and surgical care. In addition to regular subscribers, Blue Cross served 8.3 million of the elderly enrolled in Medicare, who needed coverage beyond the Medicare level of benefits. As an intermediary in various capacities in Medicare, Medicaid and other public programs in the United States, Blue Cross plans served an additional 26.0 million persons. Altogether, the combined range of private and public Blue Cross plan services in the United States reached more than 110.0 million persons in 1976–or approximately 50 percent of the nation's population.[13] In addition to the "Blue" organizations, there are about 1,000 commercial insurance companies which write health insurance policies covering 99.5 million persons for hospital care. There are also some 400 other plans with 10 million persons insured for hospital care. Among these are plans which offer health services on a prepayment or insuring basis to the subscribing public of their general area. Also included are benefit programs of welfare funds, employers, employee benefit associations or unions.[14] The diversity and array of the plans and benefits available was best described by one health authority who stated:

"To begin with, we have not even made up our minds about the name of the game. Some call it insurance and seek to replace financial losses that people incur when they need medical care. Others call it prepayment and seek to share the predictable expenses of care. From there on, the dichotomies proliferate. We have plans that regard their responsibilities as essentially financial and believe that once they have paid the amount prescribed by their policies their responsibility is discharged. We have plans that believe that their responsibilities go further into a concern with the availability, cost and quality of care they finance. We have plans that cover specified segments of care. We have plans that reimburse people a level of expenditure.

We have plans that regard the degree and content of protection the province of the patron—if he wants less he gets less; if he want to invest in extra accident benefits instead of laboratory services, that is his choice. We have plans that believe that it is their duty to provide all subscribers with a constellation of benefits designed to maximize their health. We have plans that believe in preventing illness and intervening if possible before a disease becomes grave. We have plans, on the other hand, that do not believe in the inclusion of provisions for the prevention of disease and maintenance of health in insurance. We have plans that pay the physician a separate fee for each service on the theory that such fee-for-service payment is essential to good care and that it rewards the physician only for what he does. We have plans that pay the physician a set amount over a period of time for each person in his care, believing that this encourages the physician to keep people well or at least diminishes the pecuniary incentive in prescribing more service. We have plans that regard it as their mission to preserve the conventional methods of practice. We have plans that regard it as their function to change the mode of practice. We have plans that serve a closed constituency. We have plans that try to cover as many people as possible. We have plans that believe that no one should make a profit in providing health protection. We have plans that expressly seek profit, although many, in fact, have not found it in the health field.

These are but some of the major differences in approach that have thus far shaped our plans." [15]

In light of the variety and complexity of health insurance plans presently in existence, it is not surprising that even the most sophisticated purchasers of this product can find themselves shortchanged, in terms of the benefit protection which they thought they had purchased originally, when the time comes to use the insurance.

Shortcomings of Insurance

There are many reasons why insurance carriers have problems in providing the kind of broad protection the public seeks but cannot obtain, regardless of the kind of insurance plan which may be purchased. One is that the general public does not always clearly perceive its health insurance needs. Thus, there may be little demand for a particular kind of coverage which, in turn, causes comprehensive health insurance to grow slowly. Another reason pertains to the method by which health insurance is developed. Before a new coverage can be widely sold, administrative techniques, methods of reimbursing providers of services, feasible benefit packages and data on probable utilization and costs must be developed. Experimentation is required and this takes time. A third reason relates to custom, tradition and inertia. Certain health insurance coverages have become well accepted by the public, and health insurance organizations have become used to offering them. Only gradually are the limitations of these coverages recognized, and only slowly are new and broader coverages offered and accepted. There are other reasons why insuring organizations may sell restricted coverage. They do not do so because they are unwilling to offer comprehensive benefits. Rather, individual employee groups, business corporations or unions have only so much money available to purchase health insurance and thus are limited in the scope of coverage they can obtain.

In some instances, existing legislation can also hamper or slow down an insuring organization from developing and offering new health insurance benefits to the public. For example, Blue Cross and Blue Shield plans generally operate under enabling acts which define the benefits they may offer; amendment of such legislation is frequently required before new types of benefits can be sold to the public. However, once the plans have determined that they really wish to offer these new benefits and obtain the endorsement of groups representing hospitals and physicians, for example, the desired legislation usually can be achieved.

Purchasing Private Health Insurance

Present state laws are almost completely silent on the adequacy of the benefits which private health insurers should offer the policy holder. As a result, insurance carriers are presently writing an infinite variety of policy combinations, as already noted. Because of the silence of states on benefit adequacy, it is easy to see why benefit coverage may be inadequate in terms of such basic services as hospitalization, the promotion of one-disease-only policies, the lack of uniform standards in regard to such areas as length of stay and surgical schedules, and allowing the combination of health service benefits with other benefits such as income coverage for loss of time incurred because of accident or illness. It is extremely difficult, if not impossible, for the purchaser of health insurance to compare benefits and costs and to shop intelligently among those policies which are available. And, even if he had the time to shop around, he would be overwhelmed by the fact that there are probably 10,000 kinds of insurance policies being written in the United States today, while the combinations of these policies are infinite.[16] As numerous as today's policies may be, the questions which even the most sophisticated buyer of insurance may ask and wish to explore prior to his purchasing health insurance are even more so. Who, other than an expert, perhaps, has the foresight or even the time to ask and explore such questions as the following, and to understand their implications in considering whether to seek to include or exclude certain features in the policy provisions:

- What inpatient hospitalization benefits are covered? Is deductible payment required? How much? Are benefits provided for intensive care?

- What outpatient hospital services are covered?

- How many days of hospital care are covered for each illness? Are the covered days limited to one period of hospitalization? Are there limitations on readmission to a hospital for the same illness? Are there any policy limits on payments of daily hospital room charges?

- Are there any limits on choice of hospital or other place of care?

- Does coverage provide for payment based on surgeons' and physicians' usual and customary fees? Are there any policy limits on surgical expense payments?

- Are surgical procedures covered wherever performed? If payment is subject to a schedule of benefits, what provisions are there for operations not specifically listed? Are fractures and dislocations covered? Oral surgical procedures? Is the cost of a second surgical opinion covered? What percent of its cost?

- Are there any limits on choice of physician?

- What benefits are provided for daily hospital visits by the attending physician?

- Are there provisions for office or house visits? Is deductible payment required for these visits?

- Are there provisions for concurrent services of more than one physician?

- What provisions are made for radiation therapy, diagnostic X-rays, laboratory tests, anesthesia services?

- How soon after family membership begins are maternity benefits effective? What are the benefits for normal delivery? For abnormal or complicated delivery? For out-of-hospital birth?

- In a major medical contract, does the deductible amount apply per illness, or is it based on the calendar year? Is coinsurance payment required? How much?

- What is the maximum amount payable for each illness? Can maximum benefits be restored after recovery from an illness?

- Is coverage provided for services of a registered nurse? Of a licensed practical nurse? Are nursing benefits limited to periods of hospital confinement?

- What benefits are provided for services in an extended care facility? What is the maximum number of days? Must this follow hospitalization within a specified period of time?

- Are hospital benefits provided for nervous and mental disorders? Are there deductible or co-insurance amounts? Are there benefits for psychiatric treatment in a doctor's office? In a hospital outpatient facility?

● In a prepaid group practice plan, what benefits are provided? What provisions are made for out-of-area emergency care?

● What family members are covered under a family plan? Are newborn babies covered from birth? To what age are dependent children covered? Are there provisions for older dependent children? For full-time students? Is a child covered if married?

● Can an individual apply for separate coverage after becoming ineligible for dependent coverage? Is there a time limit on this application? What provisions are made for continued coverage of dependents if the primary insured is over age 65? If the primary insured dies?

● Is there a waiting period before accident benefits begin? Before coverage of certain illnesses or operations? Are these periods acceptable in light of the family's medical history?

● Is there a waiting period following discharge from a hospital before eligibility for readmission is restored?

● Is coverage provided for injuries or illnesses which occurred or began prior to the contract's effective date?

● Are there provisions for chronic diseases?

● In a group contract, can the insured convert to another form of coverage on termination of employment?

● Are there any restrictions on conversion for any circumstances? Is there a time limit?

● Can the contract be cancelled? By whom? Under what conditions?

● Are there any exclusions other than the common ones?

● If covered under more than one contract, are benefit payments restricted?

● Is the insuring organization authorized to do business in your state?

● Does coverage apply equally to health care services anywhere in the United States? What benefits are available for health care received outside the United States?

● Does your insurance contract provide service or indemnity benefits? The "Blue" plans generally provide service benefits making payments directly to the providers of care such as hospitals on the basis of a negotiated reasonable cost figure rather than paying the charges of the covered service. Under an indemnity contract, the health provider generally bills the patient who submits proof to the insurer he has paid the charges and is then reimbursed by the health insurer in the amount of the covered charges. Most commercial health insurers operate in this manner. Any uncovered expenses are paid by the patient himself.[17]

Even if you ask such detailed questions and analyze their importance to your family, yourself, or organization, what else do you know about the policy which you are purchasing? For example, what kind of company is selling you the health insurance? An excellent policy in terms of its benefit coverage is not very useful if the insurance carrier may no longer be in business when the time arrives to collect the benefits. Therefore, you should examine and find out about the insurance company. One of the best ways to do so is in *Best's Insurance Reports—Life/Health.* The higher the rating (A+ or A) which the insurance carrier receives from *Best's,* the less likely is the insurer about to go out of business.[18] Another way to check upon the insurance firm is to ask your state insurance department if it has had any reason ever to take action against the company. It is also important that you find out if your insurer is licensed in your state. If you have trouble with an insurance company which is not licensed in your jurisdiction, your state insurance department will not be able to help you very much with your problem. Another important subject which you should investigate is whether the company has a good history of paying claims or whether it has a history of consumer complaints in this respect. State insurance departments or even your friends may have information or experience in this area. Also, try and find out about a company's loss ratio. The loss ratio is the percentage of premiums which the company pays back to its policy holders in the form of benefits. For example, the non-profit Blue Cross and Blue Shield plans have a loss ratio of about 95 percent. This means that for every dollar paid to them, they give back 95¢ to their policyholders. Commercial insurance companies average about 55¢ for each dollar, partly because they pay sales costs and state taxes while the non-profit organizations do not.[19] But the loss ratio is not the sole factor which you should use in judging an insurance firm. Older companies may have a low loss ratio because they only accept low-risk customers. A company with a high loss ratio may not be keeping enough cash in reserve and could go bankrupt. But, in general, the percentage of returned benefits can tell you whether an insurer is selling high-value policies. Most experts agree that a good company should have a loss-ratio which is at least 50 to 60 percent. You can also ask your insurer about the loss ratio on the specific health insurance policy which you are purchasing. The company may not be willing or able to give you the figure, but it will not hurt to ask.[20]

When you are thinking of buying health insurance, you should look at a company which offers a wide variety of health service benefits. You cannot predict what kind of accident or illness may put you in the hospital—therefore you should avoid buying a policy which does not cover many services which you may need. Some policies, called "dread disease" policies, are so limited in scope that they pay only if you get a specific illness like cancer. In addition, try to find a company which will give you an insurance package. Buying one big health policy is usually less costly than purchasing several smaller ones. An expensive policy may not always provide good coverage but a cheap policy will almost always be inadequate for your needs.[21]

Another area to explore when purchasing health insurance is the treatment of premiums. Can the company raise your premiums, that is, the monthly or yearly payments you make for the policy? If so how and for what reasons? Many policies allow the insurer to raise premiums only if it raises those of everyone in the same class, that is, usually everyone in the same state or age group with the same policy. This restriction prevents your insurer from raising your premium just after you file a claim. Also, in order to save on premium costs, think about the size of the deductible you are paying, that is, the amount of money which you pay for health services before the company will pay all or part of the remaining cost of the covered services. The more-the-deductible and the less-you-buy policies which cover very small charges of $15 or $20, such as those for a physician's office visit, the smaller may be your health insurance premiums. Of course, all of these decisions as to whether you purchase or forego certain kinds of health insurance coverage depend to an extent upon whether you can afford to pay such costs out of your own pocket.[22]

Finally, remember that health insurance is available, both on an individual basis and also for groups, such as at your place of employment. Group insurance is usually less expensive and is usually more comprehensive than an individual policy at the same price. Moreover, if you join a group at your place of work, your employer will probably pay most of the cost. The reason why group insurance costs less is because a group represents a cross section of the community—some sick, and some healthy. Because the odds are against most of the group members making a claim, the risk is reduced and the insurance company is likely to profit. In addition, a group policy means sharing paperwork, agent's fees and other management activities and, thus, results in savings. However, when you leave the group, you usually can convert your policy to individual coverage but the price will go up and the coverage probably will decline. One of the reasons for the higher costs of individual coverage is that many insurers believe that someone who has not found a group policy is likely to be a higher risk client. But whether you purchase group insurance or individual health policies try to protect yourself against as many risks as you can on one policy. This cannot be emphasized sufficiently. You will get more for your money—and probably better coverage—than you would with several small limited policies which will tend to overlap and cost more.[23]

Costs and Inadequacy of Insurance Protection

In view of the problems in providing, determining and purchasing adequate health insurance protection, it is not surprising to learn that there are not only gaps in health insurance protection today but also there are a significant number and percentage of Americans who have no health insurance coverage at all. As of December 1975, the percent of people under 65 years of age who did not have any health insurance protection against the costs of hospital care as well as the various services which constitute physician care (as noted in figure 12) ranged from 18 percent to about 36 percent, and for the entire American population in these same categories the percentages ranged from 20 to 40 percent. In addition, according to the Social Security Administration, about one-third of the American people of all ages still do not have any health insurance protection against the costs of out-of-hospital prescription drugs, private duty nursing, visiting nurse service and almost two-thirds have no protection against the costs of nursing home care. The Congressional Budget Office underscored the necessity of having health insurance coverage in this country by predicting that in fiscal year 1978, an estimated 2.4 million persons under the age of 65 will incur medical expenses which exceed $5,000. Also, 6.9 million families will have out-of-pocket expenses totalling more than 15 percent of their income. Most of these (4.1 million) are low-income families. Finally, an estimated 18 million persons in this country will be without any protection whatsoever under either private health insurance or public programs. In fact, the Congressional Budget Office has estimated that 37 million Americans who have health insurance are covered by plans which do not adequately cover high expenses or long hospital stays.[24] Consequently, as the public becomes more aware of these deficiencies in its health insurance coverage, pressure has begun to grow upon the insuring organizations to broaden their benefits but at a decreasing cost. The insuring organizations are perplexed, in turn, as to how they can accomplish this task without forcing society to seek other parties, such as government, to fulfill its health care needs through a national health insurance system which would supercede and replace the function, in whole or in part, of the private health insurance industry.

Of the many pressures in our society which are being brought to bear upon the insuring organizations to expand their benefits but at reduced costs, one emanates from the major labor unions. Organized labor has been very instrumental in securing better health coverage for the working people and continues to set the pace in bargaining for better health benefits with large industries. The cost of health insurance both to the unions and management is but a microcosm of the costs which must be borne today by society-at-large. For example, if an individual bought a new General Motors car in 1975, he would have paid about $160 toward the cost of health insurance for the auto workers and their families. If he bought a 1975 Ford, about $119 of the price he paid went to finance the same item.[25] Without major increases in benefits, health insurance rates rose between 20 percent to 34.4 percent for the automakers in 1975, while wages increased between 7 percent and 9 percent. One of the reasons the benefits rose so dramatically is that the costs of health care services themselves have been rising about 50 percent faster than the other items in the Consumer Price Index since wage and price controls were lifted in 1974. In 1976, Chrysler, Ford and General Motors spent an estimated $1.4 billion for the health insurance benefits of their workers, or an average of $1,600 per family. By 1978, General Motors alone projected expenditures well in excess of $1 billion for covering each of their active employees and retirees and their families in the United States or about $2,300 per person. From 1960 to 1976, health care costs at General Motors rose more than 2,000 percent compared to a 95 percent rise in the overall cost of living as measured by the Consumer Price Index, a 369 percent increase in hospital semi-private room rates, and a 30 percent increase in the prices of new General Motors automobiles during the same period of time. Ford Motor Company's experience with health care costs is even more illustrative. At present, Ford purchases health care services for nearly one million hourly and salaried employees, retirees, surviving spouses and their dependents. Since 1965, health care costs at Ford have doubled every five years and there is every indication that this trend will continue, if not accelerate, in the future. In 1965, Ford's health bill totaled $68 million. In 1977, Ford projected costs of over $450 million or $2,100 per active employee and by 1979 the company forecasts costs of over $630 million, or $2,700 per active employee. Hospital expenses account for over 60 percent of the total Ford bill. These costs increases must be recovered either through higher prices to the consumer or increased productivity. In fact, the consumer is paying. In 1965, health care costs represented $22 per unit produced and in 1977 they will total about $120 per unit—an increase of nearly $100 per vehicle in slightly more than a decade.[26] In contrast to these per capita expenditures, this country spent about $163 billion for health care in 1977—an amount equal to 8.8 percent of the Gross National Product, or about $737 for every man, woman, and child in the United States. In 1977, a representative of the United Automobile Workers Union gave even a more specific description of the impact which the costs of health insurance are having upon the automobile industry:

"The cost of our negotiated health care programs with the big three auto companies is now 95¢ to $1 per hour and each penny of this is worth about $8 million at General Motors alone. This is money which is being diverted from wages and other benefits to pay hospitals and doctors. Most of the increases our union has been able to negotiate have gone to pay increases in health care premiums for benefits for which we have bargained . . . We have to run to keep up. All the increases are going to cover inflation. Even though our union negotiates hundreds of millions of dollars of health insurance benefits, we have found private industry to be very unresponsive to consumer needs. The insurance companies are mostly concerned about profits, and Blue Cross and Blue Shield plans have been dominated by doctors and hospitals."[27]

If the 1976 settlement reached by the United Automobile Workers and the Ford Motor Company is any indication of the trends in any future health insurance negotiations, then the costs borne by the American public in purchasing automobiles are not likely to abate when the auto makers put their health insurance costs into their 1979 automobile price tags. Rather than being able to cut back on health insurance benefits, as Ford had hoped at the beginning of the 1976 bargaining sessions, the United Automobile Workers was able to broaden the benefit package for its workers. Included among the new benefits was the first nationwide vision care program, a pioneering hearing aid benefit and improved benefits in the dental care program. So the question arises, how can health care costs be contained as the consumer pays more and more either for his own health insurance or in the higher costs of consumer goods which include the benefit costs resulting from union-management collective bargaining negotiations. The unions, which have been the most vocal advocates of cradle-to-grave national health insurance, say the answer lies in federalizing the predominately private system, setting fees and enforcing controls which are on the books but not often used. The companies contend that government confuses things, that the answer lies in the willingness of the community-at-large-workers—hospitals, doctors and industry to pay a little more or to make sacrifices. As an official of the Ford Motor Company said, "there is only so much a corporation can cover through its productive efforts. We have reached that point. We want relief."[28] What the company wants relief from is the cost of a broad range of health services it buys for its employees through Blue Cross and Blue Shield plans across the country. These include hospital care, extended nursing home care, drugs and dental services, in which the workers share the costs, and diagnostic services.[29] And the very expansion of benefit protection to cover the rising prices of health services will only add more costs to those which the companies already must bear in providing this fringe benefit. In fact, the U.S. Commerce Department reported that in 1976, private industry spent about $29.9 billion on group health insurance. Billions more went to corporate medical programs and other health and safety efforts.[30] Health policy-makers generally agree, as already noted, that this rapid growth in private health insurance has generated increased spending because it makes both the physician and consumer alike less sensitive to the true cost of medical treatment. According to Martin S. Feldstein, Harvard University economist:

"There is now substantial evidence ... patients, guided by their doctors, demand more services and more expensive services when a large part of their costs are offset by insurance ... In 1950, when the average cost per patient day was $16, private insurance paid 37 percent of hospital bills. That meant on the average the net cost to a private patient was $10. In 1974, the average cost per patient day jumped to about $125, but private insurance was paying 77 percent of the private hospital bill, leaving a net cost to the patient of $28.50. But $28.50 in 1974 really only bought $13 worth of goods and services based on 1950 prices. So in real terms, the net cost to the patient has hardly changed during that 25 year period."[31]

But the costs, whether they are expressed in 1950 or 1974 dollars, are significant to the company which is paying the bills. As an official of the General Motors Corporation has stated, "everytime the union asked us to add something that was supposed to save money—outpatient psychiatry, home health care, convalescent care—it always adds up costing more."[32]

Health Insurance Carrier Costs

One of the reasons why business firms are paying more and more for health insurance is because the insurance carriers are experiencing medical care price increases which are larger for the most part, than those of 1971 before former President Nixon imposed a wage-price freeze on the economy. The increases in health care costs are being translated into premium hikes which range from 10 percent to 60 percent for employers who offer their employees group health insurance. One of the most oft-cited explanations which insurance carriers give for the sudden premium rise relates to the malpractice insurance crisis. Insurance companies attribute to it the increase in physician fees and the rise in the utilization of services as practitioners turn to so-called "defensive medicine," and the insurers are not wrong. The American Medical Association reports that in 1975 each visit to a doctor cost an average of $1.24 for medical malpractice insurance. The cost of protecting a doctor from malpractice suits amounted to 8.1 percent of the total cost of the office visit compared to an average of 30¢ or 2.4 percent of the doctor's bill two years earlier in 1973.[33] The Health Insurance Association of America has estimated that malpractice lawsuits have added as much as $1.5 billion a year to the public's bill for health insurance. The U. S. Department of Health, Education, and Welfare estimates that unnecessary "defensive medicine" — procedures not medically indicated but practiced to guard against the possibility of malpractice suits — adds between $3 - $5 billion to our health expenditures.[34] These increasing costs have been so severe that Blue Cross and Blue Shield reported a loss of more than $400 million in the first half of 1975. Beginning in the fourth quarter of 1975, hospital charges began to escalate rapidly along with physician charges and professional service utilization. The Blue Cross plans reported that per diem hospital costs were up from about 15 percent to 25 percent, with a median increase of 18.3 percent. By the beginning of 1977, Blue Cross plans were being allowed sharp premium increases up to 35 percent from state regulators. Nor has the commercial insurance industry been immune from sharply rising health care costs. Between 1969 and 1976, the 20 largest group health insurance companies, which have about 70 percent of the business in the country, reported losses in 4 years. An Aetna Insurance Co. vice president noted that in one recent year his company's net earnings were $19 million on premiums of $1,365 billion. The profit record of many smaller health insurance companies has even been worse. Therefore, the health service providers were not wasting any time in making up for the cost controls which were imposed upon them by the Economic Stabilization Program and which ended in April 1974.

Aside from the malpractice problem, another explanation for the dramatic rise, especially in regard to hospital costs, is that the products and services upon which hospitals depend are still subject to inflation. Included in the list of items are salaries, supplies—especially petrochemicals and derivatives—energy and fringe benefits. Still yet another explanation is that health care providers may be anticipating another round of price controls and are building up their financial bases. Such is the irony of the health care field. By increasing its prices, and, hence, the costs of its services to the public, the health care provider becomes the source of the inflationary spiral which could cause another set of price controls to be imposed upon the field. The fear of this possibility causes the provider to act financially in a way which may bring on the very government actions about which he complains and is trying to avoid. Perhaps, the health care provider should take heed of Pogo's famous statement, "We have met the enemy and he is us." No declaration more aptly summarizes what the health care field is inflicting upon itself and what it is inviting others to do to it.

Private Enterprise Cost Initiatives

Private enterprise is not waiting for government to take steps in controlling health care costs. Both private industry and labor unions have begun to adopt their own measures in an attempt to control their health expenses. A whole host of ideas is being utilized, ranging from the development of alternative delivery systems such as health maintenance organizations to the utilization of self-insurance mechanisms.

One corporate idea growing in popularity is the concept of self-insurance. This means that the benefit plan does not pay premiums to an insurance company for health coverage but pays the bills of health providers directly. The concept can save costs, such as taxes—which an insurance company must pay but a benefit plan need not—and other relatively small administrative costs. It also gives benefit plan administrators direct control of reimbursing health care providers and thus puts the administrators in a position to work with the providers in controlling costs. For example, Chicago's Commonwealth Edison Company has set up its own health insurance trust fund and subsequently held its cost increases to 27 percent despite increased benefits. At present, the company gains an estimated $200,000 a year—$100,000 on the premium money now gathering interest in Commonwealth Edison's own trust fund and $100,000 in underwriting fees which the company no longer pays to Aetna Life & Casualty, the previous carrier.[35]

Next to self-insurance, claims monitoring is the most common corporate device for controlling health care costs. Monitoring seeks to ensure that the health provider actually gave the care he billed for, that both the care and the bill were appropriate and that the company policy covered the care in question. Its single most important task is spotting excessive hospital stays and reporting them to utilization review committees. Sometimes the insurance carrier will serve as the monitor while, at other times, an outside consultant will perform the service. For example, AMF, Inc. carried out four audits in 1975 of the regional claims offices of its insurance carrier, Equitable Life. This was done to trace trends in high fees and overutilization associated with individual physicians; and to ensure that employees who were out sick or injured for exceptionally long periods were given medical examinations to verify their conditions. Extended work leaves were scrutinized and examinations called for, although the review process is, of course, time consuming. AMF claims that the project, which covered some 20,000 employees, resulted in net savings of $6,115,000.[36]

Another approach which business firms are using is encouraging employees and their physicians to use less costly forms of care. Typically, this means providing benefit coverage for a procedure normally performed in a hospital, when it is performed outside the hospital or in a hospital outpatient clinic. For example, through its insurance carriers, Proctor & Gamble has extended coverage of various types of less expensive, out-of-hospital care to 34,000 hourly and salaried employees. In an effort to contain costs, the company has extended coverage to outpatient and doctor's office testing, licensed nursing and convalescent home care following hospitalization, and home coverage of medical services and supplies when provided by a qualified home health agency.[37]

Still another idea which is gaining popularity is the establishment of health maintenance organizations by either industry or labor unions. One of the more successful attempts in this area is that of R. J. Reynolds Industries. The company built its own health center at a cost of more than $2 million and established a prepaid group practice plan only for its employees. As of the fall of 1977, after one year of operation, the plan had grown to 17,000 members and had a waiting list of 13,000. The health maintenance organization now enrolls about one-third of R. J. Reynolds workers and the company estimates that in five more years 80 percent of the company employees and their families will be HMO members. Thus far, the company has found that HMO members are off the job because of hospitalization about half as much as persons covered by traditional insurance plans. The company recommends the HMO approach only if the majority of a corporation's workers are in one location.[38] Going hand in hand with the HMO approach is the offering to workers of a dual choice as to whether they wish to join a health maintenance organization. The Communications Workers of America negotiated a nationwide HMO dual choice option (in 1971) for all 480,000 employees of the Bell Telephone System. The project was initiated jointly with the Bell System, which itself administers the health benefits and the dual choice option. Twenty-three prepaid group practices across country are offered under the dual choice option. The Bell System contributes the same amount which it would otherwise pay for coverage under the Basic Medical Expense Plan and employees make up the difference. The project went into operation in January, 1972 and has since enrolled some 32,000 employees.[39]

Corporations are also using other methods in order to reduce their health costs and some of these already have been examined in previous discussions. These include involving corporate executives in the health planning activities of their communities; the establishment of in-house corporate health education programs relating to personal health maintenance; providing employees with preventive care programs, such as health screening examinations and annual physical examinations in order to detect illness as early as possible; sponsoring the establishment of peer review organizations in a community to monitor the necessity of employee hospital admissions as well as the appropriateness of the treatment given and the length of hospital stay; the use of second opinion surgical programs; and the development of dental review programs which are designed to spot cosmetic or unnecessarily expensive dental procedures before they are performed. Under such a program, the third party can refuse to reimburse all or part of the cost of these procedures if a less expensive and professionally adequate alternative dental procedure is available. Thus, the dental review permits the patients and the dentists to know in advance what the benefits will be so that they can decide how to proceed. But whatever approaches are adopted, it appears that the private sector—whether it be private industry or labor unions—in cooperation with the insurance carriers, have a long way to go before they can begin to reduce substantially the vast sums of money which health care is presently costing their operations.

Conclusion

No industry is more aware of the limitations of its product and the distance it must travel to make it more effective than the health insurance industry. Despite the efforts of health insurers to broaden their benefit plans and provide more protection to more people than ever before in its history, the fact remains that full comprehensive coverage is not commonplace, and most non-hospital services call for substantial deductible and co-insurance payments by the insured. Buyers of hospital insurance also frequently encounter age-limit restrictions or the termination of insurance benefits after stated ceilings are reached. Their hospital coverage may be of limited duration, some kinds of illness may not be eligible for treatment and care, they face waiting periods before they are eligible for benefits, or they find that, because of pre-existing conditions, they are excluded from coverage. While it was previously noted in figure 12 that an estimated 35 million Americans under age 65 have no private hospital care insurance and 37 million have no surgical insurance, not all of these people are without any economic protection against health care bills. Some who can afford to purchase private health insurance choose not to do so. Others receive assistance for their health care expenses through such public programs as Medicare, Medicaid, the civilian health and medical care program of the uniformed services (CHAMPUS), the Veterans Administration programs, state temporary disability insurance programs and Workmen's Compensation. But despite the existence of these other programs, and regardless of the source of protection, their lack of comprehensive coverage against the skyrocketing costs of medical care is the unresolved problem.

The basic question, which now faces the private health insurance business, is whether or not it is too late for the industry to preserve its place in the health care system of the future. The crisis which the industry now confronts and the outside challenges to which it must respond have not changed very much from 1970. At the time Senator Charles Percy told the Health Insurance Association of America that "while the Administration is grateful for the insurers' efforts to provide health care to the nation, unless you do more and soon, the government may move in."[40] That statement is as true today as it was then. An official of the General Electric Corporation in 1970 expressed remarks to the health insurance industry, which are relevant today for the message they bear. This official stated:

"I don't know whether it is too late now or not. The lack of innovation and strong tendency of the industry to keep busy just tending shop may have been fatal here in the United States. The passive attitude has generally extended to new fields. In many of these the industry, I believe, should have made studies and had positions ready, as, for example, in optical costs, visiting nurses, dental expenses, etc. Instead, it is dragged reluctantly into such fields, all too often, unprepared with anything except negatives. Recently, group medical practice is attracting some interest, and a few of your members are getting into it gingerly. But this is 1970 and how long has group been around?

I am worried because of the trends I see which seem to indicate the end of a fine era of private development, whose death seems to be coming by lassitude when there should be aggressive enterprise by those most closely involved."[41]

Since these latter comments were addressed to the health insurance industry in 1970, the industry has introduced its own national health insurance proposal in Congress, has recommended the adoption of cost and quality control procedures, such as prospective rate review of institutional charges, hospital utilization review and peer review of professional services, and has sponsored the development of health maintenance organizations, to name but a few initiatives. In addition, in January 1977, the Aetna Life and Casualty Company started a two year experiment in the Washington, D.C. area to cut health costs by eliminating unneeded surgery by offering its subscribers another doctor's opinion on suggested surgery without additional charge. According to Aetna, if getting second opinions cuts down on surgery, the company will make the benefit permanent.[42] Given these activities by the insurance industry, one question surfaces quickly—have these measures come too late? As the country begins to scrutinize the issue of national health insurance under a Democratic Administration, whose 1976 election Party platform espoused such a program, does the health insurance industry still have time to demonstrate that is is far more capable of financing health care under a national program than the federal government? What is being witnessed today in a free enterprise society is an industry whose concept of operation is under public debate. Its large consumers, namely labor and management, expressing doubt as to its future viability, the U. S. Congress expressing deep concern over the industry's inability to control the costs of its premiums, and social planners seeking to demonstrate the inability of the industry to deal effectively with the health care problems which beset the nation. The task which lies ahead will be difficult. The industry must continue to change from its traditional conservative character to one which is innovative and aggressive and strict in its administrative procedures to reduce health costs. The social and economic conditions which are pressuring society to call for a change in the manner by which the nation finances and provides health care is not giving any group or organization much time to reflect philosophically upon the course of action. While the health insurance industry has introduced its own national health insurance plan in Congress, it is competing for attention with other plans which seek to replace, in whole or in part, the traditional role which the private health insurance industry has enjoyed in our society up to now. This is what is taking place today. The consumer has become increasingly aware of what constitutes adequate health care and is questioning the kind and cost of the care he is now receiving. Thus, the situation which confronts the private health insurance industry is but one element of the larger health care picture in which other providers of service are confronted by similar issues but of varying degree. The health care field, in turn, is but one element of the larger picture of the social and economic revolutions which are sweeping this nation. What makes the insurance element of particular significance is that the industry, as a representative of the American free enterprise system, is being given notice that if it cannot sufficiently and economically meet and serve society's needs then the public will turn to and seek assistance from its own representative—namely, government—to perform private industry's function. Private health insurance vs. national health insurance is the battleground upon which the issue will be settled.

Figure 11

DEFINITION OF
HEALTH INSURANCE PLANS

A. **Hospital Expense Plans**—provide b enefits for all or part of the costs of hospital rooms, board, and other charges.

B. **Surgical Expense Plans**—benefit payments made according to a schedule of surgical procedures listing the maximum amount of benefits for each type of operation covered.

C. **Regular Medical Expense**—provides benefits toward payment of physicians' fees for non-surgical care given in the hospital, home or at the physician's office. Some regular medical expense plans also cover for diagnostic X-ray and laboratory expenses.

D. **Major Medical Expense**—benefits paid for virtually all kinds of health care prescribed by a physician. These policies assist in covering the cost of treatment given in and out of the hospital, special nursing care, X-rays, prescriptions, medical appliances, nursing home care, ambulatory psychiatric care, and many other health care needs.

E. **Loss of Income Protection**—loss of income (or disability income) protection is designed to provide wage earners with regular weekly or monthly cash payments in the event that wages are cut off as a result of illness or accident. (Short-term policies are those with maximum benefit periods up to 2 years; long-term plans are for periods greater than 2 years.)

Source: *1976–1977 Source Book of Health Insurance Data,* Health Insurance Institute, New York, 1977, pp. 24-29.

Figure 12

ESTIMATE OF NET NUMBER OF PERSONS NOT COVERED UNDER
PRIVATE HEALTH INSURANCE PLANS, BY AGE AND BENEFIT,
AS OF DECEMBER 31, 1975

INSURANCE BENEFITS	ALL AGES		UNDER AGE 65		AGE 65 AND OVER	
	%	Number (000)	%	Number (000)	%	Number (000)
Hospital Care	20.7	43,928	18.7	35,469	37.3	8,459
Physician Services						
surgical services	22.3	47,390	19.6	37,176	45.0	10,214
in-hospital visits	24.3	51,626	20.4	38,640	57.2	12,986
x-ray & laboratory examinations	26.2	55,659	21.8	41,381	62.9	14,278
office & home visits	39.9	84,641	36.1	68,440	71.4	16,201
Dental Care	83.8	177,929	82.2	155,834	97.2	22,065
Prescription Drugs (out-of-hospital)	29.7	63,100	23.9	45,339	78.2	17,761
Private Duty Nursing	31.3	66,449	25.7	48,678	78.3	17,771
Visiting Nurse Service	33.3	70,815	28.2	53,575	75.9	17,240
Nursing Home Care	67.0	142,230	65.4	123,988	80.4	18,242
HIAA Estimates[a]						
Hospital Care	16.2	34,396	12.3	24,317	44.4	10,079
Surgical Services	20.5	43,481	16.4	31,156	54.3	12,325
Total Population[b]	212,376,000		189,674,000		22,702,000	

a. The HIAA is the Health Insurance Association of America and represents the commercial health insurance industry in the United States.

b. Based on the Bureau of Census estimate as January 1, 1976.

Source: Derived from Marjorie Smith Mueller, "Private Health Insurance in 1975: Coverage, Enrollment and Financial Experience," Social Security Bulletin, June, 1977, p. 5.

CHAPTER 8

National Health Insurance: The Beginning of the End?

IS NATIONAL HEALTH INSURANCE the *parriah* or *savior* of our health care system? Will it increase or diminish the quality and cost of care which we receive in future years? The arguments have been going on since the turn of this century. Only a decade ago this nation heard the following words:

"What this country needs is a universal, nationally financed, national health insurance program related to the Social Security system which will make health care available and accessible to all Americans."[1] So spoke the late Walter Reuther of the United Automobile Workers Union in the late 1960s at a news conference launching the Committee of 100 for National Health Insurance. Almost concurrently, a Congressional advisory committee reported to the health committee of the Senate Special Committee on Aging that "a comprehensive, compulsory health insurance program for all age groups—a program with built-in cost controls, standards for quality care, incentives for prepaid group practice and other badly needed reforms—offers the best hope this nation has for living up to the often expressed declaration that good health care is the right of every man, woman and child who lives in this land."[2] Since these admirable exclamations, our nation has entered the latter part of the 1970s with the following affirmation.. "I want to have a comprehensive health-care program fully established in this country in four years, but how much we do each succeeding year will have to be determined by what we have available."[3] The latter pronouncement was made in 1976 by Jimmy Carter, then President-Elect of the United States.

However, by the beginning of 1978, the Carter Administration's enthusiasm for enacting a national health insurance program was in a state of flux. For example, until November 1977, President Carter had promised repeatedly to send a phased-in, universal and comprehensive national health insurance proposal to Congress in early 1978. By mid-November, the Presidential pledge had been reduced to submitting only the "principles" of such a plan in 1978. By the early winter of 1978, there was still another change of emphasis. President Carter stated he expected to send a national health insurance bill to the Congress late in its second session. Thus, for all practical purposes Congress could not begin to act upon and complete the passage of such a bill until 1979. The proponents of national health insurance wanted a bill introduced during 1978, arguing that eventual passage will take two or three years. If President Carter wanted a national health insurance plan passed before the 1980 elections he had to begin marshaling his forces in 1978 to get it enacted. By the spring of the year this political activity became visible.

Thus, national health insurance has become an issue in which the government's activity, once again, has resembled a magician's sleight of hand of "now you see it and now you don't." In the early 1970s, like the latter part of the same decade, national health insurance always seemed just around the corner. The only question then was whether it would be a comprehensive and publicly financed program sponsored by Senator Edward M. Kennedy, or the more limited catastrophic approach sponsored by Senator Russell B. Long and Senator Abraham A. Ribicoff, or the mixed public-private approach advocated by the commercial health insurance industry. In contrast to past years, opposition to such a program from within the health care field as well as from outside politicians had practically disappeared. Even such one-time strong opponents as the American Medical Association were now having their own national health insurance bills introduced into the U.S. Congress.

What happened? Why is so popular a measure in terms of the diversity of its sponsors still lingering around the halls of Congress when so many groups within the health care field seem to endorse its necessity? Two reasons for this situation are apparent. One is politics, the other is economics. First, 1978 was an election year. It must be remembered that Congress had voted huge Social Security taxes in 1977, was expected to increase taxes even more during 1978 with the passage of the national energy bill, and had just received President Carter's record-breaking $500 billion budget for fiscal year 1979. Even with a prospective income tax reduction in 1978, Congress was not likely to enact another social program which would increase the tax burden of the voting public, especially since national health insurance is expected to cost even more than our present expenditures on medical care services. In 1977, this nation spent $163 billion for health care services, as already noted. In addition, as 1978 began, there was no consensus in the Congress, even after years of debate, as to the shape a national health insurance plan should assume, or who should pay for such a program and how much they should pay. Even without a new health program, the American taxpayer saw more and more of his tax dollars allocated to HEW whose budget—$181 billion for fiscal year 1979—was growing at rate of $17 billion a year. And, more specifically regarding the health insurance issue, Medicare and Medicaid were growing at a rate of $5 billion a year without any new benefits.[4] Additionally, during 1977 the Carter Administration was unable to get its hospital cost containment bill enacted into law—a program which the Administration considered to be an important prerequisite prior to the passage of any national health insurance plan. In fact, except for the passage of the Medicare-Medicaid Anti-Fraud and Abuse Amendments in 1977, the Administration did not see any measures enacted for containing the costs of health care services. (These latter Amendments were passed, in part, because of the huge cost overruns and financial scandals in Medicare and Medicaid, leading to fears that any national health insurance plan modeled after such programs would suffer similar abuses and drive taxes up sharply.) Also, Congress had other social legislation to consider, including welfare reform. Finally, in view of President Carter's promise to balance the budget by 1981, some even question how so costly a program as national health insurance could be enacted at all during the Administration's first term of office, even if it was phased in over time. Regardless of how the issue is examined, national health insurance does not seem to be an idea whose political time has come, at the moment. But no one disputes the fact that it is an idea which will become a reality at some point in the future.

Consequently, in view of the fact that national health insurance will once again become the subject of congressional debate and public dialogue in the forseeable future, this chapter will review various facets of the issue. For example, what kinds of programs are presently being advocated in Congress? What does the public want in terms of a national health insurance program? What kind of changes would national health insurance bring to the health care field, in general, and to the practice of medicine, in particular? What do these national health insurance proposals mean to you as both a patient and consumer? Does President Carter's call for a universal, mandatory and comprehensive benefit system, including preventive care services, financed by a combination of employer-employee payroll taxes and general revenues with built-in cost and quality controls seems to agree with any specific proposal introduced into past Congresses? Before analyzing these and other issues, I would like to explore the historical development of national health insurance giving a proper perspective to the following discussions.

Origin of Concept

The concept of a national compulsory health insurance system for the United States is not new. Although many consider the idea to have originated in the late 1930s when it achieved the prominence of congressional debate, a universal compulsory system of medical care insurance was actually first advocated in the United States before

World War I. In fact, the principle of compulsory participation is even older than that, for in 1798 the U. S. Government set up a Marine Hospital Service (forerunner of the Public Health Service) and required the owners of merchant ships to contribute 20 cents per month into a sickness fund for each seaman in their employ.

Historians of social welfare often cite the German compulsory health insurance program, inaugurated by Chancellor Otto Von Bismarck, as being the historic seed of modern Social Security programs. However, the German program itself was just a step in the long evolutionary process through which our modern social welfare programs evolved.

The basic principle of individuals pooling their resources in order to spread their economic risks actually can be traced to the so-called funeral societies of ancient Greece. Originally established to pay members' funeral costs, the societies ultimately came to have a variety of social and relief functions. Similarly, medieval craft guilds, the forerunners of modern labor unions, often set up welfare funds for the assistance of sick or needy members. As the industrial revolution gathered momentum in the 19th century, a number of labor unions and individual employers required that their workers join relief funds, many of which eventually came under government regulation.

The idea that the government should share some of the responsibility for health care can also be traced back at least as far as the Greek city-states. Greek citizens enjoyed the services of tax-supported public physicians.

The first broad-based compulsory health insurance law was enacted in Prussia in 1854. Twenty-nine years later, when Bismarck united Germany and became its first Chancellor, he was able to draw on this precedent when, in 1883, he persuaded the German Reichstag to extend compulsory health insurance to workers throughout the German nation. When Bismarck's program proved highly successful, it soon spread to other European countries, notably Great Britain.

Eventually it expanded into the comprehensive system of worker protection we know today as "social insurance".

At the beginning of the twentieth century, Great Britain was at the height of her power and the center of a great empire. She was greatly admired and emulated in the United States. It is not surprising that the British scheme of social insurance soon developed some advocates for a similar program in this country. This early advocacy of 1910-1920 originally was supported by the American Medical Association. However, professional opposition soon developed and, at its meeting in New Orleans in 1920, the AMA House of Delegates reversed that stand.

A number of conferences were called in 1925 and 1926 to formulate plans for a study of the structure of medical services in the United States. As a result of the conferences, the Committee on Costs of Medical Care (CCMC) was established, funded by six foundations. The final report of the Committee was published in 1932. Positions were soon taken. The majority of the Committee members held that medical service, both preventive and therapeutic, should be furnished largely by organized groups of physicians, dentists, nurses, pharmacists, and other associated personnel; and that the costs of medical care be placed on a group payment basis through the use of insurance, taxation or both. The minority report, supported by the American Medical Association, objected to the proposal for group practice and the adoption of insurance plans, unless sponsored and controlled by organized medicine.

After the CCMC report was issued, a movement began for the enactment of a national health insurance program Originally, it was supposed to have been part of the Social Security Act of 1935. But for various political reasons it was omitted. In 1939, the late Senator Robert Wagner introduced his first national health insurance bill with the Administration's approval. Subsequently, additional attempts were made via the Murray-Wagner-Dingell bills of 1943, 1945, 1947 and 1949 to secure passage of this program. Despite considerable interest and support, these bills never passed either the House or

Senate. Realizing that a universal national health insurance program could not be enacted in the foreseeable future, organized labor and other interested groups retreated and revised their strategy. It was then that the long, successful fight began for Medicare, a program which now provides financing for much of the medical care of more than 22 million elderly Americans.[5]

Renewed Interest

The enactment of the Medicare and Medicaid amendments to the Social Security Act in 1965 served as the catalyst for bringing about renewed interest, impetus and agitation for a more adequate and more comprehensive system of financing and delivering health care to the American people through such mechanisms as a national health insurance program. Although intended to alleviate, in part, the medical care access and cost problems of the American elderly and poor, Medicare and Medicaid and other programs brought new stresses and burdens to a health system already under strain.

The growing insistence that there should be further governmental involvement in the health care area derives from two major influences. First, the very existence of Medicare has demonstrated to the nation that a broad-based public compulsory health insurance program is feasible. Despite its weaknesses, Medicare has brought some financial relief, broadening the access to health care services for many millions of the elderly. In addition, the Medicare program appears to be popular among its recipients and providers of care. Second, there is growing pressure to extend such a service to those whose economic circumstances differ little, if at all, from the mass of the elderly. This feeling has been reinforced by the 1972 Amendments to the Social Security Act. The 1972 law extended coverage for the first time to individuals under age 65 who require hemodialysis or renal transplantation for chronic renal disease and who are currently or fully insured, those entitled to monthly Social Security benefits, or are the spouses or dependent children of such insured or entitled individuals. The Amendments also extended

Medicare protection to people 18 years and older who are receiving Social Security or Railroad Retirement monthly benefits based on disability, and who have been entitled to such benefits for at least 24 consecutive months. So the question arises—if Medicare benefits can be extended to certain groups within our population who are under 65 years of age and, thus, create for them a mini-national health insurance plan, why can't we have a national health insurance plan covering the rest of our population as well? Answers to this question have not met with much success since 1969-1970 when national health insurance bills were introduced in the 91st Congress. Their introduction has continued through the 95th Congress which ended in 1978. The bills introduced in the 95th Congress, like those of the four preceding ones, represented a whole range of political philosophy and thought. Some of the bills were designed solely to reorganize the present system of financing health care; others dealt essentially with the financing system with slight alteration of the delivery system; and others proposed changing both the financing mechanism and the delivery system. With all the present buildup and pressure as well as President Carter's interest in the subject, it is likely that within the next several years some major extension of governmental supported insurance will be enacted into law. But what kind of extension is not, as yet, clear.

The American People Speak

Not only is there a lack of a clear consensus in the Congress as to the eventual contents of a national health insurance program, but also there is no singular opinion among the American people as to its format. The findings of a 1977 Louis Harris public opinion poll, released in January 1978, showed mixed desires. While most Americans would like to keep the nation's health care system without a major change, a significant minority preferred that Congress pass a comprehensive national health insurance program. The survey also showed that considerable public support existed for filling three existing gaps in our present health system. These include:

- a requirement that all employers provide health insurance to all employees;
- government-provided health insurance for the unemployed;
- extended coverage in the private sector to take care of a long and serious illness.[6]

According to the Harris survey, 62 percent of the American people find acceptable the present health system, defined by the survey as consisting of Medicare and Medicaid, as well as coverage purchased from private insurance companies. Fifty-four percent of the people would be happy if the present system was reinforced by a law requiring employers to provide health insurance to all of their employees, and the government to provide insurance to everyone who is not employed. Fifty-five percent of the people would not only like the present system to contain the two previous changes but also that the benefit coverage of the employer's health insurance be broadened to encompass catastrophic illness. In addition, 51 percent of the people surveyed favor a national health insurance program covering all medical and hospital expenses paid for by federal taxes. Under such a program, the government would control hospital costs, physicians' fees and other charges—a concept which sounds very similar to the Kennedy—Corman national health insurance bill. Also, 39 percent of the people would accept a national health service under which everyone would receive health care paid for by public taxes. In such an arrangement, doctors would work for salaries which are paid for by the government, and hospitals would be government managed.[7] In a society which continually and vigorously opposes government's intrusion into the free enterprise system, we have seemingly reached a point in terms of our health care problems where 39 percent of our population would now find it acceptable if our health care system was to be nationalized or socialized. This is an approach which not even the Kennedy-Corman national health insurance bill—as radical as some may consider it to be—has dared to suggest. Under the Kennedy-Corman bill, which proposes public financing, physicians not only have the choice of being paid on a fee-for-service, salary or capitalization basis (that is, the physician is paid a fixed per capita amount for each patient whom he treats regardless of the actual number or nature of the services to the patient), but also the bill never even proposes that the government take over the management or ownership of the nation's hospitals or other health care enterprises. While the figure of 39 percent may represent a minority statistic, is it really so insignificant when we are speaking of nationalizing a specific industry within a society whose primary characteristic is its capitalistic nature?

Not Like Other Countries

However, regardless of whether the public opinion polls show that the American people are satisfied or dissatisfied with their health care system, or whether they want a national health insurance plan to retain the status quo or render mild or radical changes, the Carter Administration is developing its own concepts. One point which should be emphasized is that it will be an American plan, not a foreign one. According to Hale Champion, Undersecretary of HEW, who is supervising the development of the Carter Administration's national health insurance program:

"It will be informed by idealism but shaped by pragmatism . . . Our proposal must lead to a significant restructuring of the way care is delivered and must change the perverse incentives now at work . . . We cannot and will not accept an inflation rate two and a half times that of the general economy, and thus accept a situation in which health uses up all our national resources while education, social services, housing and other urgent needs go unmet . . . We will end up with a typically American solution, built on what now exists, aspiring toward what—given human fraility—will never be."[8]

One way in which the Carter Administration is developing its concepts for an American health plan is by visiting foreign countries to learn how their own national health insurance plans operate. One of the countries, England which HEW Secretary, Joseph A. Califano, Jr., and other Administration representatives visited in the fall of 1977, has a plan which would be quite acceptable to 39 percent of the American people cited in the 1978 Harris poll. Whenever we talk about national health insurance in this country, it is couched in terms of being socialized medicine. Whenever we hear about Senator Edward M. Kennedy's "Health Security" national health insurance plan, it is described as socialized medicine. Whenever we talk about the good or the evil of socialized medicine, we hear about England. But except for clichés or generalities, how much, as laymen, do we know about the English health system? The following overview is intended to be a brief account of the British system so that we can compare its socialized medical system to our own way of delivering and paying for health care services.

The idea of medical care as a basic right was institutionalized in England when the British Parliament passed the National Health Insurance Act in 1911. Under this Act, all manual workers whose income was below a certain level were protected by mandatory health insurance.[9] Both employers and employees contributed to the insurance payments. Government provided the funds for administering the program and for covering very low income and indigent persons. A worker's dependents did not have to be covered by the insurance but could purchase health insurance through a mutual aid society on a voluntary basis.[10] These societies were created throughout Europe in the 19th century to enable lowly paid workers to look after themselves by providing disability and sickness care insurance to these persons. Over the next 35 years, the income threshold for health insurance increased until the National Health Service Act was passed in 1946 and became effective as a program in July 1948. To the surprise of some, voluntary health insurance did not disappear in England when the National Health Service became operational. A small percentage of the British population still seeks care through private arrangements outside of the official government structure. In fact, in the mid-1970s about one percent of the hospital beds in England were reserved for private patients. As of 1969 private health insurance enrollment only numbered about 883,000 people or less than 2 percent of the total English population. Despite the fact that long waiting lists for hospital treatment of elective conditions are still a problem (though the length of the lists has declined, and no difficulty is experienced with emergency case admissions,) it appears that most patients are not displeased with the other limitations of the National Health Service to the point where they would rather pay for medical care.[11]

From 1948-1974 the structure of the British National Health Service remained as it was originally established. Its foremost achievement was the elimination of financial barriers to health care so that no one can be bankrupted by illness or left to die if unable to pay market prices. But patients, with some exceptions, continue to pay a certain amount for prescribed drugs; for prosthetic dental services; for private beds in National Health Service hospitals—a private bed system which, as of 1977, was being phased-out; for special eye glasses; and other miscellaneous items. During this 26 year period, the administration of the National Health Service was divided into three major separate sectors: general practitioner services; hospital and specialist services; and local authority public health services.

Under the National Health Service the general practitioner is paid a fixed amount every month for each person who is registered on his patient list, regardless of whether the patient uses or does not use his services. By 1970, about one-half of the general practitioner's income came from various fees rather than just from capitation payments. These other income sources included fees for such services as certain office procedures and home calls as well as grants for the engagement of allied health personnel. Under the National Health Service, a patient can change to another general practitioner at any time, whereupon his name would be transferred to the other doctor's list. In order to protect the quality of care, the maximum number of persons originally permitted on the general practitioner's list was 3,500. In recent years the average has been about 2,200.[12] A network of executive councils was established throughout England and Wales to administer the health services of the total population. On the average, each council administered the ambulatory services of about 350,000 people. In addition, these councils were responsible, among other duties, for the capitation payments to and the monitoring of general practitioners.

The second major element of the National Health Service was a network of regional hospital boards covering England and Wales. With the nationalization of the English health system, the government acquired all the property of the hospitals and assumed all their debts and obligations. Overnight, Britain's 2,700 hospitals with about 480,000 beds (about 80 percent municipal) attained financial stability.[13] The nationalization included all mental, tuberculosis and other chronic disease facilities, as well as general hospitals, but not elderly people's homes or convalescent units. The hospital regions were designed to contain about two or three million people and about 30,000 hospital beds of all types.[14] As a result of Britain's postwar financial difficulties and competing interests for housing, schools, roads, construction and other obligations, both within and outside the country, new hospital construction was not undertaken until quite recently. Capital expenditures went for renovating old structures. As a result, most British hospitals have antiquated features. Funds for both the operation and capital costs of all hospitals within a region were allotted by the central government to the regional hospital board, which, in turn, distributed the monies to the hospital management committees which the regional board appointed to administer the hospitals. These committees were typically responsible for institutions containing a total of between 1,000 to 2,000 beds. This might mean two or three large units or as many as fifteen or twenty smaller ones.

In terms of medical staff, British specialists in medicine and surgery are attached mainly to the hospitals. About 60 percent are on salary and about 40 percent spend part of their time in outside private practice. General practitioners, however, who constitute about one-half of Britain's doctors, seldom have hospital appointments under the National Health Service, nor did they have such appointments before its creation. In other words, the patient requiring hospitalization (except in emergencies) is referred by his general practitioner to a hospital outpatient department, where the examining specialist decides if he should be admitted. Likewise, the patient may be referred to the hospital's outpatient department simply for a diagnostic workup. In either case—whether admitted to a bed or not—a report is sent to the referring practitioner on the hospital specialist's findings. Thus, the separation of general practice from the hospital is quite unlike the situation in the United States where nearly all physicians, generalist and specialist, have hospital ties. The British system is not unique to that country, but prevails in most of Europe, and in most other countries of the world.[15]

The final major branch of the British National Health Service was the network of local health authorities in England and Wales, responsible for the traditional preventive public health services. While the National Health Service took away the responsibilities of local health authorities for public hospitals, these authorities were given new functions in such areas as ambulance services, visiting nurse services, homemaker care services for the chronically ill, and the operation of long-term care facilities for the aged or chronically ill not needing hospitalization, as well as responsibilities for maternal and child health services.

As a result of these separation of powers, the British health system was beset with powerful contesting interest groups, overlapping areas of responsibility, lack of coordination, fragmentation, redundancy in services, and poor health services planning and policy-making. In 1974, therefore, the British National Health Service was reorganized to integrate the administration of services. Hospitals, ambulatory services and public health organizations are now united under the Department of Health and Social Security. The country is now divided into regional, district and area authorities, each representing varying population sizes. The reorganization has weakened the power of each interest group, thus strengthening the National Health Service and hopefully its ability to improve services. It is expected that this reorganization will enable the British Health Service to have a broad planning perspective and the ability to produce specific programs for local needs. For example, while the area health authorities are responsible for all types of services— ambulatory, hospital and preventive—including the functions of the former hospital management committees to administer the hospitals), the regional health authorities retain the former responsibilities of the regional hospital boards for planning the construction of facilities. Only time will be the ultimate judge as to whether this reorganization will improve the British health care system. As of the winter of 1978, the prognosis was more negative than positive.

In view of the contrast between the American and British health systems, the information available from the early 1970s demonstrate some interesting findings when both systems are compared. In 1976, the per capita expenditure on personal health care in England was $165 versus $638 in the United States and whereas we allocated 8.6 percent of our Gross National Product for health care services, England spent 5.6 percent. The British infant mortality rate of 16.9 per 1000 live babies and the maternal mortality rate of 11.2 per 100,000 live births in 1973 was better than America's figures of 17.7 per 1000 live babies and 14.1 per 100,000 live births in these respective categories. Surgery rates in England are about one-half that of the United States, but the ratio of surgeons to the English population is also about one-half the level in the United States.[16] Whereas most surgeons in the United States practice on the fee-for-service principle and thus have an economic incentive to perform surgery even if it may not be necessary, surgeons in England do not have such an incentive since they practice medicine on fixed salaries based on merit. Lastly, only 56 million people live in Britain.

These are the essential features of the British National Health Service, whose funding is derived from several sources. The contributions from these sources vary proportionately from year to year. For example, in 1970-1971, the funding sources included: central government general revenues (80 percent); social insurance contributions (9 percent); local government revenues (6.5 percent); and payments by patients (4.5 percent).[17] In many respects, the British National Health Service is far different than our own health system. Yet, at the same time there is a small amount of similarity. With the passage of a Medicare law providing mandatory health insurance for a small segment of our population on a national basis; with the development of comprehensive health planning and the establishment of Health Systems Agencies with their regional planning responsibilities; and with the increasing involvement of our federal government in the affairs of organized medicine, this country has slowly begun to adopt some of the philosophy of the English system. This is a system which views health care as a right, not a privilege, and which has in the past and continues at present to influence social planners in many nations, including those who are helping to restructure our own health systems. Whether or not you agree or disagree with the philosophy or intent of the British National Health Service, the system is significant enough as a model for the inspection and observation of the Secretary of HEW in his formulation of an American plan.

View of the American Physician

If there is one model which the American physician would prefer our government not consider, it is the British National Health Service. A group of American physicians who visited England in 1977 to observe the National Health Service were not very pleased with the system, except for one feature. Patients know that they don't have to worry about costs if they get sick. As one physician stated, "the psychological benefit for the patient is the only exemplary feature of the system."[18] Those aspects of the National

Health Service not appealing to the physicians included: antiquated hospital buildings; the lack of intensive care units in hospitals; the fragmentation of patient care; the lack of financial incentives to keep high caliber British doctors in England; the failure of the system to redistribute medical resources in terms of facilities or personnel; the long waiting lists to get into hospitals; and the high per capita costs and high taxes which are levied to maintain the system. One physician summarized his observations by stating:

"I'd like to import their pubs, their transportation system, and the graciousness of the English people, but I'll leave their medical system with them."[20]

Well, what kind of system would the American physician prefer if there is no alternative to resolving our health care problems except to enact a national health insurance plan in this country? Answers to this question were partially revealed by a poll the American Medical Association carried out among its membership in 1977. Of 158,000 questionnaires sent out, 47.5 percent were returned and revealed the following profile. More than half of the physicians believed that national health insurance participation should be on a voluntary basis; the program should be handled by private insurers rather than by the federal government; the plan should include both basic and catastrophic health insurance coverage; physicians should be paid under a usual, customary and reasonable fee basis; deductibles should be incorporated into such a plan; almost half believed that employer participation should not be mandatory; and the national health insurance plan preferred by physicians more than any other is that supported by the American Medical Association in Congress. This program is one which individuals would purchase private health insurance policies, with the federal government paying the premiums for the poor, and contributing partial payments (based on each family's taxable income) for other groups.[21] Needless to say, the health care system is adequate from the physicians point of view and does not require any alterations as proposed by other national health insurance proposals.

Physicians are quite apprehensive about the establishment of national health insurance in this country. They realize that their freedom to practice the kind of medicine they deem best, rather than what others may determine is appropriate, is at stake. In a 1976 poll of 2,000 physicians across the country, the American Medical Association reported the following findings as it relates to this issue:

- 92.6 percent of the doctors thought that national health insurance would not improve the quality of medical services;
- 86.7 percent of the physicians said that national health insurance would overtax the health care system;
- 82.2 percent of the doctors said it would establish complete socialized medicine;
- 83 percent of the physicians said it would result in the rationing of medical care;
- 95.5 percent of the doctors said it would cause the ultimate cost of health care to the average citizen to vastly increase through taxation and inflation.[22]

The findings of this poll demonstrate that physicians fear any future national health insurance plan will assume the characteristics which critics attribute to the British National Health Service. These include the rationing of medical care, the socialization of medicine, and a decline in the quality of medical services. Yet, as already mentioned, there is no proposal in Congress of a major special interest group such as the AFL-CIO, commercial health insurance industry, or the medical profession which advocates that our health care system be nationalized. In other words, no major interest group advocates the establishment of a national health insurance plan in which the government under this single program would at the same time own and manage the facilities, employ all the personnel, and manage all the finances of the health care system. Yet, the myths and the fears persist that national health insurance will lead to the destruction of our health care system and the quality of the medical care it provides. These fears often cloud logical and rationale debate on the subject. They not only hinder the development of a plan equitable to those who finance and provide health services, but also to those who receive this care as well.

View of American Business

In addition, the nation's business leaders also do not favor a program which is compulsory, comprehensive, and federally financed. In 1975, Louis Harris and the Wharton Business School of the University of Pennsylvania conducted a poll of 1,140 business decision makers. Of those surveyed 63 percent opposed such a comprehensive program while 30 percent favored it. In addition, 63 percent even opposed a proposal for a mixed employer-employee-government health insurance program while only 28 percent favored it. However, the survey showed that, at the time, 94 percent of the companies had not made any studies of the impact of national health insurance on their costs, though 59 percent of those surveyed believed that employer-employee financed coverage under national health insurance would cost their company more money. Among medium-sized and large business establishments, employees are almost universally covered by health insurance. On the other hand, the survey showed that among smaller businesses with 10-19 employees in such fields as contracting, retail light manufacturing industries, scarcely more than 74 percent of all employees were covered by health insurance.[23] Two years later, in 1977, when HEW was conducting hearings throughout the country soliciting the public's views on national health insurance, the attitude of American business did not seem to have changed very greatly. According to a spokesman for the General Motors Corporation, "In our opinion, General Motors employees and their families and other Americans in similar positions would be better served by a strong coordinated effort to contain escalating health care insurance costs than by a broad program of national health insurance."[24] While a representative of the National Association of Manufacturers added:

"We believe that implementing national health insurance is premature at this time. Without demonstrating workable controls to slow rising costs and assure quality services, there is reason to believe that current proposals to expand coverage are likely to only add to the problem . . . Rather than blanketing the whole country, national health insurance coverage should be targeted to those who need it—the unemployed, people between jobs and those marginally covered."[25]

But the opposition of physicians and businessmen to various national health insurance proposals represents the opinions of just two of very many constituencies in our society.

National Health Insurance Plans

Since the 91st Congress in 1969, a whole variety of national health insurance proposals have been introduced in Congress, representing the viewpoints and thoughts of interest groups of all political, social and economic hues. In fact, the Social Security Administration counted at least 18 bills introduced in the 94th Congressional session, which ended in 1976. The bills fell into four broad categories—catastrophic protection, tax credits, mainly public, and a mixed public-private approach. In addition to bills which were supported by individual Congressmen and Senators, there were also bills introduced on behalf of such groups as the American Medical Association, the American Hospital Association, labor's AFL-CIO, and the Health Insurance Association of America (the commercial health insurance industry). Just as the Carter Administration designed its own bill, past Administrations formulated their own bills, (including former President Ford, who retained the Nixon Administration's proposal of the 93rd Congress as his own measure).

The various Congressional legislative proposals, regardless of origin or sponsor, collectively have certain basic objectives in common. These include: universal coverage (but not necessarily compulsory); comprehensive coverage (extent varies); holding health costs to a minimum; equal access to health care services; and holding administration costs to a minimum.[27] And containing health costs has proven to be a very difficult task for the U.S. Congress, even though this body has expressed its concern on this issue in various ways through such measures as the enactment of the Social Security Amendments of 1972 and the Health Maintenance Organization Amendments of 1976. But Congress is also sensitive to pressure from the health care industry. For example, it refused to accept the Nixon Administration plan to continue health cost controls after the expiration of the Economic Stabilization Act in 1974 and it has responded sympathetically to the hospital lobby's strong objection to Medicare cost controls.[28] Legislators rarely hear from any other force except the Administration on the subject of cost control. Virtually all Congressional witnesses testify in favor of expanding federal subsidies, not controlling them. In this environment, legislators find few incentives to support controls. "When we proposed controls we stepped on the toes of every interest in the industry; the ensuing pressures were relentless," said a former member of the House Interstate and Foreign Commerce Subcommittee on Health and Environment.[29]

Most of the proposed bills, introduced in the 95th Congress and past sessions, have attempted to correct some of the major complaints about Medicare and Medicaid. These are that Medicare does not provide catastrophic insurance and that both programs have significantly contributed to the inflation of health costs. Medicaid is abolished in many proposed national health bills because of the inequities between the states, due to the wide differences in standards for coverage and eligibility. The Medicaid program is thus absorbed into the national health insurance framework.

In testimony before the House Ways and Means Health Subcommittee in the summer of 1975, health experts summed up what had to be accomplished to build a solid framework for national health insurance. Medicare and Medicaid had to be reformed; the public sector had to gain control over the physician's fee structure; greater concentration was needed on preventive medicine and ambulatory care; stricter controls had to be instituted for physicians and hospitals; and financial assistance had to be provided for catastrophic illness.[30]

While some of the national health insurance measures address themselves to these problems, the various bills differ from each other on a number of key issues, especially in regard to the character that any national health insurance program should assume. The following are some of the major ways and questions by which the various bills differ from each other and raise in terms of public debate:

- The role of the federal government in administering and financing a national health insurance program;
- Who should be covered;
- The range and depth of benefits;
- The method of payment (Social Security taxes, income tax credits, or premiums);
- The use and amount of deductibles, copayments and co-insurance;
- The extent of private insurance involvement;
- Reimbursement methods;
- The extent of catastrophic illness coverage;
- Whether or not to federalize Medicaid;
- Incentives to health care providers for greater efficiency, management and innovation;
- How to foster other methods for improved health care delivery such as health maintenance organizations;
- Methods for keeping health care costs down,
- How to structure overall organization and delivery of health care services;
- Health maintenance and public health education;
- Methods for training and providing health manpower and care in rural areas and inner cities.[31]

Consequently, national health insurance is the ultimate program. It is the umbrella, depending upon the plan being reviewed, under which all the topics which we have discussed thus far come together and coalesce in a single program. It is the umbrella under which state hospital cost commissions are established in greater numbers; the financing of health resource development is institutionalized in a single fund; the growth of health maintenance organizations is fostered even more than at present; PSRO review activities are extended to our entire population rather than being limited to certain groups; health planning assumes added importance in controlling the growth and finances of health resources in a community; the private health insurance industry either flourishes or disappears as a viable economic entity; the costs of prescription drugs are controlled through the establishment of national drug lists called formularies; and ambulatory health care centers are developed. However, in order to witness how some of these changes may occur in more specific terms, let us examine three major national health insurance proposals introduced in the 94th Congress and reintroduced in the 95th session. One, sponsored by the American Medical Association, is mainly a mechanism for financing health care services. The second, sponsored by the Health Insurance Association for America (the commercial health insurance industry) is a mixed public and private approach which finances health care services and alters the delivery system to a small degree. The third, sponsored by Senator Edward M. Kennedy and Representative James C. Corman, is mainly a public approach which finances health care and greatly alters the delivery system. Wherever changes relevant to our discussion were made in the three bills from the 94th to the 95th Congressional sessions, these alterations will be noted in our examination of these proposed plans.

Restructuring the Health Care Field

One of the basic philosophical as well as practical questions inherent in all of these national insurance plans is whether or not our present health care system needs restructuring, and if so, to what extent. The proposal of the American Medical Association takes the following position.[32] Our health care system is basically sound, along with the present system of claims and peer review. Accordingly, the American Medical Association bill, as noted in figure 15, is addressed almost entirely to the fact that a number of people do not have adequate health insurance coverage for their medical expenses. Thus, the American Medical Association's plan covers the entire U. S. population in a two-part program. The first component requires employers to offer private health insurance to their employees. The second part makes private health insurance available for low-income families, the unemployed and the self-employed, with the federal government subsidizing the premium through income tax credits or subsidy certificates. The private health insurance industry provides the health insurance and is supervised by the states under regulations issued by a federal government board. Thus, as far as the American Medical Association is concerned, the only problem with our health care system is that our nation needs better health insurance coverage. This is the intent of their bill.

The commercial health insurance industry offers a middle-of-the road approach to national health insurance. Its bill, as noted in figure 16, involves a three part program including a voluntary plan for employers and employees, a plan for individuals, under which the contributors would receive tax advantages, and a state plan for the poor. The private health insurance industry administers these plans all of which provide the same benefits. One of the premises of this bill is that health care costs can be reduced by a slight alteration of the health care system, including the following changes:

● Payments of benefits are denied to facilities which are required but do not have certificate-of-need.

● The PSRO program is expanded to include all patients with the provider of health services rather than the patient paying for this review expense.

● The National Health Planning and Resources Development Act (P.L. 93-641) would be changed to provide that insurers be guaranteed representation on Health Systems Agency boards; that Health Systems Agencies be empowered to recommend the decertification of existing health care facilities, that is, be empowered to order the closing of beds or entire institutions such as hospitals which are judged to be underutilized or surplus; that federal funds be provided to finance the closing of unnecessary hospital facilities; and that ambulatory health care centers and diagnostic centers (but not physicians' offices) be subject to certificate-of-need legislation.

The latter proposals are included for the first time in the National Health Care Act of 1977. This bill was introduced in the 95th Congress by Senator Thomas J. McIntyre and Representative Omar Burleson. In addition to the latter recommendations, the health insurance industry included in its bill of the 94th Congress the following proposals:

- Approval from a health planning agency would be required before capital expenditures would be recognized for reimbursement;
- HMOs must be made available as an option to persons enrolled in the state health insurance plan;
- Grants, loans and loan guarantees are to be made available for the construction and operation of ambulatory care centers;
- Loans and grants for health students would be increased, with special provisions for shortage areas.[33]

However, the most far reaching proposal in terms of restructuring the health care delivery system is the Kennedy-Corman "Health Security" bill, as noted in figure 17. This legislation has the support of organized labor. The federal government would administer the program and finance the plan from federal general revenues and levying special taxes on earned and unearned income.[34] A special five member Health Security Board would be created within HEW and would administer the program, with 10 regional and 100 area offices being established throughout the country. Within each health service area a local Health Security office and any necessary branch offices would be set up. Based upon the previous year's expenditures plus estimated cost increases, each region would decide how much money was going to be needed for health care in the ensuing year and allot such sums among the local areas. Development grants, construction loans and payments to offset operating deficits would foster the growth of health maintenance organizations. In cooperation with state governments, HEW would also be responsible for health planning. Priority is given to the development of comprehensive care on an ambulatory basis within this new system.

The Kennedy-Corman bill also creates a Commission on the Quality of Care—a quasi-independent board reporting to the Health Security Board. This Commission would develop cost control features within the program, including national standards for health care providers. Hospitals, skilled nursing homes, home health agencies, specified free-standing centers, medical or dental foundations and health maintenance organizations can participate in the program if they meet the national standards established by the Health Security Board. For example, in order to upgrade the level of nursing home care, the Health Security program requires that facilities providing this care meet the same standards as is presently required by the Medicare program, meet the requirements of the Life Safety Code of the National Fire Protection Association, and have an affiliation with a hospital or HMO whose medical staff assumes the responsibility for professional services in the nursing home. Thus, the bill attempts to bring nursing homes into the mainstream of American medicine by having their operations affiliated with health care institutions whose medical staff will oversee the quality of the nursing home's medical services. Perhaps, at that time, books on nursing homes as by former Senator Frank Moss won't be titled *Too Old Too Sick Too Bad*. (And if you are seeking nursing home care either for yourself or a loved one, you should also check and find out if the facility meets the standards required by Medicare and set forth by the National Fire Protection Association, if for no other reason than personal health and safety.)

In addition to the previous changes, the Health Security bill calls for consumer participation at all levels of policy formulation and program development. For example, a majority of consumers would be represented on the National Advisory Council to the

Health Security Board and on regional and local councils. The membership of the councils would reflect the composition of the state and community. There would be public control of the program's basic policies and full public accountability of its finances and operations. The program would encourage consumer organizations to establish health care plans such as health maintenance organizations. The significance to the practice of medicine of consumer participation in program policy, development and administration on the national, state, and local levels cannot be distinctly discerned. But some of the negative experiences gained by physicians in their association with consumers on the boards of local Health Systems Agencies may be harbingers of events to come.

As a final example of the Health Security's restructuring of our health care system, let us look at prescription drugs. This program would establish a national drug formulary and would only pay for those drugs which are on this list. This formulary would apply to patients in a hospital or persons enrolled in a comprehensive health plan such as an HMO who receive their prescription medicines from the institution's pharmacy or a community pharmacy providing services under contract to these institutions. In addition, there is a second formulary which would apply to those prescription medicines required for chronic illness and conditions necessitating long and costly drug therapy as prescribed by physicians in private fee-for-service practice. Again, the program would only pay for those drugs ruled as being appropriate for a given illness.[35] Also, the special five member board created within HEW under this bill would be authorized under the program's regulations, with the approval of the Secretary of HEW, to furnish all professional practitioners with information concerning the safety and efficacy of drugs appearing on either formulary along with indications for their use as well as their contraindications. Thus, the Kennedy-Corman proposal would greatly alter the way medicine is practiced and financed in this country.

Physician Reimbursement

Payments for physician services under some of the national health insurance proposals will not differ very greatly from present methods, except that a physician will receive more of his income from third party payments. In the Comprehensive Health Care Insurance Act of 1977, introduced by Senator Clifford P. Hansen and Congressman Tim Lee Carter, the American Medical Association modified its concept of reimbursement as outlined in its bill of the 94th Congress. In the 1977 proposal, usual, customary, and reasonable charges was changed to specify that physician reimbursement will be based on current charges calculated at least twice a year (on January 1 and July 1). Each calculation would be based on actual charge data from the preceding 6 month period. The commercial health insurance industry would restrict the physician's payments of the 75th percentile of usual and customary charges, a method of reimbursement which is used by the Medicare program.

However, under the Kennedy-Corman bill, physician reimbursement is not only slightly more complex but also may be designed to alter the pattern of medical practice in this country. First, physicians have a choice of payment. They can be reimbursed by salary, full or part-time, through agreement with the program; or on a capitation basis for the number of persons enrolled with them to receive the mandated comprehensive care; or on a fee-for-service basis according to an established fee schedule formed after consultation with representatives of the profession. Based upon the expenditures of the previous year plus appropriate cost adjustments, the government would allocate monies to each region in the country. Each region, in turn, would allocate its sum to its local health service areas, which would reimburse the physician for his services. The budgeted per capita amount for each type of covered service would be divided between the categories of providers according to the number of individuals who elected to receive care from those providers. For example in a city of 100,000 people, 25,000 may be enrolled in health maintenance organizations. If the amount budgeted for physician services in that area is $65 per capita, the HMOs would be paid $1,625,000—or $65 x 25,000—for physician services. Since the other 75,000 individuals elected to receive care from solo-fee-for-service practitioners, the program's Health Security Board would create a fund of $4,875,000—or $65 x 75,000—to pay all fee-for-service bills submitted by physicians in the community.[36] Also, remember under this program health providers would have to agree not to charge individuals for all or part of any service provided. Payment in full would be made directly by the program to the health provider or to the agency representing him. There would be no billing of the patient or an indemnity payment to him.

What do these previous procedures mean for the physician in solo fee-for-service practice? The implications are very great. The physician who elects to be paid on a fee-for-service basis would not make any more money than the physician who elects to be paid on a capitation basis. In fact, because of the additional burden of paperwork—submitting claims for each and every service—the physician who elects fee-for-service reimbursement would have higher administrative costs. The doctors who are practicing in such delivery systems as health maintenance organizations could make more money by delegating such functions as multi-phasic screening, medical history taking, well-baby care and management of chronic disease to physician assistants, pediatric nurses and other paraprofessional personnel.[37] Also, remember it is to the advantage of the prepaid group practice plans to operate as efficiently as possible because whatever savings they may achieve from their operations may be retained by the organizations and, perhaps, increase the physician's income even more. As a physician under this Health Security program, you cannot send your fee-for-service patient a supplemental bill for all or part of the unlimited comprehensive services provided to him in order to absorb your high administrative costs. You are totally dependent upon the amount of money the program allocates to your area. Therefore, if, as a group of physicians, you all submit bills adding up to more than the total amount of money allocated to your area, as a group you would have to absorb the loss. The program would still pay you individually for your services but the payments would be reduced proportionately. The effect of this reimbursement system is very significant. As a physician you can choose to practice medicine whichever way you wish whether it be in solo-fee-for-service practice, or in health maintenance organizations, or any other manner of medical practice. You are also free to choose the way you wish to be paid. But under the fee-for-service method, your annual income may not be as high as those physicians who are on capitation payments. This is unlike present day practice where the reverse of this situation may be true. Such a situation under Health Security creates the financial incentive for physicians to practice on a capitation basis as in an HMO. It also gives HMOs a greater potential pool of medical manpower to draw upon for their development and it could, over the long term, curtail what this program perceives as the excesses of the present fee-for-service private health insurance system. In addition, the program's per capita budgeting also has another goal. Areas which are over-doctored would receive a somewhat lower budget, on a per capita basis, than under-doctored areas. Use of the budget in this manner would hopefully provide an incentive for the better geographical distribution of physicians.

Patient's Payments

As far as the patient is concerned, most of the national health insurance plans require some kind of cost sharing by the patient, whether it is paying a deductible and/or a coinsurance amount, generally on an income-related scale, prior to his becoming eligible for the program's benefits.[38] The purpose of this cost sharing is to deter the excess use of health care services. This rationale, as previously discussed, is part of our present health insurance system.

Again the one exception to the way medical care is purchased under national health insurance is the Kennedy-Corman "Health Security" plan. Here coverage is universal and mandatory. All basic benefits are immediately available without any cost sharing by the patient. This idea is also known as "first dollar coverage." The sponsors of the plan believe that deductibles and copayments have no place in a genuine national health insurance program. All benefits in the Kennedy-Corman bill are without limit, except for nursing home care, dental care, which is phased in by age, mental health services and prescription drugs. Proponents of this proposal do not believe that the lack of cost sharing devices will lead to excessive or burdensome utilization of health care services. They cite the experience of health maintenance organizations and the Canadian National Health Insurance System as the evidence for their beliefs.

Financing National Health Insurance

All the principal national health insurance bills rely in varying degrees on employer-employee contributions. Although an employer is required to offer his employees health insurance under the American Medical Association plan and has the choice to do so under the commercial health insurance bill, the employee under both plans has the choice of accepting it or not. Also, every measure would use the general revenues of the federal Treasury, mostly to finance coverage for the poor and the elderly. The American Medical Association plan, which in years past provided that everyone who purchased health insurance receive income tax credits for the purchase, now limits these credits to low-income families, the self-employed and the unemployed. The insurance industry plan allows both employers and employees to tax-deduct their premium payments. In contrast with other bills designed to subsidize basic private health insurance, the Kennedy-Corman plan stands apart from all the rest in financing national health insurance. Under the Kennedy-Corman plan, the federal government would raise and disburse all the money, one-half of the monies would come from general revenues and the other half from payroll taxes plus a special tax to be levied on unearned income and the self-employed. The sponsors of the bill believe that a key element in controlling health care quality and its costs is financing national health insurance through the creation of a Health Security Trust Fund, similar to the Social Security Trust Fund. In short, they do not want any private insurance carrier collecting the money and paying the claims.[39] In the words of Dr. I. S. Falk, professor emeritus of public health at Yale University School of Medicine and one of architects of the Health Security plan:

"Massive national experience shows that the insurance industry adds billions in cost and distorts sensible patterns of service and expenditure, while contributing little in administration and less in quality and cost control that could not be done at least as well and probably better and at lesser cost by public administration."[40]

In contrast to this opinion, many other leaders within and outside of the health care system want the private sector to have as large a role as possible within a national health insurance system to serve as a buffer between the providers of health care and the government.

Professional Standards

Earlier in this book we noted the problems of professional incompetency as it related to the practice of medicine. The national health insurance proposals address themselves to this issue as well. Most plans require the same professional standards for health service providers as presently required by the Medicare program. These Medicare standards relate to licensing, records, utilization review and other requirements. In addition, a physician's assistant in some plans must meet federal standards established by the national health insurance plan in order to treat patients. But the Kennedy-Corman bill goes a lot further than other proposals in its impact on medical practice. First, the plan will not allow hospitals to refuse staff privileges to qualified physicians. While physicians and other professionals would be eligible to participate in the program if licensed in a state before the program begins, they would have to meet continuing education requirements established by the plan in order to maintain their qualification. The continuing educational requirements would take into consideration those prerequisites issued or approved by professional organizations. Reports on compliance with these requirements would be filed. Practitioners who failed to comply could be suspended or terminated from participation in the Health Security program. If a professional is licensed after the program begins, he would attain eligibility by meeting its national standards. If he meets these standards, the professional would then be qualified to practice in any state, in addition to the jurisdiction where he received his license. Finally, if a health provider renders services in a hospital not participating in the program, then the program would not pay for his services. Hence, it would be to his financial advantage to use institutions certified by the Health Security plan. This situation places pressure on nonqualified institutions to meet the program's standards if they want to attract physicians to their staff and patients to their beds.

A great amount of discussion is underway concerning the amount of unnecessary surgery taking place in this country. In October 1976, a Harvard University study reported that too many operations are being performed by doctors who are not specialists in surgery, while at the same time the nation's surgeons do not have enough work to keep them busy. According to *The New England Journal of Medicine,* a review of 285,000 operations performed by 2,700 physicians in four metropolitan areas across the country revealed that the average workload of surgical specialists was modest compared to what they could handle. On the other hand, general practitioners were performing operations whose relative volume was small. Among the procedures were appendectomies, tonsillectomies and obstetrical deliveries.[41] The Kennedy-Corman bill also deals with this issue. First, the program only pays for major surgery and other specialized services designated by the plan's regulations. The services must be performed by a specialist upon referral by a physician in general or family practice. Certain kinds of surgery as specified by the program's regulations would require prior consultation and approval by other specialists. For these specified types of surgery, the program's regulations could also require the submission of a pathology report and clinical abstract or discharge report. If the surgery is not approved under these provisions, then the program would not cover the costs of hospital care and other services related to the surgery. Except for the requirement of a clinical report, the previous standards would not apply in the case of emergency services. For these requirements, a physician would be considered a specialist if he is board certified or board eligible; meets specified standards established by regulation; and where appropriate, is recommended by a hospital participating in the program.[42]

These requirements are not solely significant because they are attempting to improve the quality of surgical services while concurrently reducing the number of unnecessary procedures. The regulations are also meaningful because they demonstrate that social planners are well aware of the problems existing in the practice of medicine. The surgical regulations were written long before the Congress addressed itself to the unnecessary surgery question in 1976 and before Harvard University made public the findings of its surgical study the same year. Thus, the social planners are writing regulations into law through official government programs to correct the deficiencies in medical practice which organized medicine either cannot or will not correct itself. If the surgical practice regulations are considered a precedent of government interference in the doctor-patient relationship, then the question arises as to what other medical specialities have problems requiring government resolution when the specialty cannot solve these problems on its own initiative. It is not the inference of these comments that government regulations, as in the case of surgical services, will necessarily result in lower quality medical services. Obviously, in view of the Harvard University findings, greater controls on qualifications are needed in the medical field for those who perform surgical procedures. The Kennedy-Corman bill seeks to strengthen and upgrade the quality of such surgical services in this country. But that is not the entire issue.

The point to be stressed is that such government regulations might not be necessary at all if organized medicine itself effectively prevented physicians from deliverying services for which they are not qualified. This is the significance of the Kennedy-Corman surgical provision. This is one of the reasons why government is entering the doctor-patient relationship. If organized medicine cannot effectively control the competency of physicians who deliver various services and if government, as a representative of the public, also will not do so—as some of government's critics advocate—then who will look out for the public's welfare? Who has the authority of law to perform this task? Who is left to do so?

The Politics

In view of this brief review of the kinds of national health insurance proposals which have been introduced in the Congress, let us return to one of the questions posed earlier in this discussion. Does President Carter's call for a universal, mandatory and comprehensive benefit system, including preventive care services, financed by a combination of employer-employee payroll taxes and general revenues with built-in cost and quality controls sound like any specific proposal introduced thus far into Congress? Does the statement, mentioned earlier, by Hale Champion, HEW Undersecretary, that our proposal must lead to a significant restructuring of the way care is delivered and must change the perverse incentives now at work sound like any proposal introduced into the 95th Congress? The answer is yes. It sounds like many of the elements in the Kennedy-Corman bill which stresses these principles. It could also sound like any other national health insurance bill which might be introduced at some later date and meet these criteria. Remember, the American Medical Association plan is simply a financing mechanism while the commercial health insurance plan is not mandatory. Also, the cost control mechanisms incorporated in the commercial health insurance industry's bills are not as extensive as that of the Kennedy-Corman legislation. Also, be mindful that the

Kennedy-Corman program has the support of organized labor. But just as organized labor can generate considerable financial and political power in the election arena, it can also generate powerful opposition in the Congress to the legislative reforms it seeks to enact. To some, therefore, there were no surprises when HEW Secretary, Joseph A. Califano, Jr., announced on July 29, 1978 the *Principles* upon which the Carter Administration will develop a national health insurance plan for submission to Congress (see figure 18). According to Secretary Califano, the aim of the program, in eventually providing universal and comprehensive coverage, is to obtain the broadest possible congressional support, protect the general economy and not increase inflation. In not supporting the Carter approach, Senator Edward M. Kennedy, organized labor and other allied groups claimed the *Principles* were too vague, too cautious, the plan's implementation was too fragmented and subject to conditions of the economy, and was not a complete and single program which could be phased-in over time. In view of these sharp political differences, the Carter plan will become but one of the alternatives which Congress will consider along with bills sponsored by such other groups as Senator Kennedy and organized labor, the American Medical Association and the private health insurance industry. However, one point should be stressed. Given the diversity in political philosophies of those concerned with the national health insurance issue, together with the political compromises and pressures attending the writing of a law, it is not unusual to observe that a law eventually enacted is not always the same as the original bill. However, even a compromise bill becoming law can contain some of the philosophy and provisions of the original legislation. For this reason, it is advantageous to be aware of and understand the meaning of the various provisions of all the proposed national health insurance bills.

Conclusion

For the past several years national health insurance has appeared to be more of a dream than a coming reality, despite the number of bills introduced into Congress advocating the establishment of such a system. Of course, with the election of Jimmy Carter as President of the United States, national health insurance is, once more, a viable possibility. This is especially true since the Democratic platform upon which President Carter campaigned called for its enactment. The social and economic conditions which exist in this country will, of course, determine whether this promise becomes a law, and if so, the kind of program and the degree of involvement government and the private sector of society will have in such a plan. Health authorities say that certain conditions must continue to exist for government to have greater control over the health care system than it has at present (and to which many groups and organizations may not be willing to accede.) They state that as long as:

- The costs of medical care continue to outsoar the Consumer Price Index;
- Physicians become more and more the targets of public and Congressional criticism;
- Medicaid problems worsen instead of improve;
- Public complaints against the high costs of medical care intensifies;
- Congress reacts with more and more investigations into the abuses of the system by those who provide the health services;
- Business believes that the health insurance which it purchases does not adequately cover health care services due to rising costs and as long as the health insurance contributions on behalf of its employees reduce its own profit margins;

then the convergence of all these aforementioned forces may impel Congress to enact a program which, it believes, will ameliorate the conditions about which the public, big business and labor are most vocal, namely, the high costs of paying for ill health. And the public may not be too discriminating as to the methods used to accomplish this task, as long as its own personal pocket book is helped by such a measure and the medical costs which it must bear are controlled, if not reduced, over time. Even Robert D. Kilpatrick, president of Connecticut General Insurance Company has had to admit:

"If the private sector cannot show that it is able to control these rapidly rising costs, business managements, unions, and everyone else concerned may well throw in the towel and seek a government takeover out of despair."[43]

Thus, social planners in the interest of national health insurance may have to reorder the approach of the health care field, including that of organized medicine, assign new roles and develop new kinds of organizations for delivery the highest quality of care at reasonable costs.

Our discussion of national health insurance has given us a small glimpse of our future health care system. If a single characteristic may describe its central feature, it would be, perhaps, the word *control*. If we examine the debates which are taking place today whether they be concerned with the kind of measures which must be enacted prior to the establishment of a national health insurance system or the kind of measures which such a program should embrace, these measures are controls. They regulate the quality of care which is delivered and the costs of such care to the patient. These measures may be the mandatory revenue ceilings which the Carter Administration wishes to impose on the hospital industry or the voluntary controls which the industry wishes to impose upon itself—but nonetheless they are controls. They may be the certificate-of-need laws which apply to hospitals or health maintenance organizations, but still they are controls. They may be the use of public funds to induce physicians financially to practice in underdoctored areas in this country and to leave areas of a physician surplus, but nevertheless they are controls. They may be the development of state hospital commissions through the present planning law or through a proposed national health insurance system, but these bodies are still systems of controls. They may be formulas of prospective reimbursement to health care providers, but they are nonetheless methods of control. They may be participation requirements in a national health plan that nursing homes must have hospital affiliations, and that the hospital medical staff oversee the quality of care delivered in these nursing facilities, but they are a system of control. They may be standards for performing surgical or other medical procedures, but nonetheless they are an order of controls.

To be sure there will be new kinds of delivery systems developed in the future whether they be called health maintenance organizations, or ambulatory care centers or other innovative mechanisms which have yet to be devised. Also, allied health professionals will assume more responsibility in assisting in the delivery of health care services and be paid for their services whether they be nurse practitioners or physician's assistants. But the underlying tenet of our health care system as it evolves in the future will be controls whether they be by state government, or the federal government, or a combination of both. Thus far, voluntary controls over the costs of health care or even monitoring the quality of care of those who deliver such services have not been very successful in the view of those who advocate controls. Perhaps, the industry can achieve such success if it feels its operations are sufficiently threatened by government intervention. Usually, the cliché, "only time will tell," could be used as a concluding point but as we have seen in our discussions of national health insurance and the politics involved, there may not be too much time left from a practical viewpoint. The concept of public controls over the health care industry may not as yet affect the entire American population in terms of the costs or quality of care they receive or all the health providers in terms of the kinds and costs of services which they deliver, but the concept certainly has begun to affect some. And this impact is more than likely to expand rather than contract in future years if recent political history in the health care field is any criterion by which to make such a judgement. It was only in 1972 that Professional Standards Review Organizations were enacted into law, followed by the Health Maintenance Organization Act in 1973, still followed by a new comprehensive health planning law in 1974, and still followed by a new health manpower act in 1976. The pace is beginning to quicken and the pieces for solving various aspects of the health care puzzle are falling into place. They are part of the revolution which is sweeping this country. It is a revolution to bring about social change so as to achieve the premise that health care is a right and not a privilege. Forty years after national health insurance proposals were introduced into Congress during the 1930s, this mechanism has again been chosen as the possible panacea for bridling our nation's health care problems and for bringing them under control in some kind of orderly and organized manner. It is only a matter of time before such a program is enacted into law. Whether or not it will be the ultimate answer to our nation's ills, only history will be the ultimate judge. But one point is for certain—there are now many powerful forces in our society who now believe it to be true.

Figure 13
THE CATASTROPHIC HEALTH INSURANCE AND MEDICAL ASSISTANCE REFORM ACT,
Introduced by Senators Russell B. Long and Abraham A. Ribicoff and by Representative Joe D. Waggonner
(Catastrophic Illness Approach)

Subject	Provisions		
General concept and approach	Proposal includes (1) a catastrophic illness insurance program for the general population provided through a federally administered plan or alternatively under approved private plans and (2) a Federal medical assistance program for the poor and medically indigent. Also includes provisions for Federal certification of qualified private basic health insurance.		
	Catastrophic insurance		**Medical Assistance Plan**
	Government plan	Private plans	
Coverage of the population	All U.S. residents, except persons under private plans.	Employees (and their families) of employers who voluntarily elect private plan. Self-employed who voluntarily elect.	Without regard to age or employment, low-income families and families qualifying under "spend-down" provisions.
Benefit structure	After person spends 60 days in the hospital, following benefits become available: Additional hospital days, skilled nursing facility (100-day limit), and home health services. After family spends $2,000 on medical expenses, following benefits become available to all members of family: Physicians services, laboratory and X-ray, home health services, medical supplies and appliances. No limit on amount of services (except SNF) and no cost sharing.		No limits on services and no cost sharing except as indicated: Institutional services: Hospital (60 days), skilled nursing and intermediate care facilities. Personal services: Physicians ($3 a visit for first 10 visits), laboratory and X-ray, family planning, maternity, and exams for children. Other: Medical supplies and appliances.
Administration	Similar to Medicare program.	Employers and self-employed purchase approved private insurance from approved carriers. DHEW supervises program.	Similar to Medicare program.
Relationship to other Government programs	Catastrophic benefits payable without regard to coverage under other government programs or private plans. Medical assistance benefits secondary to all other programs and plans. Medicare program continues and Medicaid abolished.		
Financing	Payroll tax of 1% on employers, including Federal, State, and local governments; employers allowed a credit against their Federal income tax of 50% of the tax. Similar provisions for self-employed.	Employers are subject to regular 1% payroll tax, but this tax is reduced by the actuarial value of their private coverage; also receives the 50% tax credit. Similar provisions for self-employed.	Financed by Federal and State general revenues. State share is fixed annual amount based on State cost under Medicaid for types of services under new program, with some additions and subtractions.
Standards for providers of services	Same as Medicare.		
Reimbursement of providers of services	Same as Medicare.	Determined by carrier.	Same as Medicare, but physicians must accept plan's payment as payment in full.
Delivery and resources	Government catastrophic program and medical assistance plan incorporate HMO and PSRO provisions now applicable to Medicare.		
Encouragement of basic insurance	Under provisions designed to encourage improved basic health insurance, DHEW would certify private policies meeting specified standards (including coverage of 60 hospital days and first $2,000 in medical services). States would arrange marketing of this insurance through pools and reinsurance arrangements. DHEW would offer certified insurance in States where not available.		

Source: U.S. Department of Health, Education, and Welfare, "National Health Insurance Proposals: Provisions of Bills Introduced in 94th Congress as of February, 1976", Social Security Administration, Washington, D.C., March, 1976, p. 19.

Figure 14

THE NATIONAL HEALTH CARE SERVICES REORGANIZATION AND FINANCING ACT,
Introduced by Representative Al Ullman
(Mixed Public and Private Approach)

Subject	Provisions	
General concept and approach	A 3-part program including: (1) a plan requiring employers to provide private coverage for employees, (2) a plan for individuals, and (3) federally contracted coverage for the poor and aged. State establishes a health care plan, supervises carriers and insurers, and promotes a system of health care corporations (HCC). Supported by American Hospital Association.	
	Private plans	Plan for low income and aged
Coverage of the population	Employees of employers under social security and of State and local governments. Also, individuals who elect coverage.	Low-income and medically indigent families, and aged persons.

Benefit structure	Benefits phased in over 5-year period. Final benefits:
	  Institutional services:
	    Hospital: 90 days, $5 copayment per day.
	    Skilled nursing facility: 30 days, $2.50 copayment per day.
	    Nursing home: 90 days, $2.50 copayment per day.
	  Personal services:
	    Physicians: 10 visits per year, $2 copayment per visit.
	    Laboratory and X-ray: 20 percent coinsurance.
	    Home health services: 200 visits per year, $2 copayment per visit.
	    Dental services: Children age 7-12: 1 exam per year, other services, 20 percent coinsurance.
	  Other services and supplies:
	    Prescription drugs: Limited to specified conditions, $1. per prescription.
	    Medical equipment and appliances and ambulance service: 20 percent coinsurance.
	    Eyeglasses: Children to age 12, 1 set per year, 20 percent coinsurance.
	  Catastrophic coverage: Payable when certain noncovered expenses reach a specified limit, which varies by family income and age; would remove the cost sharing on all benefits and the limitation on number of hospital days and physicians' visits.	

Administration	Administered by private insurance carriers under State supervision, according to Federal guidelines.	Federal Government would contract with private insurance carriers who issue policies to eligible persons.
Relationship to other Government programs	Medicare: Abolished. Medicaid and other assistance programs: Would not pay for covered services. Other programs: Mostly not affected.	
Financing	Employee-employer premium payments, with employer paying at least 75 percent. Federal subsidy of premium for low-income workers and certain small employers, and 10 percent subsidy for HCC enrollees. Individuals pay own premium.	Financed in part by premium payments by medically indigent, but with no premium for lowest income group. Balance of cost financed by Federal general revenues and the payroll taxes of the present Medicare program.
Standards for providers of services	All institutions and HCC's must meet Medicare standards. Skilled nursing facilities must be under supervision of a hospital medical staff or have its own organized staff. Use of paramedical personnel must meet Federal standards. All providers and HCC's must establish systems of peer review, medical audit and other procedures to meet Federal-State requirements on quality and utilization of services.	
Reimbursement of providers of services	Institutions and HCC's: State commission would establish prospective payment methods and review proposed charges. Physicians and other professionals: Reasonable fee, salaries, or other compensation, as approved by State commission.	
Delivery and resources	State health commission: Establishes a State health plan, including provisions for regulation of providers and insurance carriers. Takes responsibility for health planning and must approve, in advance, proposed capital expenditures of providers. Health care corporations: State commissions would incorporate system of HCC's, approved to operate in designated geographical areas. HCC must furnish all covered services through its own facilities or affiliated providers (and permit all qualified practitioners to furnish services for it). Would be required to hold open enrollment for public and eventually offer services on a capitation basis. Federal grants provided for HCC's for planning, development, outpatient centers, medical and data equipment, and to cover initial operating deficits.	

Source: U.S. Department of Health, Education, and Welfare, "National Health Insurance Proposals: Provisions of Bills Introduced in 94th Congress as of February, 1976", Social Security Administration, Washington, D.C., March, 1976, p. 4.

Figure 15
COMPREHENSIVE HEALTH INSURANCE ACT OF 1975,
Introduced by Representative Richard H. Fulton
(Tax Credit Approach)

Subject	Provisions	
General concept and approach	A 2-part plan including (1) a plan requiring employers to offer private health insurance to employees and (2) a plan making available private insurance for the nonemployed and self-employed, with Federal subsidies of the premium provided through tax credits or subsidy certificates. Supported by American Medical Association.	
	Employee plan	**Plan for nonemployed and self-employed**
Coverage of the population	Full-time employees of private employers and of Federal, State, and local governments (including persons under Medicare) and workers receiving unemployment insurance.	Low-income families, self-employed, and all others not under an employee plan (including persons under Medicare).
Benefit structure	No limits on benefits, except where indicated: Institutional services: 　Hospital inpatient and outpatient. 　Skilled nursing facilities: 100 days. Personal services: 　Physicians services. 　Dental care: Initially for children age 2-6, later extended to age 17. 　Home health services. 　Laboratory and X-ray. 　Health exams, maternity care, and well-child care. Other services and supplies: 　Medical supplies and equipment. 　Cost sharing: 20% coinsurance, with maximum limit of $1,500 for individuals and $2,000 for families; cost sharing reduced or eliminated for low-income and unemployed families. Medicare beneficiaries: Same benefit coverage, but policy excludes the benefits provided by Medicare.	
Administration	Insurance provided through private carriers, supervised by the States under regulations issued by a new Federal board.	
	Employers purchase insurance from carriers.	Family purchases insurance from carriers.
Relationship to other Government programs	Medicare: Continues to operate. Medicaid: Would not pay for covered services.	
Financing	Employee-employer premium payments, with employer paying at least 65% of cost. Special maximum limit on amount of premium costs for small employers. Federal subsidies for all employers with large increases in payroll costs. Premium for unemployed persons paid by Federal Government.	Federal subsidy of premium ranging from 100% to 10% of premium costs, varied according to annual tax payment of family; this subsidy is taken as income tax credit or by obtaining a subsidy certificate from DHEW. State insurance pools established to assure coverage.
Standards for providers of services	Standards could be issued by a new Federal board.	
Reimbursement of providers of services	Hospitals: Reimbursement determined by State governments, based on prospective payment or other methods. Physicians: Payment on basis of usual and customary or reasonable charges.	
Delivery and resources	Studies to be conducted by new Federal board.	

Source: U.S. Department of Health, Education, and Welfare, "National Health Insurance Proposals: Provisions of Bills Introduced in 94th Congress as of February, 1976", Social Security Administration, Washington, D.C., March, 1976, p. 14.

Figure 16

THE NATIONAL HEALTH CARE ACT OF 1975,
Introduced by Representative Omar Burleson and Senator Thomas J. McIntyre
(Mainly Public and Private Approach)

Subject	Provisions	
General concept and approach	A 3-part plan including a voluntary employee-employer plan and a plan for individuals, under which contributors would receive tax advantages, and a State plan for the poor. All plans administered through private insurance carriers and provide same benefits. Supported by the Health Insurance Association of America.	
	Private plans	**State plan**
Coverage of the population	Employee-employer plan includes employees (and their families) of employers who voluntarily elect a qualified plan. Individual plan includes persons who voluntarily elect.	Low-income families.

Benefit structure	Benefits phased-in over a 8-year period, final benefits as follows:
	Deductible of $100 per person and 20% coinsurance, except where noted.
	  Institutional services:
	    Hospital.
	    Skilled nursing facility: 180 days.
	  Personal services:
	    Physicians.
	    Dentists.
	    Home health services: 270 days.
	    Laboratory and X-ray: No cost sharing.
	    Health exams and family planning. Well-child care with no cost sharing.
	  Other services and supplies:
	    Medical appliances.
	    Eyeglasses.
	    Prescription drugs.	

	Annual limit for all cost sharing of $1,000 per family.	Reduced cost sharing and family maximum, according to family income.
Administration	Insurance administered by private carriers under State supervision. Treasury Department determines tax status of plan.	Insurance administered by private carriers under agreement with the State. Regulations for program established by DHEW.
Relationship to other Government programs	Medicare: Continues to operate. Medicaid and other assistance programs: Other programs: Most not affected.	Would not pay for services under these programs.
Financing	For employee-employer plan, premium paid by employers and employees, as arranged between them, but contributions of low-income workers limited according to their wage level. For individual plan, policyholder pays entire premium. Employees and individuals who itemize deductions can take entire premium as deduction on income tax return.1/ Employers can take their entire premium as normal business deduction as under present law (but contributions to nonqualified plans would not be deductible).	No premium required for lowest income group; for others, premium paid by enrollees, varying according to family income. Federal and State governments pay balance of costs from their general revenues, with Federal share 70 to 90 percent, depending on State per capita income.
Standards for providers of services	Same as Medicare.	
Reimbursement of providers of services	Hospitals and other institutions: Prospectively approved rates for various categories of institutions. Hospitals prepare budgets and schedule of charges which are reviewed by a State commission which approves or disapproves charges, subject to DHEW review of rate levels. Physicians and dentists: Reasonable charges, based on customary and prevailing rates.	
Delivery and resources	Health planning: Planning agency approval required for capital expenditures to be recognized for reimbursement. Health maintenance organizations: Must be made available as an option to persons enrolled in State plan. Ambulatory health centers: Grants, loans, and loan guarantees for construction and operation of centers. Health manpower: Increases loans and grants for students, with special provisions for shortage areas.	

1/ Under present law, deduction of premium is limited to one-half the premium cost up to a maximum of $150.

Source: U.S. Department of Health, Education, and Welfare, "National Health Insurance Proposals: Provisions of Bills Introduced in 94th Congress as of February, 1976", Social Security Administration, Washington, D.C., March, 1976, p. 5.

Figure 17

THE HEALTH SECURITY ACT,
Introduced by Representative James C. Corman and Senator Edward M. Kennedy
(Mainly Public Approach)

Subject	Provisions
General concept and approach	A program administered by Federal Government and financed by special taxes on earned and unearned income and by Federal general revenues. Supported by Committee for National Health Insurance and AFL-CIO.
Coverage of the population	All U.S. residents.
Benefit structure	Benefits with no limitations, except as noted. No cost sharing by patient. Institutional services: Hospital. Skilled nursing facility: 120 days. Personal services: Physicians. Dentists: For children under age 15; scheduled extension to age 25; eventually to entire population. Home health services. Other health professionals. Laboratory and X-ray. Other services and supplies: Medical appliances and ambulance services. Eyeglasses and hearing aids. Prescription drugs needed for chronic illness and other specified diseases.
Administration	Federal Government: Special board in DHEW, with regional and local offices to operate program.
Relationship to other Government programs	Medicare: Abolished. Medicaid and other assistance programs: Would not pay for covered services. Other programs: Most not affected.
Financing	Special taxes: On payroll (1.0% for employees and 2.5% for employers), self-employment income (2.5%) and unearned income (1.0%) Income subject to tax: Amount equal to 150% of earning base under social security (i.e., $22,950 in 1976). Employment subject to tax: Workers under social security and Federal, State, and local government employment. Federal general revenues: Equal to amount received from special taxes.
Standards for providers of services	Same as Medicare, but with additional requirements: Hospitals cannot refuse staff privileges to qualified physicians. Skilled nursing facilities must be affiliated with hospital which would take responsibility for quality of medical services in home. Physicians must meet national standards; major surgery performed only by qualified specialists. All providers: Records subject to review by regional office. Can be directed to add or reduce services and to provide services in a new location.
Reimbursement of providers of services	National health budget established and funds allocated, by type of medical services, to regions and local areas. Hospitals and nursing homes: Annual predetermined budget, based on reasonable cost. Physicians, dentists, and other professionals: Methods available are fee-for-service based on fee schedule, per capita payment for persons enrolled, and (by agreement) full- or part-time salary. Payments for fee-for-service may be reduced if payments exceed allocation. Health maintenance organizations: Per capita payment for all services (or budget for institutional services). Can retain all or part of savings.
Delivery and resources	Health planning: DHEW responsible for health planning, in cooperation with State planning agencies. Priority to be given to development of comprehensive care on ambulatory basis. Health resources development fund: Will receive, ultimately, 5 percent of total income of program, to be used for improving delivery of health care and increasing health resources. Health maintenance organizations: Grants for development, loans for construction, and payments to offset operating deficits. Manpower training: Grants to schools and allowances to students for training of physicians for general practice and shortage specialties, other health occupations, and development of new kinds of health personnel. Personal care services: Demonstration projects to provide personal care in the home, including homemaker, laundry, meals-on-wheels, transportation, and shopping services.

Source: U.S. Department of Health, Education, and Welfare, "National Health Insurance Proposals: Provisions of Bills Introduced in 94th Congress as of February, 1976", Social Security Administration, Washington, D.C., March, 1976, p. 10.

Figure 18

────── **PRINCIPLES OF PRESIDENT CARTER'S** ──────
NATIONAL HEALTH INSURANCE PLAN
JULY 29, 1978

● The plan should assure that all Americans have comprehensive health care coverage, including protection against catastrophic medical expenses.

● The plan should make quality health care available to all Americans. It should seek to eliminate those aspects of the current health system that often cause the poor to receive substandard care.

● The plan should assure that all Americans have freedom of choice in the selection of physicians, hospitals, and health delivery systems.

● The plan must support our efforts to control inflation in the economy by reducing unnecessary health care spending. The plan should include aggressive cost containment measures and should also strengthen competitive forces in the health care sector.

● The plan should be designed so that additional public and private expenditures for improved health benefits and coverage will be substantially offset by savings from greater efficiency in the health care system.

● The plan will involve no additional federal spending until FY 1983, because of tight fiscal constraints and the need for careful planning and implementation. Thereafter, the plan should be phased in gradually. As the plan moves from phase to phase, consideration should be given to such factors as the economic and administrative experience under prior phases. The experience of other government programs, in which expenditures far exceeded initial projections, must not be repeated.

● The plan should be financed through multiple sources, including government funding and contributions from employers and employees. Careful consideration should be given to the other demands on government budgets, the existing tax burdens on the American people, and the ability of many consumers to share a moderate portion of the cost of their care.

● The plan should include a significant role for the private insurance industry, with appropriate government regulation.

● The plan should provide resources and develop payment methods to promote such major reforms in delivering health care services as substantially increasing the availability of ambulatory and preventive services, attracting personnel to underserved rural and urban areas, and encouraging the use of prepaid health plans.

● The plan should assure consumer representation throughout its operation.

Source: The White House, Washington, D.C., July 29, 1978. A directive issued by President Jimmy Carter to Joseph A. Califano, Jr., Secretary of Health, Education, and Welfare.

CHAPTER 9

A Final Word:
Gulliver Travels to America

A FINAL CHAPTER SHOULD IDEALLY tie together all the preceding loose strands and thoughts into a neat package and lucidly point out to the reader the happy or unhappy denouement. But this book does not really have a definitive conclusion for the issues are still evolving as you read these words.

The central questions in today's health care crisis concern the fate of the American physician. Will the physician survive all the political, social and economic pressures which he presently faces? Will he continue to practice the kind of medicine he has in years past, in the same manner and with the same freedoms he has always enjoyed? Or, will his manner of medical practice, the patient's medical treatment and the system through which the doctor delivers his care, be changed forever by elements—both public and private—operating outside of the medical profession? These questions raised at the beginning of this book are certainly pertinent at its end.

When the physician takes the oath of Hippocrates upon graduation from medical school he swears, in part, that *"according to my ability and judgement I will keep this oath and stipulation that:*

"I will follow that system of regimen which according to my ability and judgement I consider for the benefit of my patients."

But, how many physicians today practice "defensive medicine" by ordering treatments not required by the patient in order to protect themselves against the possibility of medical malpractice lawsuits?

"I will not cut persons laboring under the stone but I will leave this to be done by men who are practitioners of the work.

But, how many physicians perform procedures today for which they are not qualified?

"Into whatever houses I enter, I will go into them for the benefit of the sick."

But, where are the house calls of yesterday?

"And [I] will abstain from every voluntary act of mischief and corruption."

But, how many doctors are defrauding and abusing public programs?

"Whatever in connection with professional practice or not in connection with it, I see or hear in the life of men which ought not to be spoken of abroad, I will not divulge as reckoning that all such should be kept secret."

But, is the confidentiality of the patient-physician relationship threatened by public programs such as PSROs?

"While I continue to keep this oath unviolated, may it be granted to me to enjoy life and the practice of the art, respected by all men in all times. But should I trespass and violate this oath, may the reverse be my lot."

Are we now observing, "the reverse of the physician's lot?" Has the public indeed lost its respect for the American physician? The violations of the ideals of Hippocrates bear witness to the crisis in health care today.

The theme of this book originated a long time ago in Jonathan Swift's ageless work, *Gulliver's Travels*. As you may recall, Gulliver, in one part of his travels, is captured by the miniature Lilliputians. While lying on the ground, his captors swarm all over him, entwining and tying down his body with a multitude of strings. The American physician can be likened to Gulliver—a giant among those who provide health services to the 218 million Lilluputians in American society. The physician is the Gulliver, or giant, of the health care field because around his decisions such entities as corporations, institutions, and allied health personnel exist and depend. The Lilliputians are analogous to the patient population, expressing their displeasure of the physician through the strings of government—or laws.

But Jonathan Swift wrote fiction and by the stroke of his pen he could free Gulliver from his bonds and his captors. The American physician is not so lucky. No author writes his script. The ties that bind are legal ones with which the body politic is immobilizing him. The physician's world is real, not fiction. What strings are we talking about? Many of these already have been discussed:

- *Drug programs* and *laws* named *Maximum Allowable Cost* and *antisubstitution;*
- *Professional Standards Review Organizations* which watch and examine his manner of medical practice;
- *Health Maintenance Organizations* which try to encourage the physician to enter into and practice with a prepaid group practice;
- *Health planning laws* which will affect the institutions in which the physician treats his patients;
- *Medical malpractice laws* which affect his legal protection and, ultimately, the way the physician practices medicine;
- And, of course, the never ending spectre and anticipation of the biggest string of all, *national health insurance* and all its unknown implications for medical practice in this country.

If one conclusion is clear, it is that our American "Gulliver" must use the courts to free himself from the binding legal strings. As long as the courts uphold the laws and rulings tying him up, medicine, as we have known it, will never be the same again. In this latter sense the physician will not survive. The facts that:

- the federal government legislates physicians to have minority representation on the boards of health agencies which plan a community's health facilities;
- government threatens physicians with even more stringent review programs if PSROs are not successful in achieving their goals;

- the American Bar Association does not endorse policy recommendations which might alleviate the medical malpractice crisis;
- government must establish through law harsh penalties for physicians and other health providers who defraud public medical programs;
- President Jimmy Carter denounces the American Medical Association as being the major obstacle to better health care in this country;
- allegations of professional incompetency, unnecessary surgery, overprescribing of drugs and other accusations of medical malpractice are being made in public forums against the physician;

and more, are all omens that the physician's customary climate of practice is now threatened with extinction. Again, in this sense, the physician will not survive. Of course, there will always be physicians to practice medicine, but not in the manner they have always known. Margaret Mitchell described it best when she wrote of the changes war brought to the social, economic and political climate of the Old South. In every sense, the same description applies to the social, economic and political war in which the physician is engaged. What happened to the Order of the Old South is descriptive of what happened to the Old Order in which the physician has practiced medicine. In Margaret Mitchell's words, *Gone With The Wind*.

As previously indicated, American medicine is in the throes of a revolution. It is a revolution bringing about profound and lasting changes in the way the physician is publicly perceived and privately practices. Although some of the programs are still in their embryonic stage of development and some of the concepts, such as national health insurance, are still unborn as legal entities, all the signs point to at least one serious conclusion. It is the possibility that American medicine one day will *not* be regarded as a profession but rather as a business trade or regulated public utility as other U. S. businesses are regarded. This is especially true in view of the Federal Trade Commission investigations into organized medicine and the ramifications which may emanate from its findings. A glimpse into medicine's future may have been provided in May 1978 when the

Federal Trade Commission approved new rules permitting the advertising of prices and other information pertaining to eyeglasses, contact lenses and eye examinations. One of the major provisions of the ruling requires consumers to have copies of their prescriptions so that they can shop and compare the prices and quality of eyeglasses and lenses. Since opthalmologists are affected by the ruling, then the precedent may have been established to broaden these requirements to other forms of medical practice. In addition, the Carter Administration, a year earlier, proposed that Congress enact legislation permitting the federal government to limit the increase in hospital income from one year to the next from all sources— Medicare, Blue Cross, commercial insurers and individuals. An annual figure of 1½ times the inflation rate, or 9 percent, for 1978 was initially suggested. In view of the federal government's active role in promoting cost containment and competition among health providers, what is to prevent government from recommending legislation to regulate increases in physician fees as well? While the latter proposition is a serious possibility, the changes occurring in a physician's prescribing habits is an everyday reality. State governments, in ever increasing numbers, are repealing their antisubstitution drug laws and more prescription medicines are coming under the aegis of the federal government's Maximum Allowable Cost drug program. Even the very operation of the physician's private office at some future point may be subject to the controls and legal authority of Health Systems Agencies (if the legal precedent for governing physician offices under the certificate-of-need law in Hawaii is any indication of events to come). While subject to the legal controls of non-physician authority, a physician's manner of prescribing therapy will come under the ever increasing scrutiny of his physician peers. Perhaps, physician reviews by Professional Standards Review Organizations one day will include a doctor's entire patient population rather than just those qualifying for Medicare, Medicaid and child health programs. And as his manner of medical practice comes under the increasing review of his professional peers, the physician's private fee-for-service practice may become more circumscribed. This may be especially true as new delivery systems, such as health maintenance organizations, grow in number and through competition enroll some of the patient population (as predicted in the case of Medicare and Medicaid beneficiaries qualifying for such programs). The situation is analogous to the independent "mom and pop" grocery store which could not compete successfully with the new chainstore supermarket down the block.

These are some, but not all, of the mini-revolutions taking place or beginning to occur in medicine today. However, their implications are not as yet clearly discernable. The guidelines from such national programs as health planning are just beginning to appear on the national scene and no one can foretell with certainty what kind of impact investigations by government will have upon the medical profession. But when these mini-revolutions are examined as a totality, they represent a significant revolution bringing about dramatic changes in American medical practice and health care service delivery. Such is the nature of today's crisis in American medicine. It is a social, economic, and political revolution.

Although the preceding discussion centered on the physician, these laws also apply to other elements in the health field as well such as hospitals, HMOs and the pharmaceutical industry. Hopefully, if the laws are applied in a judicious and equitable manner to all they concern, they will be able to check the runaway increases in the costs of health care. So far, the cost issue has eluded voluntary solution, although the hospital industry in 1977 did embark upon a voluntary program to hold down the rise of institutional charges. However, the cost problem did not elude the attention of the federal government when it instituted, for a short period during the early 1970s, price controls over the health care field and held down price increases by administrative fiat from Washington, D. C. But placing controls over prices did not deter physicians in California from getting around the program and increasing, for example, the costs of the Medicare program from 1972-1975. According to a study of the Urban

Institute in Washington, D. C., 5,000 California physicians, unable to raise their charges because of the federal Economic Stabilization Program, sharply expanded the quantity of services to Medicare patients. When the price controls were removed, the increase in services fell off.[1] Thus, despite the imposition of wage and price controls, ways can be found to avoid them and increase personal income by other means. Whether or not the rise in services to Medicare patients would have occurred if Professional Standards Review Organizations existed to review the necessity of such treatments as well as their payments is not known. PSROs were not functional entities during that period. But this illustration does demonstrate why government believes it must enact programs to contain health care costs because the physician does not appear to be restraining himself in holding down such expenditures. Consequently, while many may hope that various laws will lead to a reduction in health costs in the future, that day does not appear to be imminent.

Attempting to control health care prices is a cost-benefit experience—a benefit to one group and a cost to another. For example, a two year study of PSRO activity in New Mexico, as reported in October 1976, found that the physicians gave 60 percent fewer injections to patients when their treatment was monitored by their physician peer group. This is good for the patient and his medical bill, which did not contain needless drug charges, but bad for the company making the injectionable drug product which was not used.[2] But, this is what free enterprise is supposed to be all about. One group's gain is another group's loss and the public's well-being should be the ultimate focus for all segments of the health care field. Unfortunately for the public, health care is one of the few market places where the consumer has very little choice as to whether or not he wishes to purchase its services.[3] An individual can forgo many products in an economy without having the self-denial affect the state of his personal welfare since alternative products and services exist. Thus, if a consumer cannot afford a new automobile, there are used autos, auto rental agencies, public transportation, bicycles or other modes of transportation. If an individual cannot afford certain kinds of foods, there are alternatives which may be cheaper and equally nutritious. However, in the instance of ill health, there is no generally no choice. If a consumer does not wish to use the products or the services of those health providers who may help him recover, then he must either depend upon the healing processes of nature or become, perhaps, even fatally ill. Most patients wish to get well no matter how much of a financial burden this decision may impose upon them or their family. For argument's sake, if a drug is priced at $20 per bottle or tube and your life literally depends upon its use, then you will find some way to obtain it even if it requires the sacrifice of some other item in your personal standard of living. If a physician wants you hospitalized for diagnostic tests, you will enter the hospital. If a physician or group of physicians decide that an operation is necessary for your future well-being, you will accept that judgement, especially when the alternative to that decision may be fatal.

Unlike most market services and products, the patient participates in a system over which he has little control and even less knowledge and understanding. This lack of understanding contributes much to the criticism directed toward various health providers, especially the physician. While the patient may not understand the scientific processes allowing a certain drug, a physician's judgment, or the mechanical technology of a hospital to alleviate or cure his illness, he is quite aware of the costs such care requires. The patient does not understand why a physician's office visit or treatment is a certain price or how such charges are derived; why the daily costs of hospital care have risen so rapidly in the past decade; and why a prescribed drug, though low in unit cost, can vary so widely in price from one retail pharmacy to another. The consumer-patient has every justified reason to suspect whether there is some kind of secret collusion when he hears of price-fixing among products or services or kick-backs among health providers. When these and other revelations are made public, the consumer begins to question the extent of these practices throughout the entire health care field. The consumer-patient begins to feel that he is a captive of the health providers because these providers know that ultimately people must come to them for assistance if they wish to remain in good health. Thus, it is easy for some consumers to conclude that the health providers are taking advantage of their unique position by charging the public whatever the "traffic will bear." This conclusion is reinforced in some of the public's mind when it hears of personal incomes or profit levels ranging far higher than those of other professions or non-health industries. And the public may not understand the reasons for this situation. Feeling powerless to exert some control over the prices he must pay for health care, the consumer becomes agitated and begins to demand that someone do something to make this most indispensable service affordable for all. Hence, in the past several years we have witnessed both industry and government establishing such programs as second surgical opinions, rate review agencies and prepaid group practice plans. Meanwhile, government investigations result in rulings allowing health providers to advertise, bringing more competition into the field and, hopefully, lowering the prices of the services and products which the consumer-patient purchases.

However, these and other programs, as well as laws, have a potentially negative aspect as well as a positive side. Hopefully, they will not immerse the physician in endless red tape. No one wins when the physician must begin to spend more of his time concerned about the business aspects of his practice instead of the treatment of his patients, passing the costs on to his patients in the form of higher medical bills (costs resulting from red tape). Indications already exist that the patient is paying the penalty for these administrative expenses. An HEW study conducted in 1977 found that administrative costs in a physician's office amounted to $2.45, or about 15 percent of a $15 office visit.[4] The average physician spends about six hours per week filling out insurance forms and on a variety of other administrative tasks. Yet, if the free enterprise system of American medicine does little voluntarily and effectively to police its own house and improve the quality of care while controlling its costs, then what other alternatives does society have except new government programs and regulations? If government, as a representative of the public, also will not do so, then who will look out for the public's welfare? Who has the authority of law to perform this task? Who is left to do so? How much of a financial burden can the American public bear in terms of rising health costs, in addition to all the other areas of an inflationary economy? When does the burden break the proverbial camel's back?

The consumer alone pays these costs either directly from his own pocket or indirectly through higher premium payments to health insurance companies or through taxes to government for supporting public medical care programs (in which his participation may be restricted or prohibited). As long as health care reforms and programs come along in a piecemeal and unorganized fashion, then the costs of health care are likely to continue their rise. The escalation results from duplication, mismanagement and inefficiency of programs and efforts.

The piecemeal attempts to resolve the cost and quality of care problems within the health care field is termed by Senator Edward M. Kennedy as the "Control of the Month" approach. When a control is legislated and then tried out but does not work fast enough, another control is then created. Hence, the health care system is filled with a myriad of concepts and programs by both public and private organizations whose development is uneven, fragmented and not in operational harmony. Some of these developments include Professional Standards Review Organizations, health planning agencies, hospital cost commissions, and prospective reimbursement programs. The core of the health system may begin with the doctor-patient relationship but their interaction eventually affects other segments of the health care field. The following examples illustrate these ramifications:

- whether or not a health insurance company pays benefit claims for the patient's visit;
- whether or not a laboratory is utilized to assist in the patient's diagnosis;
- whether or not other specialists—medical or paraprofessional personnel—are called in for consultation;
- whether or not a short-term acute or long-term institution is utilized in his treatment;
- whether or not a pharmaceutical firm's drug product is prescribed for his ailment.

It must be remembered that the various elements making up our health care system are not isolated entities but rather are interlocked and interrelated with all the other activities. When a reform to improve the system is addressed to one group within the industry, its impact eventually has a ripple effect on other groups. Consequently, the problems besetting the health care system must be viewed and resolved as an organic whole rather than as isolated entities. For this and other reasons there is now a drive to reorganize and restructure the health care system by means of a national health insurance system. The national plan is designed to shake up the old system of cottage industries and put into its place a coherent, organized and integrated system. In this fashion, the system hopefully will become more accessible to those who are underserved while its quality will be controlled, and it will be delivered at prices fair to both the consumer and its providers.

However, not everyone believes our present health system requires reorganization. If you believe that the health system should remain as it is, then consider the organization where you are employed, especially if it operates on the profit motive. Look at your organization and ask yourself the following questions: Are the management functions of your establishment integrated and coordinated? Does your business have a department whose sole purpose is corporate planning? Does your department operate within a defined budget determined in advance of the business year? Is there a chart defining the lines of departmental authority and responsibility as well as interdepartmental relationships throughout the organization? Do you know the specific purpose of your department as well as that of others within your company? Does your establishment maintain some kind of training program for new employees and encourage taking educational courses outside of employment hours to keep abreast of developments in the field? Does your Board of Directors oversee your business operations and give guidance and direction towards its future operational goals? Does your establishment strive for management efficiency and economy in its operations? Does your organization maintain an affiliation with other companies which are part of its overall corporate structure?

These same questions defining the structure of your organization's operations have great relevance to the health care field, but, in some instances, the concepts to which they refer have different names. They are called prospective reimbursement, rate review, cost commissions, prospective budgeting, health care planning, institutional affiliation, continuing education, and more. If your organization operated with an open-ended budget, with duplicative departments and services, without an organizational chart as to functional responsibilities, without interdepartmental support, without organizational planning as to its future goals, without hierarchal oversight or direction as to its future operations, your organization and its stockholders would go out of business and become bankrupt quickly. Because of the latter characteristics, the health care system, as we know it, also appears to be going out of business. Its stockholders (the American consumer-patient whose finances support the system) are becoming bankrupt because of its present methods of operation. If it is not fair to ask your organization's stockholders to lose their money because of the way your company operates, is it any more fair to ask the American patient to lose his?

Perhaps, if the system could become organized and integrated then the cost of health care can truly be brought under control and its quality improved. No other measures seem to be working at the moment. Then, and only then, will the American public benefit from all the strings which are being placed on the American physician. At that moment these strings will cease to be the ties that bind. Rather, they will become links to those changes which move society forward to realize its fullest potential for quality health care at reasonable cost.

REFERENCES

CHAPTER 1

1.) "Medical System Blasted", *The Washington Post,* Washington, DC, July 13, 1969, pp. A1 & A2.

2.) Robert M. Gibson and Charles R. Fisher "National Health Expenditures, Fiscal Year 1977", Health Care Financing Administration, *Health Note,* May 1978, p.3.
During the Administration of President Lyndon B. Johnson, a great deal of significant health-related legislation was enacted into law. In addition to the Social Security Amendments of 1965, which established the Medicare and Medicaid programs, there were the Heart Disease, Cancer and Stroke Amendments of 1965, under which the Regional Medical Programs were established; the Comprehensive Health Planning and Public Health Service Amendments of 1966, and the Partnership for Health Amendments of 1967 (later to be replaced and superceded by the National Health Planning and Resources Development Act of 1974, which also replaced the Regional Medical Programs); the Economic Opportunity Act of 1964 which was the legal basis for the Johnson Administration's "War on Poverty"; and the Appalachian Regional Development Act of 1965. Additionally, other bills, though lesser known but equally important, were also enacted into law. These included the establishment of the National Center for Health Services Research and Development, which was an offshoot of the 1967 Partnership for Health legislation; and the massive manpower push embodied in the Health Professions Educational Assistance Act of 1963, the Nursing Training Act of 1964, the Allied Professions Personnel Training Act of 1966 and the Health Manpower Act of 1968.

3.) U.S. Department of Health, Education, and Welfare, "Forward Plan For Health, FY 1978-1982", Public Health Service, Washington, DC, August 1976, p.48.
Between 1965 and 1975 our total national health expenditures rose from $38.9 billion to $122.2 billion. As a proportion of these totals, federal spending increased from 12 percent to 28 percent; private health spending decreased from 75 percent to 58 percent; and state and local government health spending remained at about the same level of 13-14 percent.

4.) Lester Breslow, "The Urgency of Social Action for Health", *American Journal of the Public Health Association,* January 1970, pp. 11 & 12.
In fiscal year 1977 (October 1976 through September 1977) local, state and federal spending ($68.4 billion) represented 42 percent of all 1977 money ($163 billion) spent for health care in the United States. Of this amount, $46.5 billion was federal funds. (Robert M. Gibson and Charles R. Fisher, "National Health Expenditures, Fiscal Year 1977", Health Care Financing Administration, Health Note, May, 1978, p.1.)

5.) Robert M. Gibson and Charles R. Fisher, op. cit., p.1.
The amount of health care dollars expended by or on behalf of each individual in the United States during fiscal year 1977 was approximately $737, according to estimates of the Health Care Financing Administration in HEW, or almost 3½ times the $197 figure recorded in 1965, and this per capita expenditure is still rising on a national basis.

6.) Edward M. Kennedy, "A Bill to Establish a Transitional System of Hospital Cost Containment", *Congressional Record,* April 26, 1977, p. S6401.

7.) U.S. House of Representatives, "National Health Insurance Resource Book," Committee on Ways and Means, Washington, DC, 30 August 1976, p. 13.

From 1966 to 1971 hospital prices, as measured by semi-private room charges, had an annual rate of increase of 14.6 percent. During the Economic Stabilization Period of August 1971 to April 1974 when price controls were imposed upon the health care industry, including hospitals, this rate was reduced substantially to 5.7 percent. Since controls were lifted, hospital prices have risen at a record rate of 15.5 percent annually.

8.) Edward M. Kennedy, op. cit., p. S 6401.

Americans spent an estimated $103.2 billion for personal health care in fiscal year 1975. Personal health care expenditures include all health services and supplies received directly by individuals. Together with spending for medical research and medical facilities' construction, administrative costs of government programs, government public health activities, philanthropic organization fund raising activities for health, and the net cost of private health insurance, they make up the total national expenditures for health—$118.5 billion in fiscal year 1975, a figure that was revised to $122.2˙ billion by the Social Security Administration in December, 1976. Between fiscal years 1965 and 1975 personal health expenditures rose from a figure of $33.5 billion to $103.2 billion, or an increase of $69.7 billion. Of this ten year rise:

* *about 53 percent, or $36.9 billion, could be attributed to higher prices.*
* *another 9 percent, or $6.1 billion, was the result of population growth.*
* *the remaining 38 percent, or $26.7 billion, was due to the public's increased use of services and to a wide variety of lifesaving, but often costly, medical techniques.*

9.) "Outrageous Hospital Charge", *Congressional Record,* July 11, 1977, p. 4319.

Expenditures for hospital care, including both inpatient and outpatient care in public and private hospitals, represented 40 percent of total spending and reached $65.6 billion in fiscal year 1977. Hospital spending from private sources increased at a greater rate than government—15.5 percent compared with 13 percent. All third parties combined—including private health insurers, philanthropy and industry, as well as governments—financed over 94 percent of hospital care in fiscal year 1977.

(Robert M. Gibson and Charles R. Fisher, "National Health Expenditures, Fiscal Year 1977", Health Care Financing Administration, Health Note, May, 1978, p.1.)

10.) "Gloom Pervades Talk on Carter's Cost-Cut Program", *Medical World News,* October 31, 1977, p. 34.

11.) "AHA Says Hospitals Would Cut Services If Cost-Containment Plan Is Enacted", *Health Planning and Manpower Reports,* October 17, 1977, p. 6.

On April 25, 1977, Representative Paul Rogers and Representative Daniel Rostenkowski introduced into the Congress the Carter Administration's bill (H. R. 6575) to limit the growth of annual hospital expenditures at a proposed rate of 9 percent per year or 1½ percent of whatever the inflation rate might be in the general economy and on an annual basis. On April 26, 1977 Senator Edward M. Kennedy, together with Senator Hathaway and Senator Anderson, introduced the same bill (S. 1391) into the U. S. Senate. Specifically, this bill, the Hospital Cost Containment Act of 1977, will:

—Limit the in-patient reimbursements of acute care hospitals, excepting new hospitals, federal hospitals and Health Maintenance Organization (HMO) hospitals.
—Provide an automatic formula to adjust the nine percent limit for moderate changes in expected patient load. The formula will contain strong incentives to discourage unnecessary hospitalization.
—Include an adjustment for hospitals which provide wage increases to their non-supervisory employees.
—Provide an exceptions process for the small percentage of hospitals which will undergo extraordinary changes in patient loads or major changes in capital equipment and services. The program will require the Department of HEW to respond to any application for an exception within 90 days.
—Disallow in the computation of a hospital's base cost any unwarranted expenditures made in anticipation of the implementation of the program.
—Allow states which operate cost containment programs, and are capable of meeting the federal program's criteria, to continue their own regulatory approaches.

This bill, if enacted into law, was projected to save about $2 billion in fiscal year 1978—over $650 million in the federal budget, over $300 million in state and local budgets and almost $900 million in private health insurance and payments by individuals. In fiscal year 1978, total savings were projected at more than $5.5 billion.

The legislation will also impose a limit on new capital expenditures for acute care hospitals. With the assistance of local planning agencies each state will determine which facilities merit new capital expenditures. The program will fix a limit nationally for such capital expenditures below that of recent years and allocate new capital spending among the states by formula.
(Congressional Record, *"Proposed Improvements In The Health Care System—Message From The President", Washington, D. C., 25 April 1977, p. S 6314.)*

12.) Council on Wage and Price Stability, "Physicians: A Study of Physician Fees", Executive Office of the President, Washington, DC, March 1978, p. 56 (percent derived from Table II-6).

Physician fees during the Economic Stabilization Program rose at about three-fifths the rate of the 7-8 percent increase which was recorded between 1966-1971; during the post Economic Stabilization period, as of 1975, these increases accelerated to annual rate of 13.4 percent.
("The Size and Shape of the Medical Care Dollar", Social Security Administration Washington, DC, 1975, p. 16.)

13.) Robert M. Gibson and Robert R. Fisher, op. cit., pp. 1 & 3.

In fiscal year 1977, $32.2 billion was spent on physician services in this country—2½ times that of $13.1 billion in 1970 and about 4 times the amount of $7.5 billion in 1965.

14.) Robert M. Gibson, Marjorie Smith Mueller and Charles F. Fischer, "Age Differences in Health Care Spending, Fiscal Year 1976", *Social Security Bulletin*, August 1977, p. 5.

In fiscal year 1976 the personal health expenditures of the American public amounted to $120.4 billion. Of this amount, almost one-third (28.9 percent) was spent by or on behalf of the elderly who make up only one-tenth of the population. In fiscal year 1966, the year before Medicare became operational, the expenditures of the elderly represented only one-fifth of the total amount. According to the Health Care Financing Administration in HEW, $142.6 billion was spent for personal health care in fiscal year 1977 (excluding spending for research, construction, public health and administrative costs).

15.) Marjorie Smith Mueller and Robert M. Gibson, "Age Differences in Health Care Spending, Fiscal Year 1975," *Social Security Bulletin*, June 1976, p. 18.

The differences among expenditures for those over 65 years of age, those between 19-64 years and those under 19 years of age during fiscal year 1976 varied greatly by health service category. For example, per capita hospital care expenditures for the aged ($689) were almost eight times those for a young person under 19 years of age ($90) and close to 2½ times those for individuals between 19-64 years of age ($268). For physician services during fiscal year 1976 the average expenditure for an aged individual ($256) was more than three times that for a young person under 19 years of age ($77) and twice that for a person in the intermediate group ($121). Also, the elderly spent twice as much for drugs and drug sundries ($121) as did those between the ages of 19-64 ($51) and seven times as much as for those under 19 years of age ($30). Finally, the elderly spent almost 18 times as much for nursing-home care ($351) as did those between the ages of 19-64 ($20) and 170 times as much on a per capita basis than those under 19 years of age ($2). The latter expenses, that is, out-of-hospital prescription drugs and drug sundries are not covered to any significant extent by private health insurance. In fact, Medicare does not cover out-of-hospital prescription drug expenses at all and the program only paid 3.6 percent of the elderly's nursing-home expenses in fiscal year 1976.
(Robert M. Gibson, Marjorie Smith Mueller and Charles F. Fischer, "Age Differences in Health Care Spending, Fiscal Year 1976", Social Security Bulletin, August 1977, p. 10.)

16.) "Age Differences in Health Care Spending, Fiscal Year 1976", op. cit., p. 3.

When public and private dollars are considered together, they differ considerably in the services that they purchase. In fiscal year 1976, thirty-five percent of the private medical care dollar was spent for hospital care compared to 63 percent of the public medical care dollar that was purchasing this same service. On the other hand, 14 percent of the private health care dollar was spent on drugs, whereas only 2 percent of the public medical care dollar went for this purchase. Also, nursing-home care represented 6 percent of private expenditures compared to about 12 percent from

public outlays. As a final example, 40 percent of the private health care dollar, compared with about 16 percent of the public medical dollar, purchased the services of such health professionals as dentists and physicians as well as other professional service providers.
(The aforementioned data were derived from Table 1 entitled "Estimated Personal Health Care Expenditures, By Type of Expenditure and Source of Funds, For Three Age Groups, Fiscal Years 1974-1976 as cited in Robert M. Gibson, Marjorie Smith Mueller and Charles F. Fischer, "Age Differences in Health Care Spending, Fiscal Year 1976", Social Security Bulletin, August 1977, p. 4.)

17.) "Causes of Social Security's Financial Problems", *Congressional Record*, October 1 1977, p. S 18383.

In 1973, when the Congress last enacted major social security legislation, the estimates of the cost of the cash-benefits programs were based on demographic and economic assumptions which no longer appear realistic. At that time, social security cost projections assumed that the ultimate fertility rate would be 2.55 children per woman. Subsequent cost estimates were based on lower fertility rates. The initial reduction came in 1974 when a rate of 2.1 was assumed and a further reduction was made in 1976 when an ultimate fertility rate of 1.9 was used for the 1976 assumptions.

As for the economic assumptions made in 1973, the most significant were that after 1977 average earnings would increase at an annual rate of 5 percent while the CPI would increase at 2¾ percent a year. As early as the end of 1973, these projections were perceived as unrealistic. Therefore, the 1974 estimates were based on the assumption that the annual rise in the CPI would average 3 percent a year. The effect of this change, however, was offset to some degree by eliminating an 0.375 percent additional cost which had been included as a "safety factor" for years prior to 2011 in the 1973 estimates. By 1976, the assumptions had been changed to a 5.75 percent annual increase in average wages and a 4 percent annual rise in the CPI.

The long-range economic assumptions used for the 1977 estimates are basically those used for the 1976 estimates. Significant changes, though, were made in the mortality and fertility assumptions. Mortality was assumed to improve, thus raising the cost of the program by 0.64 percent of taxable payroll. This increase in cost was offset by assuming that the fertility rate would rise to 2.1, the approximate rate at which the population eventually would neither grow nor decline.

The social security benefits formula also is the source of much of the long-term deficit. In 1972, the social security benefit formula was made too sensitive to changing economic conditions. The benefit formula was intended to keep future benefits on a par with those benefits being received by present beneficiaries, but it in fact has not worked that way. Future benefits are increasing more rapidly than intended. This is because the formula for calculating future benefits is tied to increases both in prices and wages. Because wages go up partly as a reflection of prices, workers retiring in future years receive double adjustments for inflation.

This problem has become known as over-indexing or double-indexing. Without corrective action by Congress, future retirees could receive social security benefits exceeding the highest wages they earned before retirement. This factor alone causes one-half of the long-term deficit.

18.) The Congress of the United States, "Catastrophic Health Insurance", Congressional Budget Office, Washington, DC, January 1977, p. 15.

19.) "Doctor Loses Suit For Delaying Care", *The Washington Star*, Washington, DC, February 13, 1978, p. A6.

20.) Robert M. Gibson and Charles R. Fisher, op. cit., p. 4.
In addition to the $20.7 billion spent for Medicare and the $9.2 billion for Medicaid by the federal government in fiscal year 1977, the states spent another $7.1 billion under Medicaid for a total outlay of $37 billion for both programs in that year. In fiscal year 1976, Medicare expended $16.9 billion and Medicaid spent $14.6 billion or a total of $31.5 billion of which $6.6 billion constituted state funds.

21.) "Age Differences in Health Care Spending, Fiscal Year 1976," op. cit., p. 10.
In 1976, Medicare benefits paid only 43 percent of all health expenses of the aged. If premiums are deducted, the Medicare benefit share is reduced to 38 percent. According to the Health Care Financing Administration in HEW, for each person receiving Medicare benefits in fiscal year 1977, Medicare spent $1,442; for Medicaid, each beneficiary received an average of $753.

22.) "Physician Heal Thyself . . . Or Else!", *Forbes,* October 1, 1977, p. 45.

23.) "Health: United States, 1976-1977 Chartbook", op. cit., p. 6.

The lack of stringent cost controls for the various health care services provided under Medicare and Medicaid has had an interesting impact on the pattern by which public and private funds have been purchasing medical care since 1960. In the early 1960s, private spending for medical care rose faster (8.3 percent) than public spending (7.1 percent). But during the second half of the 1960s, after Medicare and Medicaid became operational, public spending rose three times (24 percent) as fast as private spending (8.3 percent). Since 1970, the annual increase in public expenditures has decelerated considerably, due principally to the Economic Stabilization Program's controls over health care costs in the early 1970s. But the average public rate of increase is still higher (13.4 percent) than the private increase rate (9.2 percent) because of the continued expansion of Medicare to the disabled and to persons with chronic renal disease.

("The Size and Shape of the Medical Care Dollar", Social Security Administration, Washington, D.C., 1975, p. 8.

24.) William J. Eaton, "Doctor Glut Seen Hiking Health Costs", *Boston Evening Globe* June 29, 1977, p. 10.

25.) Lawrence Meyer, "New U.S. Problem: Too Many Doctors," *The Washington Post,* Washington, DC, July 6, 1977, p. 1.

There are a number of statistical indicators available which are leading health experts to believe that the physician shortage in this country is ending and that within a decade there actually may be physician surplus in the United States. These indicators include:

*   *A 28% increase in the ratio of physicians to population. In 1950, there were 141 doctors for every 100,000 persons. By 1975, the number had grown to 181 per 100,000 population. Future increases in the ratio of physicians to population have been variously estimated at 28%-40% over the next 13 years.*
*   *A 44% increase in medical schools. In 1950, we had 79 medical schools. In 1975, the number stood at 114.*
*   *A 121% increase in medical school graduates. In 1950-51, U.S. medical schools produced 6,135 physicians. By 1975-76, the total number of graduates reached 13,561.*
*   *A 180% increase in newly licensed physicians (including foreign medical graduates). In 1950, 6,002 new licentiates; by 1975, 16,859.*

(Robert M. Hendrickson, "Physician Supply: Shortage to Surplus?", American Medical News, November 28, 1977, Impact/p. 1.)

26.) Judith Randal, "Can Runaway Medical Costs Be Curbed?", *The Washington Star,* Washington, DC, March 1, 1970.

27.) Herman M. Somers, "Health Economics", *Public Health News,* November 1969, p. 245.

28.) Ibid.

29.) "Counterattack Launched by AMA's Dr. Sammons", *American Medical News,* June 27/July 4, 1977, p. 21.

30.) Ibid.

31.) "National Health Care Conference on Health Care Costs", *Congressional Record,* June 18, 1977, p. S 12206.

32.) "Aim at Doctors, Says Poll", *Medical World News,* June 13, 1977, p. 12.

CHAPTER 2

1.) "Health Care Ripoffs", *The Washington Star,* Washington, DC, August 4, 1976, (an editorial).

2.) "High Rating Given to Doctors in Poll", *The New York Times*, August 22, 1976; "You Through Your Patients' Eyes: How You Fare in Other Surveys", *Medical Economics*, November 29, 1976, p. 169.

According to the American Medical Association, physician's average net income by medical specialty in 1974 was as follows: all medical doctors—$51,224; general surgeons—$60,031; obstetrician-gynecologists—$58,238; internists—$51,115; anesthesiologists—$50,780; general practitioners—$43,808; pediatricians—$43,429; and psychiatrists—$39,997. (U.S. House of Representatives," National Health Insurance Resource Book", Committee on Ways and Means, Washington, D.C., August 30, 1976, p. 51).

3.) U.S. Department of Health, Education and Welfare, "Medical Care Expenditures, Prices and Costs: A Background Book", Social Security Administration, Washington DC, September 1975, pp. 52-60; *The Washington Post*, "Medical Spending Jumps; Dilemma See on Insurance", December 22, 1976, p. A2; American Medical Association, "Profile of Medical Practice". Center for Health Services Research and Development, Chicago, Illinois, 1975-1976, pp. 9-21, 61, 75 & 160; American Medical Association, "Socioeconomic Issues of Health", Center for Health Services Research and Development, Chicago, Illinois, 1975-1976, p. 6.

As of December 31, 1974, there were 379,748 physicians in the United States or one doctor for each 566 persons. Of this total number 330,266 were classified as being active and 301,238 were categorized as being patient care physicians. As of December 31, 1975, there were 8,483 medical groups in the United States whose 66,842 physicians represented 23.5 percent of the active nonfederal physician population. Of the total number of groups 54 percent were single specialty practices, 35 percent were multi-specialty practices and the remainder (11 percent) were general practice groups. Approximately 79 percent of the groups (6,721) were composed of seven or fewer physicians. The average size of a medical group has increased from 6.3 physicians in 1969 to 7.7 physicians in 1975.
There has been a tendency for physicians to specialize. For example, of the 301,238 physicians involved in patient care in the United States in 1974, more than 248,000 (or 82 percent) were practicing in one or more specialty areas. Only 53,000 physicians (or 18 percent) were general practitioners. In contrast in 1968, 201,000 physicians were specialists (77 percent) and 60,000 were general practitioners (or 23 percent). The specialty attracting the largest number of physicians—52,000 in 1974—was internal medicine. It was followed by general surgery with 31,000 doctors and psychiatry with over 23,000. These have been consistently the largest three specialties since 1968. In 1973, about 86 percent of the 295,257 patient care physicians practiced in metropolitan areas—a rate of nearly 150 doctors per 100,000 population.
In recent years, many physicians have grouped themselves into partnerships of one form or another. In 1972, the number of partnerships and partners—10,329 and 36,677 respectively—were on the decline as physicians groups began to incorporate to take more favorable advantage of the tax laws. It has also been observed that physicians who practiced in the two man or small group practices saw more patients, worked more hours per week, and earned higher incomes than either solo practitioner or those practicing in very large groups.
Finally, about nine percent of the 330,266 physicians classified as being active in December 1974 were engaged in a variety of areas other than direct patient care as theiir primary activity. These activities included administration (11,739), research (8,159), medical teaching (6,464), and other activities (2,666). Of the physicians in patient care, approximately 68 percent were in office-based practice and 32 percent were in hospital-based practice.

4.) U.S. House of Representatives, "National Health Insurance Resource Book", Committee on Ways and Means, Washington, DC, August 30, 1976, p. 53.

According to the American Medical Association, the number of physicians in patient care per 100,000 population among the states in 1974 was as follows: Idaho, Wyoming, North Dakota, South Dakota, Alaska, Oklahoma, Arkansas, Mississippi, Alabama, and South Carolina had less than 90 physicians per 100,000 population; Nevada, Montana, New Mexico, Texas, Kansas, Nebraska, Iowa, Missouri, Louisiana, Wisconsin, Georgia, Tennessee, North Carolina, Virginia, West Virginia, Kentucky, Indiana, Ohio, Michigan, and Maine had 90-120 physicians per 100,000 population; Washington, Oregon, Utah, Arizona, Minnesota, Illinois, Florida, Hawaii, Pennsylvania, Delaware, New Jersey, and New Hampshire had 121-140 physicians per 100,000 population; California, Colorado, New York, Maryland, District of Columbia, Connecticut, Rhode Island, Massachusetts, and Vermont had more than 140 physicians per 100,000 population.

(U.S. House of Representatives, "National Health Insurance Resource Book", Committee on Ways and Means, Washington, D.C., August 30, 1976, p. 47)

5.) Senator Frank E. Moss, Chairman of the Subcommittee on Long-Term Care, Senate Committee on Aging, Testimony before the Senate Finance Committee, July 28, 1976.
In October, 1977, President Jimmy Carter signed into Public Law 95,142 the Medicare-Medicaid Anti-Fraud and Abuse Amendments of 1977. Among the law's provisions were the following:
● *Medicare and Medicaid fraud was made a felony, subject to a $25,000 fine and up to 5 years in prison. Until this law, such fraud had only been a misdemeanor, subject to a $10,000 fine and one year's imprisonment.*
● *factoring arrangements—selling Medicaid—Medicare billings at a discount to factoring, or brokerage, firms for cash—are prohibited. Factoring was forbidden in 1972 but some physicians may have assigned their power of attorney to factoring firms to circumvent the prohibition; the new law prevents this situation.*
● *physicians will be suspended nationally from both Medicare and Medicaid for "program related criminal offenses".*
● *the ownership and financial structure of health care facilities—and information about prior criminal convictions of physicians involved—must be disclosed as a precondition of participation in Medicare and Medicaid. This legislation also grants federal authorities direct access to such information.*
● *professional standards review organizations (PSROs), which hitherto have been limited to monitoring the quality of care offered in hospitals and nursing homes, for example, will be authorized to evaluate Medicaid "mills," which up to now have been designated outpatient facilities since they are composed of office-based private practitioners of various disciplines working under the same roof.*
● *the comptroller general, who runs the General Accounting Office for Congress, will be given power of subpoena.*
● *any Medicare or Medicaid provider who hires an individual who had been employed by an intermediary insurance company—one that handled the federal government's Medicare claims—will have to put HEW on notice immediately of any potential conflict of interest.*
● *in the first year, the federal government will finance 100 percent of the cost of state Medicaid fraud control units. Funding decreases to 90 percent in the second year, 75 percent in the third year and 50 percent from then on.*
● *the practice adopted by some nursing homes of requiring Medicare patients' families to make financial contributions as a precondition of admission is expressly forbidden. Freely offered contributions, however, are still permitted.*
● *HEW is required to conduct a special study on how to assure quality and appropriate utilization of home health care services and ways of preventing fraud.*
● *a uniform reporting system similar to that suggested by the American Hospital Association is to be established for institutional providers.*
(Medical World News, "Medicare and Medicaid Frauds Are Now Felonies", October 31, 1977, pp. 28 & 29.)

6.) John Fialka, "HEW Opens Massive Hunt For Health Program Cheats", *The Washington Star*, Washington, DC, November 21, 1977, p. 1.

7.) "Ban on Advertising by Doctors Opposed in FTC Complaint", *The Wall St. Journal*, December 23, 1975, p. 15.
On November 14, 1976 the U.S. District Court in Alexandria, Virginia struck down as unconstitutional a Virginia statute that prohibited physicians from providing information about their services and fees for a consumer directory. The ruling is said to be the first by any court in the nation to overturn a statute forbidding doctors to advertise, and the precedent threatens the existence of similar laws in 33 other states. The court enjoined the Virginia State Board of Medicine from taking disciplinary action against physicians who furnish the information.

8.) "AMA Vows to Fight FTC Attempt to End Ban on Ads by Physicians", *American Medical News*, January 5, 1976, p. 1.
The Federal Trade Commission's complaint that the American Medical Association's Principles of Medical Ethics prohibited advertising by physicians in restraint of trade was not only directed at the American Medical Association but also included the Connecticut State Medical Society and the New Haven, Connecticut, County Medical Association as well.

9.) Ibid.

On June 27, 1977, the Supreme Court ruled in Bates and O'Steen v. State Bar of Arizona (97 S. Ct. 2691) that advertising by an attorney can deal with availability and rates but not with quality of the services to be rendered. The case only applies to lawyers but possibly could be extended to physicians. The only constitutional issue in this case is whether state government may prevent the newspaper publication of a lawyer's truthful advertisement concerning the availability and terms of routine legal services. The Supreme Court ruled simply that the flow of such information may not be restrained. The Supreme Court did not rule on the antitrust question because states are exempt from antitrust laws but any private organization within a state which restricts advertising may be subject to freedom of speech and antitrust law violations. (National Health Lawyers Association," Lawyers May Advertise Their Availability and Rates", Newsletter, July 1977, pp. 5 & 6.)

10.) Ibid.

During 1976, two medical organizations agreed to abandon relative value scales, which had been attacked by the Federal Trade Commission as fee freezing that restricts price competition. Consent agreements were signed with the American Academy of Orthopedic Surgeons and the American College of Obstreticians and Gynecologists, representing a total of some 19,000 physicians. The medical organizations agreed to stop publishing the scales and to recall those published. The Federal Trade Commission said that the relative value scales of the orthopedic surgeons and obstreticians and gynecologists have the effect of establishing, maintaining, or otherwise influencing fees charged by their members. The settlement of the case does not resolve the legal dispute on the overall relative value issue which is predicted to be settled by the courts. As in all consent agreements, all parties stipulate that signing does not constitute admission of wrongdoing.

(American Medical News, "Specialists Abandon Value Scales", July 26, 1976, p. 1.)

11.) "Physician Control of Blue Shield Plans is Subject of FTC Antitrust Investigation", *The Wall St. Journal,* February 27, 1976, p. 5.

12.) "FTC Moves into Health Area Again with Probe of AMA and MD Education", Washington Report on Medicine and Health, April 19, 1976, p. 2.

13.) "FTC Jumps on Antisubstitution Bandwagon", *PMA Newsletter,* August 9, 1976, p. 4.

14.) "Drug Substitution Laws—Problems for Physicians", *Medical World News,* August 9, 1976, p. 85.

In dismissing the suit brought against the U. S. Department of Health, Education, and Welfare by the American Medical Association, the Pharmaceutical Manufacturers Association and five physicians in regard to HEW's Maximum Allowable Cost program, the U. S. District Court for the Northern District of Illinois stated in a 74 paged opinion that "if the MAC regulations have the effect of altering present drug prescription habits in the medical profession to reflect greater cost efficiency, that effect is consistent with congressional intent."

(The Wall Street Journal, "Court Dismisses Suit To Bar HEW Limits On Drug Payments", March 10, 1977, p. 26).

15.) Ibid.

16.) "FDA Chief Says Generic, Brand Rx's Nearly Equal", *AMA News,* November 21, 1977, p. 3.

Effective in 1977, maximum allowable cost limits had been set on the amounts which Medicare and Medicaid would pay for dosages of ampicillin and penicillin. The oral liquid form of ampicillin may be priced up to 1.45 cents for each 5 ml at the 125 mg/ 5ml strength and 2.05 cents for each 5 ml at the 250 mg/ 5 ml strength. Four forms of penicillin VK were assigned limits: 5.35 cents for a 250 mg tablet and 10.25 cents for a 500 mg tablet. In the oral liquid form of penicillin, MACs were set at 1.2 cents per 5 ml at the 125 mg/ 5 ml strength and 1.6 cents per 5 ml for the 250 mg/ 5 ml strength. (Forum, Maximum Prices Set for Ampicillin and Penicillin", Health Care Financing Administration, Washington, D. C., November/December 1977, p. 38.)

17.) William R. Barclay, "Unnecessary Surgery", *Journal of the American Medical Association,* July 26, 1976, p. 387 (an editorial).

18.) "Doctor Finds 'Sickness' In Profession", *The Washington Star*, Washington, DC, August 28, 1976, pp. 1 & D-16.

19.) "Champion Supports Crackdown on Unnecessary Surgery", *The Blue Sheet*, November 2, 1977, p. 3.

In January 1978, the American Association of Professional Standards Review Organizations identified 11 surgical procedures which, it said, have significant potential for inappropriate utilization. A set of screening criteria for these procedures were sent to local PSROs. The Association stated that the surgical criteria must not be viewed as mandated national standards but rather that the local PSRO may wish to adopt or adapt the screening criteria for local use. The 11 surgical procedures included:

Abdominal hysterectomy, vaginal hysterectomy, coronary arteriography, cataract removal, dilatation and curettage, tonsillectomy and adenoidectomy, cholecystectomy, hiatal hernia repair, lumbar disc excision for rupture or protrusion, meniscectomy and appendectomy.

(American Medical News, "Potential Abuse Targets Listed", January 30, 1978, p. 7.

20.) Spencer Klaw, "Bad Medicine: When Practice Makes Imperfect", *The Washington Post*, Washington, DC, December 21, 1975, p. 4e.

21.) Ibid.

22.) Ibid.

23.) Ibid.

24.) Richard L. Peck, "What Does Society Really Want From Doctors?: Greater Accountability", *Medical Economics*, May 29, 1978, p. 105.

The National Commission on Health Certifying Agencies was established in December 1977 by 65 medical and health groups in the United States. Certifying is the process by which health professionals are examined by private, nonprofit boards of examiners on their ability in specialized fields. It is not the same process as official licensing: testing, then approval by a state government body. State laws established to license physicians will not be preempted by this commission. This agency will establish and monitor performance standards for existing health professional certifying bodies. It will create new certifying systems for emerging health occupations, recommend methods to assure continuing competence after certification and maintain a register of organizations. The commission will also collect data on cost-saving procedures, study the effect standards have on health personnel performance and, finally, encourage member professions to use common examinations nationally.

25.) "Are You Ready to Blow the Whistle on Bad Doctors?", *Medical Economics*, November 22, 1974, p. 77.

Arizona and Oregon have enacted legislation requiring health care providers to report to the state board of medical examiners any information appearing to show that a doctor is or may be medically incompetent. This includes the reporting of incidents which have not yet become the subject of   malpractice claims.

(American Bar Association, "Interim Report of the Commission on Medical Professional Liability", Chicago, Illinois, September 27, 1976, p. 17.)

26.) Ibid., p. 79.

27.) "Doctor Finds 'Sickness' in Profession", op. cit., p. D-16.

28.) American Medical Association, "AMA Supports Anti-Fraud Measure", *Legislative Roundup*, September 17, 1976, p. 2.

CHAPTER 3

1.) Marshall B. Segal, "A Hard Look at the PSRO Law", *The Journal of Legal Medicine*, September-October 1974, p. 26.

2.) "PSROs: Here They Come–Ready or Not", *Medical World News*, March 30, 1973, p 15.

3.) Stanton M. Evans, "The Lessons of PSRO", *Private Practice,* November 1974, pp. 27 & 29.

4.) Nowhere in the PSRO law is there any mention of national norms, criteria or standards. Inasmuch as those terms are used more or less interchangeably, the Office of Professional Review Standards in HEW has adopted the following definitions:
Medical care appraisal norms *are averages or medians of observed performance that are stated in numerical or statistical terms.*
Medical care criteria *are predetermined, measurable elements of health care delivery that are requisite to the delivery of care of high quality; they are developed by professionals relying on professional judgement, consensus and expertise and on professional literature.*
Standards *are professionally developed measures of the range of acceptable variation from a norm or criteria.*
Source: John R. Farrell, "PSROs and Internal Hospital Review", The Hospital Medical Staff, November 1973, p. 4.

5.) U.S. Department of Health, Education, and Welfare, "PSRO: Question & Answers", Office of Professional Standards Review, Rockville, Maryland, December 1973.
*In October 1977, President Jimmy Carter signed the Medicare-Medicaid Anti-Fraud and Abuse Amendments of 1977 into law (P. L. 95-142). In addition to dealing with the Medicare and Medicaid programs, the law also directs the U. S. Department of Health, Education, and Welfare to develop ambulatory care review methodologies for PSRO use; directs HEW to require capable PSROs to undertake ambulatory care review within two years after designation as a PSRO; makes "competent" PSRO reviews of services conclusive for purposes of federal payment, if the PSRO has entered into a memorandum of understanding regarding Medicaid administering agency. Fraud and abuse information detected by a PSRO would be provided to federal and state investigative agencies. Patient records in the PSRO would not, however, be subject to subpoena or discovery proceedings in a civil action.
(American Medical News, "Medicaid Fraud Bill Approved", October 3, 1977, p. 14.)*

6.) "The Size and Shape of the Medical Care Dollar", Social Security Administration, Washington, DC, 1975, p. 28.

7.) Senator Wallace F. Bennett, "Remarks on PSROs", *Congressional Record,* Washington, DC, September 27, 1972, pp. S16111 & S 16112.

8.) U.S. Senate, "Background Material Relating to Professional Standards Review Organizations", Committee on Finance, Washington, DC, May 8, 1974, pp. 19 & 20, 22 & 23.

9.) Ibid.

10.) "PSRO: Question & Answers". op. cit., p. 3.

11.) Ibid., p. 4.

12.) Ibid., p. 3.

13.) Ibid., p. 2.

14.) Ibid., pp. 3 & 4.

15.) Ken Rankin, "Henry Simmons' Inside View of PSRO", *Physician's Management,* November 1974, pp. 54-u & 59-u.

16.) James A. Reynolds, "You Doubt If PSRO Will Work? So Do Some Feds!", *Medical Economics,* November 25, 1974. p. 35.
An unpublished report that was submitted to the House of Representatives Commerce Oversight Subcommittee in the Spring of 1977 by John Thompson, Professor of Hospital Administration, Yale University, criticized the lack of direction and fragmentation of the Professional Standards Review Organization program. The study stated that the conflicts between the PSRO's law's intent and local and federal administration of it all combine to produce an aura of multiple conflicts so pervasive as to threaten the success of the legislation by hampering the federal government's ability to carry out the mandated programs. The study stated that the translation of the law

into a specific program is now enmeshed in a maze of conflicts. PSRO and HEW fear of an MD walkout has set the management mode throughout the various levels of the program and caused an attitude of tender treatment toward the medical profession . . . As a consequence, there is confusion as to whether the activity of the hospital or the physician is being monitored or whose behaviour is hopefully changed by negative inducements . . . The PSRO program may be accurately classified as moving in a state of critical transition. Tremendous problems exist in physician acceptance, technology and philosophy which remain to be resolved . . . Consequently, PSROs may best be viewed as ongoing experiments which, to succeed, must evolve over a number of years in an environment allowing flexibility, modification, and change". The report observes that a friction among the federal agencies administering the PSRO program is not surprising. "Understandably, the Social Rehabilitation Service and the Social Security Administration tend to emphasize the fiscal impact of review while the Bureau of Quality Assurance stresses quality issues. But the report concludes that the study of the overall cost control strategy cries for coordination. Individual pieces of legislation, however well intended, cannot have their maximum effect unless they are interdigitated with other mandated programs".
(The Blue Sheet, *"Still-Secret House Subcommittee Report Hits Fragmentation of PSRO Program; Payment Denials to MDs Seen Cutting Unnecessary Hospital Admissions", Washington, DC, July 6, 1977, pp. 13-14.)*

17.) Ibid.

18.) Ibid.

19.) Ibid., p. 19.

20.) Ibid.

21.) Ibid., p. 43.

22.) Jonathan Spivak, "Medical-Review Stirs a Fiery Debate Among U. S. Physicians", *The Wall St. Journal,* June 1974, p. 1.

23.) James E. Hague, "PSRO and Politics Dominate AMA Convention", *The Hospital Medical Staff,* August 1974, p. 29.

24.) "Delegates Refuse to Seek PSRO Repeal", *American Medical News,* July 1–8, 1974, p. 1.

25.) Jonathan Spivak, op. cit., p. 1.

26.) Fayetta Weaver, James C. Respress, and Leon Geoffrey, "Professional Standards Review Organization (PSRO): A Positive Look at the Possibilities", *Virginia Medical Monthly,* September 1973, p. 806.
Within the PSRO program, it costs from $10 to $36 to review one patient. Total PSRO program costs have grown from $48 million in fiscal year 1974 to an estimated $119 million in fiscal year 1978. When all PSROs are in place, the total is expected to be about twice that amount.
(William A. Knaus, "PSRO Update: Where We Stand Now", American Medical News, June 20, 1977, Impact/p. 5.)

27.) Ibid.

28.) Ibid., p. 807.

29.) Ibid.

30.) Ibid.

31.) "Making CME and PSRO Work Together", *Medical World News,* March 6, 1978, p. 65.

32.) "If Peer Review Won't Work, What Will?", *Medical Economics,* May 17, 1976, pp. 101-102 & 106.
In 1974, Medical World News published the findings of a survey that it conducted among a scientifically selected cross section of physicians and osteopaths in regard to their views of PSROs. The response rate to the 2,337 questionnaires was an unusually 40.7 percent or 951 returns. The following were among the survey's findings:

● *One fifth of the nation's practicing general practitioners said that they would refuse to treat Medicare and Medicaid patients rather than have a PSRO monitor their performance.*
● *One third of all practitioners feared that PSROs would trigger more malpractice suits.*
● *Slightly more than one half (53.1 percent) of all the doctors were opposed to PSROs.*
● *Most doctors who were either hospital-based, under 45 years of age, or lived in the northeast part of the country favored PSROs.*
● *Two out-of-three doctors believed that PSROs would not reduce Medicare and Medicaid expenditure outlays.*
● *57.8 percent of all doctors felt that PSROs either would lengthen or have no effect on hospital stays while the remainder felt that they would have such an effect.*
● *77.8 percent of all doctors did not believe that PSROs would change or improve the quality of present medical care, while one out of four general practitioners, general surgeons and osteopaths predicted that PSROs would impair treatment.*
● *83.1 percent of all doctors did not believe that PSROs would lower the number of malpractice suits.*
● *39.6 percent of all doctors stated that PSROs would discourage the use of new medical and surgical procedures.*
● *25.6 percent of the physicians believed that PSROs would reduce their income while 82 percent saw PSROs being extended beyond Medicare and Medicaid within five years.*
● *Another widely shared view, no percent being given, was that PSROs would jeopardize the confidentiality of medical records.*
● *One-half of all doctors said that they were willing to serve on PSROs' review panels compared with 41.5 percent of all doctors who favored the PSRO. Obviously, even if they do not like the program, quite a few doctors intended to participate.*
● *Only 36 percent of all doctors believed that PSROs would be of benefit in developing programs of continuing education.*
● *One third of all doctors feared that organized medical groups would have too little say in a PSRO.*
● *Nearly four out of five of all doctors wanted local practitioners and not national medical associations—such as the AMA and specialty groups—to set the standards and criteria with which the PSROs would judge the physician's performance.*
(Medical World News, *"Are You in Favor of PSRO?"*, October 25, 1974, pp. 71-77.)

33.) Ibid.

34.) "Patients' Rights and the Quality of Care", *Time Magazine*, December 17, 1973, p. 56 (an essay).

35.) "Care Problems, Not Politics, May Kill PSRO, Says Roth", *Medical Group News*, November 1974, p. 12.

36.) Ibid., pp. 1 & 12.

37.) Charles C. Edwards, "Can PSRO Improve the Quality of Health Care?, *Medical Tribune*, December 5, 1973, p. 4.
It is too early to assess the full impact of PSRO activities because of the short time that these organizations have been performing binding review. However, preliminary data from several conditional PSROs indicate that where PSRO review has been implemented, hospital lengths of stay have been shortened, quality has improved, and unnecessary use of services has been curtailed. A number of illustrations of the impact of PSRO review are summarized briefly below:

1.   Sacramento Foundation for Medical Care
Overall reductions in hospital utilization resulted from the review program of the Sacramento PSRO Certified Hospital Admission Program (CHAP), according to a study conducted by the Office of Research and Statistics (ORS) of the Social Security Administration. After the first year of Medicare CHAP review, patient days per 1,000 enrollees decreased by 5.3 percent in the CHAP area, while increasing by 4.6 percent in the five comparison areas. ORS estimated that CHAP review resulted in a saving of 16,500 days of care during the first year.

2.   South Carolina Medical Care Foundation
Average lengths of stay for Medicaid patients were reduced by 0.9 days, due to review conducted by this PSRO. That was. the finding of a study conducted by

the South Carolina Department of Social Services, which covered two 6-month periods; pre-PSRO, October 1974 to March 1975, and post-PSRO, October 1975 to March 1976.

3. Multnomah Foundation for Medical Care, Oregon
Average lengths of stay were reduced by 10.4 percent for Medicare patients and 23.5 percent for Medicaid patients, in a comparison between 1974 (pre-PSRO) and 1976 (post-PSRO) data for this PSRO. This represented 48,852 fewer patient days of care for a 1-year period.

4. Delmarva Foundation for Medical Care, Maryland
Results of a study at this PSRO showed a reduction of about half a day in the average length of stay for both Medicare and Medicaid patients. For this study, 1976 data for the three largest hospitals in the area were compared with 1974 and 1975 (pre-PSRO) data.

5. Wyoming Health Service
Medicare lengths-of-stay decreased almost one day, and Medicaid lengths-of-stay decreased 0.2 days in a Wyoming study showed a 24 percent reduction in the number of Medicare admissions.
(U.S. Department of Health, Education, and Welfare, "PSRO Fact Book", Health Care Financing Administration, Office of Health Standards and Quality, Washington, DC, May 1977, pp. 33 & 34.)

38.) Richard E. Thompson, "Medical Care Evaluation Studies: The Crux of Quality", The Hospital Medical Staff, September 1974, p. 12.

39.) Robert Ray McGee, "How I Became a Sloppy Doctor", Medical Economics, April 3, 1978, p. 80.

40.) Ibid., pp. 79-82.

41.) Robert Pear, "Review Boards Seen Reducing Hospital Costs", The Washington Star, Washington, DC, May 22, 1976, p. 3.
In fiscal 1976, PSROs reviewed more than one million federal admissions. When fully implemented in 1978 in all 203 designated PSRO geographic areas throughout the nation, PSROs are expected to review five million federal admissions, or one-third of the total U.S. hospital admissions. Preliminary data from conditional PSROs indicate that average length of stay has been reduced by 25 percent. As of July 1, 1976, there were 79,976 physicians affiliated with PSROs and 1,113 hospitals under review.
(American Medical News, "PSRO Program Faces Its Final Hurdle: Will it Prove Effective?". August 23, 1976, p. 11.)

42.) "HEW, Too, Says PSROs Don't Save Money", Medical World News, November 1977, pp. 15 & 16.

43.) Robert Pear, op. cit., p. 3.
In 1976, the American Medical Association's Council on Medical Service issued a list of guidelines for physician-controlled PSROs that was adopted as formal AMA policy. Specifically, the guidelines stated that control over gathering, security and release of data is a primary responsibility of the PSRO. The way the data are handled should be controlled by the PSRO itself and data reports required by law should not identify individual patients, hospitals, or physicians. Further, the AMA and other medical organizations should oppose any government controlled systems for storing or handling data for PSROs, according to the policy statement. The AMA House of Delegates adopted as policy in 1976 that physicians involved in PSRO activity should be compensated, according to what each local PSRO decides—and should not be subject to the U.S. Department of Health, Education, and Welfare's arbitrary limit of $35 per hour.
(American Medical News, "PSRO Policy Guide Adopted", December 13, 1976, p. 15.)

CHAPTER 4

1.) "The Biggest HMO Advocate Backs Off On Prepayment," Medical Economics. August 9, 1976, pp. 29 & 30.

2.) American Public Health Association, "A Guide to Medical Care Administration: Concepts and Principles", Appendix II, p. 81.

3.) "Universal 'Group Practice' Prepayment Health Plans–A Clarification and Economic Implication", *Journal of the National Association of Retail Druggists*, May 19, 1969, p. 21.

   Closed panel *of physicians is the more traditional type of prepaid group practice in which physicians work together as a group (typically as a professional corporation or partnership), pool their income, and share common facilities, support staff and medical records.*
   Open panel *of physicians refers to independent solo practitioners or small group practices who maintain their existing fee-for service practices and individual offices while agreeing to provide prepaid care to HMO plan subscribers in much the same way that they provide such services to Blue Shield plan subscribers.*

4.) American Public Health Association, op. cit., p. 76.

5.) U.S. Senate. Committee on Labor and Public Welfare, "Health Maintenance Organization Act of 1973, S. 14", Subcommittee on Health, Washington, DC, February 1974, p. 2 (explanation of Act and text of Public Law 93-222).

6.) Martin Judge, "HMOs Stimulate Competition; Bring Hospitalization Rates Down", *Forum*, September/October 1977, p. 3.

7.) Jordan Braverman, "Group Practice Prepayment Plans–Universities Give New Impetus to Old Concept", *Journal of the American Pharmaceutical Association*, November 1969, p. 564.

8.) Ibid., pp. 564 & 565.

9.) F.H. Seubold, "HMOs–The View From The Program", *Public Health Reports*, March-April 1975, p. 99.

10.) Ibid., p. 100.

11.) "Toward A Comprehensive Health Policy For The 1970s: A White Paper", U. S. Department of Health, Education, and Welfare, Washington, DC, May 1971, p. 31.

12.) Arnold J. Rosoff "Phase Two of the Federal HMO Development Program: New Directions After a Shaky Start", *American Journal of Law and Medicine*, Fall 1975, pp. 211 & 212.

13.) F.H. Seubold, op. cit., p. 100.

14.) "HMO Report", U.S. Department of Health, Education, and Welfare, Washington, DC, December 19, 1975, (a press release).

15.) "Blue Cross Plans Increase HMO Efforts", *Blue Cross Consumer Reports*, January 1976.

16.) "Health Maintenance Organization Act of 1973, S. 14", op. cit., p. 1.

17.) F.H. Seubold, op. cit., pp. 101 & 102.

   Copayment–*Requires the patient to pay a fixed amount, for example, on each prescription (e.g. 75 cents) and the insurer pays the remainder.*
   Co-insurance–*The patient pays a percentage of his medical bills (after an initial deductible is satisfied, if any.) For example, he may pay 20 percent and his insurance company pays the remaining 80 percent.*
   Deductible–*The patient is required to pay all medical costs up to a certain fixed sum (e.g. $25 or $100 per year) before he is eligible for any benefits.*

18.) Ibid., p. 102.

   The HMO Act (section 1302 (8) of the PHS Act) defines community rating as a system of fixing rates of payments for health services which may be determined on a per person or per family basis and "may vary with the number of persons in a family, but must be equivalent for all individuals and for families with similar composition." The intent of a community rating is to spread the cost of illness evenly over all subscribers (the whole community) rather than charging the sick more than the healthy for health insurance.

19.) Claudia B. Galiher and Marjorie A. Costa, "Consumer Acceptance of HMOs", *Public Health Reports*, March-April 1975, p. 108.

20.) Paul Starr, "An Experiment Designed to Fail: The New Medicine", *The New Republic*, April 19, 1975, p. 16.

21.) "Still Waiting For That Revolutionary Health Plan", *Business Week*, July 13, 1975, p. 54.

22.) Ibid., p. 53.

23.) Howard Lewis, "The Selling of HMOs: 1975", *Modern Health Care*, May 1975, p. 33.

24.) "HMOs Becoming More Competitive", *HMO & Health Services Report*, Mt. Arlington, N.J., October 1977, p. 2.

25.) Martin Judge, op. cit. p. 3.

26.) Howard Lewis, op. cit., p. 40.

27.) Martin Judge, op. cit., p. 3.

28.) Richard McNeil and Robert E. Schenker, "HMOs, Competition and Government", *Milbank Memorial Fund Quarterly/ Health and Society*, Spring, 1975, pp. 208-209.
*A number of states have restrictive provisions relating to the operation of an HMO including the following: sixteen states require the medical society to approve the furnishing of services by an HMO; nineteen states require that physicians constitute all or part of an HMOs governing body; thirteen states require supervison of an HMO by the insurance commissioner; one state requires that an HMO contract only with hospitals; one state prohibits physicians from practicing with unlicensed persons; and some states laws can put a limit on marketing expenditures or require insurance commissioner approval for marketing procedures.
(Report To The Congress by the Comptroller General of the United States, "Factors That Impede Progress In Implementing The Health Maintenance Organization Act of 1973, Washington, DC, September 3, 1976, pp. 28 & 29.)*

29.) Ibid., p. 197.

30.) Ibid., p. 200.

31.) Ibid., p. 218.

32.) Ibid., p. 202.

33.) Martin Judge, op. cit., pp. 4 & 5.

34.) Arthur Owens, "Is That New HMO A Lemon?", *Medical Economics*, February 11, 1975, p. 1.
*Under the HMO Amendments of 1976 which require federal HMO qualification for Medicaid Prepaid Health Plans (PHP), three plans had qualified in California for operation by the end of 1976. From a peak of more than 50 PHPs serving a quarter of a million welfare clients in 1974, the program in California has been reduced to 25 with less than 188,000 members. By the summer of 1977, there may be only a dozen PHPs in operation, depending upon how many of the PHPs can meet the strict new federal and state standards. California still has the largest number of Medicaid Prepaid Health Plans of any state with Maryland having seven plans; Minnesota, Pennsylvania and Washington state having four plans each and ten other states having one to three plans each.
Medical World News, "Prepaid Poverty Plans Dwindle", February 7, 1977, p. 33.*

34.) Joann S. Lublin, "Unhealthy Start", *The Wall St. Journal*, February 11, 1975, p. 1.
*In July, 1976 the Blue Cross Association, the National Association of Blue Shield Plans, the Interstudy research group of Minneapolis, Minn., and HEW's Division of Health Maintenance Organizations jointly conducted a membership and utilization census of HMOs on a national basis. Highlight of the census include the following findings:
(1) Total membership in the 175 prepaid health plans was 6,106,443. (2) 59 percent of the total membership is in consumer-sponsored plans. (3) 62 percent of the total membership is in prepaid group practice plans. (4) 70 percent of the total membership*

is in plans with 100,000 or more members. (5) 74 percent of the total membership is in plans that have been operational for at least 10 years. (6) 64 percent of the total membership is in the West—50 percent of the total membership is in California. (7) 41 percent of the prepaid plans are in the West. (8) Inpatient hospital utilization for all plans is 449 days per 1,000 members per year. (9) Physician visits per member per year for all plans is 3.8. (10) Prepaid Group Practice Plans have much lower inpatient utilization than Individual Practice Associations. (11) Plans which have been operational longer have lower inpatient utilization. (12) Plans in the West have lower inpatient utilization than plans in other parts of the country.
(Blue Cross Consumer Report, *"National HMO Census Data Released",* March 1977.)

36.) "The Kaiser-Performance Health Plan", *Congressional Record,* November 4, 1977, p. S18992.

37.) Ibid., p. 1.

38.) Arthur Owens, op. cit., p. 101.

39.) "Dual Option Boosts Certified HMOs", *Medical World News,* February 9, 1976, p. 23.
Indemnity benefit—*The patient or consumer pays directly for the services or product and is reimbursed by the third party*
Service benefit—*The vendor is paid by a third party for the service he performs or the medication he dispenses*

40.) "Amendments Ease HMO Enrollment Requirements", *Modern Healthcare,* November 1976, p. 22.
Among the more detailed provisions of the HMO Amendments of 1976 were the following:
● *The HMO Act of 1973 mandates that employers of 25 or more persons who offer health benefits to their employees must offer the option of membership in an HMO. The 1976 amdnements require that this option be offered to those employees who reside in an HMO service area (undefined by the amendments) in which 25 or more such employees reside. In addition, if the employees who are eligible for this option are represented by a collective bargaining unit or other representative, the offer of membership in an HMO must first be made to such a representative, and if accepted by the representative, then to the eligible employees. Furthermore, the amendments exempt the following units from having to offer an HMO as an alternative health benefit: the federal government, the government of the District of Columbia, or any territory or possession of the United States, any state or political subdivision, or any agency or instrumentality of any of the above, or any church and convention or association of churches.*
● *Medical groups, to qualify under the 1976 amendments, must now devote a "substantial" part of their professional responsibility to HMO duties. As explained in the House-Senate Conference Report the whole group must demonstrate that it provides over 35% of its services to HMO subscribers, although no time requirements are imposed upon group members. The 35% standard does not apply, however, for the first three years following certification of an HMO, and can be waived after the three-year period depending upon how the requirement would affect the ability of the HMO to provide service and upon the population's density and composition in the HMO service area.*
● *For the first 36 months after the HMO becomes qualified, contracts for the provision of both basic and supplemental services may be entered into by the HMO with outside health professionals. Under the old law outside contracts were forbidden except for unusual or infrequent health services. The amendments limit the amount of outside contracting to 15% of an HMO's total payment to physicians for services, or 30% if the HMO is located in a rural area.*
● *The amendments require HMOs offering services for five years or have 50,000 enrolled members, and which have not operated at a financial loss during the prior year to have an open enrollment period of the lesser of 30 days or the time it takes to enroll enough individuals to at least equal 3% of its total net increase in enrollment in the preceding fiscal year. HMOs are not required to enroll persons who are institutionalized due to a permanent injury or chronic illness, if such enrollment would cause economic impairment to the HMO. The open enrollment provisions may be waived if adherence to the principle would threaten the economic well-being of the HMO in its*

particular service area. The amendments also provide for a 90-day waiting period before benefits apply to new enrollees.
● *The Secretary of HEW is required under the amendments to prepare and update a digest that will indicate state laws and regulations that appear to be inconsistent with the intent of the 1973 Act. The Secretary is also responsible for bringing the inconsistencies to the attention of the government on at least an annual basis.*
● *As far as the certificate-of-need laws are concerned, the legislation requires that areawide and statewide planning agencies' criteria for HMOs be consistent with HMO laws and standards.*
● *Medicaid and Medicare recipients who join an HMO must still receive the benefits of these two public programs rather than the health services mandated to the HMO by federal law.*
● *Federal funding maximums were raised by the amendments: an HMO can receive $75,000 for feasibility studies, instead of the previous $50,000. Planning grant limits are now $200,000 instead of $125,000. An HMO that has already received $1 million for development can receive up to $1.6 million more for an expansion project. Initial operating loans will be provided for up to five years, compared with three years under the 1973 act. Funding for all HMO support programs (excluding feasibility studies) was stretched out to fiscal 1979 (the original law provided funding through fiscal 1977), and the total was increased by $10 million. Funding is $40 million for fiscal 1979.*

41.) Doctors May Lose Some Medicare Patients to HMOs", *Medical World News,* April 5, 1976, p. 93.
As of June 1977, only 1.5 percent or under 700,000 Medicare and Medicaid recipients were enrolled in HMOs.
(National Journal, *"Carter Wants to Heal The Long-Suffering HMOs",* July 23, 1977, p. 1147.)

42.) John K. Iglehart, "HMOs–An Idea Whose Time Has Come", *National Journal,* February 25, 1978, p. 314.

43.) Arthur Owens, "Where You Fit in With HMOs", *Medical Economics,* September 29, 1975, p. 52.

44.) Ibid., pp. 62-64.

CHAPTER 5

1.) "That Blockbusting Health Planning Act: How Will Doctors Fit In?", *Medical World News,* April 5, 1976, p. 55.

2.) South Carolina State Board of Health, "Community Health Planning", *Journal of the South Carolina Pharmaceutical Association,* September 1969 p. 16.

3.) Daniel A. Kane, "Comprehensive Health Planning: A Study in Creative Federalism", *American Journal of Public Health,* September 1969, p. 16.

4.) James D. Williams, "Comprehensive Health Planning: An Organizational Means for Transition", *American Journal of Public Health,* January 1969, p. 50.

5.) Ibid.
Planning essentially involves four basic steps:
● *the survey, during which the problems are defined, resources located and the facts obtained*
● *the analysis, including the forecasting of anticipated conditions and the relation of the central issue to those either influencing or influenced by it*
● *the plan, directed toward goals, based on needs and standards, and elaborated with cost estimates and time schedules for implementation*
● *the implementation which most planners are not inclined to ignore. They approach it by stimulating community participation in the planning process.*

6.) Health Insurance Council, "Community Health Action–Planning, Problems and Potentials", New York, March 1969, p. 2.

7.) Richard B. Froh, "The Evolution of Community Health Planning", *Journal of the American Pharmaceutical Association*, June 1969, p. 255.

8.) Ibid.

9.) Health Insurance Council, op. cit., pp. 4 & 5.

10.) Joel J. May, "Will Third Generation Planning Succeed?" *Hospital Progress*, March 1976, p. 60.

11.) Stanley H. Werlin, Alexandra Walcott and Michael Joroff, "Implementing Formative Health Planning Under P. L. 93-641", *The New England Journal of Medicine*, September 23, 1976, p. 699.

12.) Ibid.

13.) "That Blockbusting Health Planning Act: How Will Doctors Fit In?", op. cit., pp. 54 & 55.

Aside from Health Systems Agencies, other planning bodies on the state and federal levels which are of importance include:

• State Health Planning and Development Agency (usually called simply the "state agency")

These will provide the enforcement for carrying out the HSA decisions on major equipment purchases and new construction. They administer the certificate-of-need laws (that all states must enact under penalty of losing federal funds). State agencies are designated by the governor from one of the existing agencies, such as the state health department, which had previously operated the certificate-of-need program.

• Statewide Health Coordinating Council

The members of the SHCC themselves are appointed by the governor from the boards of the HSAs (at least 60 percent) and from his own sources (not more than 40 percent). The SHCC prepares the state health plan, which can supersede an HSA's local plan. They also monitor the HSA and report to Washington on its importance. All SHCC business meetings are public.

• National Council on Health Planning and Development

This advisory council helps the Secretary of HEW develop national health guidelines, implements P. L. 93-641, and evaluate anything coming along that could affect the nation's health care. Besides the HEW assistant secretary for health, the Defense Department assistant secretary for health and environment, and the Veterans Administration chief medical director, it is made up of at least five "providers of health services," at least three members of HSA governing bodies, and at least three SHCC members. This council also will probably have the responsibility of supervising, according to the law's requirements, the establishment of at least five national centers for health planning.[15]

14.) Donald F. Phillips, "Health Planning: New Hope for A Fresh Start," *Hospitals*, April 5, 1976, p. 54

15.) "That Blockbusting Health Planning Act: How Will Doctors Fit In?", op cit., p. 54.

16.) Ibid., p. 55.

17.) "Health Planning: New Program Gives Consumers, Uncle Sam A Voice", *Science*, January 17, 1975, pp. 152 & 153.

The majority of a Health Systems Agency's governing board must be health consumers, comprising up to 60 percent of the total board's membership. This majority will represent the socio-economic population within the geographic service area. The remaining members are providers, such as physicians, dentists, nurses, health care institutions such as hospitals and HMOs as well as health insurers, professional schools and allied health professionals. At least one-third of the board members must be health-care providers. Membership also includes publicly elected officials, other representatives, government agencies, the persons who reside in the nonmetropolitan areas of the health-service area.

18.) "National Health Planning: What Scares the Hell out of Gene Rubel", *Modern Health Care,* May 1976, p. 53.

19.) "Regulatory Wave Engulfing Medicine", *American Medical News,* February 2, 1976, May 10, 1976, p. 1.

20.) "'H' Withdraws Draft Guidelines for National Health Planning Policy: Fight Looms Over Goals Binding Local Providers of Health Services", *The Blue Sheet,* Washington, DC, October 13, 1976, p. 5.

21.) "AMA Criticizes Planning Regulations", *American Medical News,* May 10, 1976, p. 1.

22.) "Fight Looms on Health Planning", *Medical World News,* August 8, 1976, p. 54.
*In April 1976, the state of North Carolina, later joined by the American Medical Association, the North Carolina Medical Society and the state of Nebraska, filed a suit against the U. S. Department of Health, Education, and Welfare on the grounds that the new health planning law was unconstitutional and usurps state and local authority. HEW asked dismissal of the suit by stating that the federal government can place conditions on grants without violating the principles of federalism. According to HEW, the planning law does not infringe upon physicians' rights to practice medicine and the planning law in no way requires a physician to prescribe or refrain from endorsing any form of treatment. In September 1977, a federal court in Raleigh, North Carolina ruled the law constitutional and that Congress can attach any conditions it wants to the distribution of federal funds. The plaintiffs had argued that the law's requirement that states pass certificate-of-need legislation before receiving federal grants was an unconstitutional violation of states' rights. The AMA asserted that the planning law violates the privacy of the physician-patient relationship and forces physicians to bow to federal controls even though they may not participate in a federal program. In April 1978, the U. S. Supreme Court affirmed without opinion the ruling of the federal court upholding the constitutionality of the 1974 planning law.
(Washington Report on Medicine and Health, "HEW Seeks Dismissal of AMA Suit to Overturn Health Planning Law", Washington, DC, January 3, 1977, p. 3; National Journal, "AMA, North Carolina Join in Lawsuit", Washington, DC, April 10, 1976, p. 492; American Medical News, "Court Says No To AMA Appeal on Planning Law", April 28, 1978, p. 1.)*

23.) "Confusion Reigns at Planning Meeting", *American Medical News,* August 30, 1976, p. 31.

24.) "Government Controls: New Ground Rules for Your Hospital", *Medical Economics,* September 29, 1975, p. 93.

25.) U.S. Department of Health, Education, and Welfare, "Final Planning Guidelines Issued", *Health Resource News,* Washington, DC, April 1978, pp. 1 & 3.

26.) U.S. Department of Health, Education, and Welfare, "Health Planning Guidelines", Health Resources Administration, Washington, DC, March 22, 1978, p. 3 (a press release).

27.) "AMA Again Opposes New Planning Rules", *American Medical News,* February 28, 1978, p. 6.

28.) "Government Controls: New Ground Rules for Your Hospital", op. cit., p. 93.
On January 21, 1977, the U.S. Department of Health, Education, and Welfare announced final regulations governing the review of new institutional health services under the National Health Planning and Resources Development Act of 1974, P. L. 93-641. Issuance of the final regulations will enable states to begin drafting authorizing legislation for certificate-of-need programs that are required by P. L. 93-641. The new regulations define health facilities to include hospitals, psychiatric hospitals, skilled nursing facilities, tuberculosis hospitals, kidney disease treatment centers, intermediate care facilities and ambulatory surgical facilities. Home health agencies, outpatient physical therapy, and organized ambulatory care facilities are not covered by the rules. Essentially, new institutional services, new construction, modernization and conversions are subject to certificate-of-need review. Although the process begins with the Health Systems Agencies (HSAs), state agencies are the final authority. There are five review "thresholds", the point at which a certificate-of-need becomes a requirement:

• *construction of a new facility or Health Maintenance Organization*
• *a capital expenditure of $150,000 or more*
• *a substantial change in the numbers, categories or relocations of health facility beds. The rules define substantial to mean 40 beds, or 25 percent of bed capacity. Changes involving fewer beds are not subject to review. On April 8, 1977, this regulation was amended by the U. S. Department of Health, Education, and Welfare so that reviews would be ordered for proposed alterations involving 10 beds, or 10 percent of capacity, whichever is less, at hospitals and other health facilities. A second change made by the U. S. Department of Health, Education, and Welfare on April 8, 1977 required a written finding of the "appropriateness and efficiency" of similar existing facilities when new or expanded health services are sought. A written finding of the cost and efficiency of the proposed service will also be required.*
• *new services that have not been offered regularly during the preceding 12 month period*
• *pre-development activity costing in excess of $150,000*
Property acquisition was excluded from the $150,000 threshold requirement because institutions often inherit land or buy it for investment purposes. Predevelopment expenses, including architectural costs, are counted.
(Health Planning and Manpower Reports, *"New Certificate-of-Need Rules: Major Change in Ways States Control Health-Service Costs", February 7, 1977, pp. 9 & 10.)*

29.) "Planning Act: A Plus for Hospitals", *Modern Healthcare*, August 1976, p. 38.
   Although the federal government's health planning law does not include physician's offices within the certificate-of-need review, precedents have been established in Hawaii which brings the physician's office within the purview of the state laws—a precedent which could be followed by other jurisdictions should they so desire.
   The Hawaii law includes private physicians' offices "in any case of purchase or acquisition of equipment attendant to the delivery of health care service and the instruction or supervision therefor for any such private or clinic or laboratory involving a total expenditure of $100,000 . . ."
   (American Medical Association," Certificate of Need—State Laws", State Health Legislation Report, November 1976, p. 12.)

30.) Sheilah Kast, "Hospitals, MDs Protest Agency's Health Care Plan", *The Washington Star*, Washington, DC, November 14, 1977, pp. B1 & B3.

31.) "Healthcare Planning Gets Muscles", *Modern Healthcare*, March 1975, p. 32.
   An analysis of certificate-of-need legislation, as announced in February 1977 and prepared for the National Center for Health Services Research, revealed that certificate-of need laws did not substantially affect total hospital investment since they encouraged a shift of investment capital from bed expansion to new equipment and services. The investment in other services and facilities resulted in increased plant assets per bed, so that the estimated overall influence of certificate-of-need programs over the four year period of the study was to raise a typical state's per capita costs by 1.5 to 2.4 percent. The report was based on cost data from 48 states and the District of Columbia from 1968 to 1972. During the study period, 24 states had certificate-of-need legislation. Presently, all but two states—West Virginia and Missouri—have certificate-of need laws or conduct capital expenditure review programs under section 1122 of the Social S curity Act.
   (Health Resources News, *"CON Laws Cut Beds, Spur Other Expenses", Health Resources Administration, U. S. Department of Health Education, and Welfare, February 1977, p. 2.)*

CHAPTER 6

1.) Claude E. Welch, "Medical Malpractice", *The New England Journal of Medicine*, June 25, 1972, p. 1372.

2.) "Now Doctors Charge Insurers With Malpractice," *Business Week*, August 4, 1975, p. 40.

3.) Claude E. Welch, op. cit., pp. 1372 & 1373.

4.) "Malpractice: Who Paid What, Where", *Medical World News,* July 12, 1976, p. 52.

Of 14,074 claim reports analyzed by the National Association of Insurance Commissioners for the twelve month period of July 1975 to June 1976, 9,018 claims or 64% involved no payment of indemnity at all. These were instances in which the claims were disposed of in favor of the defendent. Of the 5,056 claim reports involving payment of indemnity, 3,181 or 63% resulted in payments of less than $10,000. Only 4.8% or 245 of these claims resulted in payments exceeding $100,000. The remainder of the paid claims, or 32.2%, fell into the $10,000 to $99,000 range.
(American Medical News, *"If I Lose Will I Lose Big?",* April 18, 1978, p. 5; (Impact section.)

5.) Ibid.

6.) Ibid.

7.) Claude E. Welch, op. cit., pp. 1373 & 1374.

8.) Ibid., p. 1375.

According to figures released by the American Medical Association in October 1976, the average doctor's malpractice insurance premium rose from $1,905 in 1973 to $7,787 in 1975 (The New York Times, *"Doctors Attend to Insurance",* December 5, 1976; Ideas and Trends section.)

9.) "Malpractice: Grim Outlook For '76", *Medical World News,* January 12, 1976, pp. 71 & 75.

In a 1976 survey of 6,600 office-based, fee-for-service physicians, Medical Economics *found that in terms of medical malpractice insurance only one doctor in 70 had paid $25,000 and up for such insurance in that year. One-half had paid no more than $3,000. For most private practitioners it still represents no more than 3 percent of gross receipts and less than 9 percent of total professional expenses. One in four surveyed physicians—and nearly one-half of the surveyed general practitioners—stated that they have stopped offering their patients certain medical services—such as radiotherapy and electricshock therapy in order to place themselves in lower-risk categories for malpractice premium purposes.*
(Medical Economics, *"How Much Have Malpractice Premiums Gone up?",* December 27, 1976, pp. 103 & 108.)

10.) "Malpractice '77:50–State Picture Improves", *Medical World News,* January 10, 1977, pp. 21 & 23.

Medical World News *found the following adjustments in medical malpractice insurance at the end of 1976. In seven states there was actually a decrease in premium costs. In 15 states, there was little or no change. In seven states, the increase was within three percentage points of the inflation rate in medical care costs (about 9 percent during 1976). In fourteen states, the premiums increased less than 50 percent. (In eight of these states, the increase was 16 percent). And in the remaining seven states, the premiums rose 50 percent or more.*

11.) "Hospitals' Malpractice Woes Worsen", *Medical World News,* March 8, 1976, p. 24.

In 1974, the nation's more than 6,000 hospitals (not counting Veterans Administration hospitals) paid a total of about $350 million for malpractice insurance. In 1975, the figure more than doubled to $750 million and in 1976 the bill ran to an estimated $1 billion.
(The Wall St. Journal, *"Medical Malpractice Insurance Crisis May End Up Improving Hospital Care",* December 27, 1976, p. 2.)

12.) Ibid.

Florida has enacted legislation requiring every hospital to establish an internal risk management program, one component of which is an incident reporting system.
(American Bar Association, *"Interim Report of the Commission on Medical Professional Liability",* Chicago, Illinois, September 27, 1976, p. 17.)

13.) American Hospital Association and Maryland Hospital Education Institute, "Controlling Hospital Liability: A Systems Approach", Chicago, Illinois, 1976, p. 23.

In order to try and resolve the malpractice insurance problem, hospital associations during 1976 in New Jersey, Michigan, Missouri, Texas, Iowa, Wisconsin, and

Washington state were setting up insurance companies. Hospitals in states such as Alabama have set up insurance pools.
(The Wall St. Journal, *"Medical Malpractice Insurance Crisis May End Up Improving Hospital Care",* December 27, 1976, p. 2.)

14.) Ibid., pp. 8 & 24.

15.) "Malpractice Poll: People Back MDs", *Medical World News,* August 11, 1975, p. 27.

16.) "Is There A Trend To Going Bare?" *American Medical News,* June 28, 1976, Impact/ p. 5.
In 1974, as the medical malpractice insurance crisis began to become worse, only one physician out of 100, under age 65, went without such insurance protection. According to a 1976 survey of 6,600 office-based, fee-for-service physicians by Medical Economics, *one in every 19 physicians under age 65 by early 1976 was going without malpractice insurance protection as the malpractice insurance rates increased dramatically since 1974. Most likely to be "going bare" today are general practitioners (one in eight), physicians 65 years and over (one in 10), and those netting less than $30,000.*
(Medical Economics, *"How Much Have Malpractice Premiums Gone Up?",* December 27, 1976, p. 104.)

17.) "Behind The Countersuit Trend: Physicians' Frustration and Anger", *American Medical News,* June 28, 1976, pp. 1 & 8.
In a review of 24,158 claims filed between July 1, 1975 and June 30, 1976 the National Association of Insurance Commissioners found that about 10 percent of the claims (2,376) were disposed of by trial, by settlement during trial, by binding arbitration, or by review panel. A total of 21,782 claims were disposed of in some other manner. Of these, 64% were victories for the defendent, and 36% were victories for the plaintiff. Of the remaining 2,376 claims, 1,704 were decided by trial. Eighty percent were disposed of in favor of the doctor-defendant and only 20% were in favor of the plaintiff. Other cases (460) also went to trial but were settled during the proceedings. Of these, 60% were settled in favor of the plaintiff and only 40% in favor of the defendant. The NAIC analysis also showed that pretrial screening panels and other review mechanisms (96 cases) now established in some states to consider malpractice claims produced about the same 80% for the doctor/20% for the plaintiff results as do the trial costs. Finally, binding arbitration (116 cases) produce more victories for plaintiffs with 47% of these cases being disposed of in the plaintiff's behalf as against 53% in the defendant's behalf.
(American Medical News, *"Will I Win If I Go To Trial?",* April 28, 1978, Im-pact/p. 5)

25.) "Is Insurance Available?", *American Medical News,* April 28, 1978; Impact p. 7.
A Joint Underwriter Association is an association created by statute which typically requires casualty insurers writing in the state to provide malpractice coverage and distribute profits or losses among the participating companies. In some states a Joint Underwriters Association may be set up to be the exclusive source of medical malpractice coverage, whereas in other jurisdictions a Joint Underwriters Association may be simply an available avenue for health providers who cannot obtain insurance in the voluntary market.
(American Bar Association, *"Interim Report of the Commission on Medical Professional Liability",* Chicago, Illinois, September 27, 1976, p. 26.)

26.) Charlotte L. Rosenberg "Can Deductibles Really Cut Malpractice Rates?", *Medical Economics,* April 5, 1976, p. 43.
Two years after the Medical Society of New York established a self-insurance plan in 1975 (when the Argonaut Insurance Company left New York State's physicians with no malpractice insurance coverage), the company is doing well. The Medical Liability Insurance Company of New York had more than 16,000 insured members in 1977 compared with 4,000 for the state-legislated alternative Joint Underwriting Association, or JUA, which is a mandatory pool of liability carriers in New York state. The Medical Liability Insurance Company has continued to provide up to $1-million/ $3-million occurrence-type policies, charging premium rates that went up only 15 percent in 1975 and 20 percent in 1976. The JUA's premiums are only slightly higher because the state denied that group its proposed increases of 100 percent and 90 percent, respectively, for those two years. Medical Liability Mutual has asked for a

one-time $1,750 contribution from each member toward a capital surplus fund, whereas the JUA requires a surcharge of 20 percent of the premium cost each year for an indefinite period. Thus, doctors who have been with the JUA for their third year will have contributed in most instances far more than those with Medical Liability, according to the company's president, and their rates have been higher.
(Medical World News, *"MD-Owned Insurer Claims Top Health"*, May 2, 1977, p. 40.)

27.) "Malpractice: Grim Outlook for '76", op. cit., p. 75.

28.) Howard Hazzard and Robert E. Cartwright, "Change For Tort System: Pro and Con", *Medical World News*, September 8, 1975, p. 60.

29.) "Malpractice: Grim Outlook for '76", op. cit., p. 83.
Eighteen states have enacted legislation providing for the mandatory review of every malpractice claim by a panel as a condition precedent to litigation, and in twelve of the states the panel's findings as to liability (and in some states instant damages) is admissable in a later court proceeding. These states include Florida, Illinois, Louisiana, Massachusetts, Nevada, New York, Ohio, Tennessee, and Pennsylvania in 1975; Arizona, Hawaii, Idaho, Maryland, Missouri, Nebraska, New Mexico and Rhode Island in 1976.
(American Bar Association, *"Interim Report of the Commission on Medical Professional Liability"*, Chicago, Illinois, September 27, 1976, p. 24.)

30.) Don Harper Mills, "Malpractice Litigation: Are Solutions In Sight?", *Journal of the American Medical Association*, April 28, 1975, p. 372.

31.) Claude E. Welch, op. cit., p. 1374.

32.) Lawrence H. Miike, "Public Policy Directions In Medical Malpractice; *The Journal of Legal Medicine*, April 1976., p. 11.

33.) Claude E. Welch, op. cit., p. 1374.

34.) Howard Hazzard and Robert E. Cartwright, op. cit., p. 61.

35.) Claude E. Welch, op. cit., p. 1375.
Since 1975, ten states have adopted malpractice arbitration laws. Alabama, Alaska, California, Illinois, Louisiana, Michigan, Ohio, South Dakota, Vermont, and Virginia have arbitration laws applying specifically to medical injury claims. Some 37 states, including all of the above, except Alabama and Vermont, have statutes sanctioning arbitration for various kinds of disputes, including personal injury; and in the remaining 13 states, binding arbitration agreements are permissible under common law.
(Medical Economics, *"Binding Malpractice Arbitration: Most Doctors Are For It"*; April 4, 1977, p. 135.)

36.) Don Harper Mills, op. cit., pp. 372 & 373.

37.) Claude E. Welch, op. cit., p. 1375.

38.) Charlotte L. Rosenberg, "Are Those Hopeful Malpractice Omens For Real?", *Medical Economics*, October 31, 1977, p. 113.
Based upon the random responses of 1,648 readers—lawyers and law students' Juris Doctor in a 1977 survey concluded that 28 percent of the attorneys believe that at least one-fifth of their fellow lawyers are not competent and 20 percent also believe that more than one-fifth of all lawyers are dishonest or unethical. As far as the medical malpractice crisis is concerned, only 12 percent of the readers listed malpractice lawyers as the primary cause of the high insurance rates, while 23 percent blamed the insurance companies and 39 percent blamed incompetent and unethical physicians.
(Juris Doctor, *"Project '77 Results: Incompetence Rising"*, July/August 1977, pp. 23-25.)

39.) Bart Sheridan and Stanley Ferber, "Malpractice: A Contract to Keep You Out of Court", *Medical Economics*, May 3, 1976, pp. 80-87.

40.) Claude E. Welch, op. cit., p. 1375.

41.) Jeffrey O'Connell and Richard Roddis, "Can No Fault Malpractice Insurance Really Work?", *Medical World News*, October 6, 1975, p. 99.

42.) Marianne G. Decker, "How Would You End the Medical Malpractice Crisis", *Medical Economics*, April 19, 1976, p. 87.
*Three out of four American physicians (75.7 percent) are now practicing "defensive medicine"—that is, ordering extra tests and procedures for patients—as a protection against potential malpractice suits, according to the results of a poll taken and published by the American Medical Association in 1977 among a statistically valid sample of 500 physicians of whom 111 doctors responded to the survey. In ordering additional tests, 58.5 percent of the 82 physicians responding to this question said they were ordering one or more extra tests—x-rays, laboratory tests, other diagnostic procedures—while 26.8 percent estimated that they were ordering three or four more tests. About one of ten (9.8 percent) said that they were ordering five or six additional precautionary tests and 4.9 percent reported that they were now ordering more than six. As far as increasing malpractice premiums having an impact on their physician fees during the last year (1976), three out of five (59.8 percent) said yes, while two out of five (40.2 percent) said no. Of those who did raise fees, almost half (47.5 percent) reported that the increase ranged from 1 to 10 percent, while another 29.5 percent said the increase was from 11 to 20 percent. About 14.8 percent stated that they increased their fees from 21 to 30 percent. Only 8.1 percent reported increases of 30 to 60 percent, and none reported increases of more than 60 percent.
(American Medical News, "Why Most MDs Practice "Defensive Medicine", March 28, 1977, p. 3; Impact Section.)*

43.) Warren Weaver, Jr. "Lawyers Shun Curbs on Suing Physicians", *New York Times*, February 16, 1978, p. 41.

44.) Ibid.

45.) Robert Ray McGee, "How I Became A Sloppy Doctor", *Medical Economics*, April 3, 1978, pp. 81 & 82.

46.) Carol Brierly Golin, "How Are My Colleagues Coping?", *American Medical News*, April 28, 1978; Impact p. 13.

CHAPTER 7

1.) "Crisis and Health Insurers", *Life Association News*, June 1970, p. 1.

2.) "Big Business Digs in Against Rising Health Costs", *Medical Economics*, September 20, 1976, p. 149

3.) Ibid., p. 154.

4.) "Who, Me? Need Health Insurance?", *Current Consumer*, January 1978, p. 4.

5.) Ibid., p. 5.

6.) "Hospital Costs: Biggest Piece of the Health Care Bill", *Medical World News*, May 2, 1977, p. 52.

7.) I.S. Falk, "Beyond Medicare", *American Journal of Public Health*, April 1969, pp. 610-611.

8.) "Private Health Insurers Plead For Chance To Prove Their Plan Works" *National Health Insurance Reports*, September 26, 1977, p. 4.

9.) *Source Book of Health Insurance Data, 1976-1977*, Health Insurance Institute, New York, N.Y., 1977, pp. 7 & 8.

10.) Inland Steel v. National Labor Relations Board, 170 Federal Second to 47, Court of Appeals, 7th Circuit 1948, Denial of Certiorari (Denial of Review), 336-U.S. 960.

11.) *1971-1972 Source Book of Health Insurance Data*, Health Insurance Institute, New York, N.Y., p. 8.

12.) Modern Health Insurance, Health Insurance Institute, New York, N.Y., 1969, pp. 9 & 36.

13.) *Blue Cross and Blue Shield Fact Book, 1977,* Blue Cross Association and National Association of Blue Shield Plans, Chicago, Illinois, 1977 pp. 3 & 12.
The "Blue" plans operate on a service benefits *basis, making payments directly to the providers of care such as hospitals and physicians on the basis of a negotiated cost figure, rather than reimbursing the insured as private health insurance carriers normally do under* indemnity *plans.*

14.) *Source Book of Health Insurance Data, 1976-1977,* op. cit., p. 21.

15.) J. Pollack, "New Approaches to Health Care Plans" as cited in *Proceedings of a Seminar on Prepaid Group Practice Health Plans,* University of Colorado, Denver, Colorado, March 20-21, 1968, p. 1.

16.) U.S. House of Representatives, "National Health Insurance Resource Book", Committee on Ways and Means, Washington, DC, April 11, 1974, p. 214.

17.) "Does Coverage Meet Your Needs?", *Today's Health,* December 1969, p. 54.

18.) "Who, Me? Need Health Insurance?", op. cit., p. 4-14.

19.) Ibid.

20.) Ibid.

21.) Ibid.

22.) Ibid.

23.) Ibid.

24.) Congress of the United States, "Catastrophic Health Insurance: Budget Issue Paper", Congressional Budget Office, Washington, DC, January, 1977, pp. xiv & xv.

25.) Nancy Hicks, "Soaring Cost of Health Insurance is Debated in Auto Contract Talks", *The New York Times,* August 22, 1976, p. 24.

26.) "GM's Outlays For National Health Insurance Exceeds $1 Billion; Ford Undertakes Pilot Programs on Health Care", *The Review,* December, 1977, pp. 27, 28 & 30.

27.) "HEW Holds Hearings on National Health Insurance", *Forum,* November/December 1977, p. 28.

28.) Nancy Hicks, op. cit., p. 24.

29.) Ibid.

30.) "Washington Business Group on Health: A Growing Force in Delivery and Cost Control", *Hospital Progress,* December 1977, p. 49.

31.) John K. Iglehart, "Health Care Cost Explosion Squeezes Government Programs, Insurers", *National Health Journal,* April 29-30, 1976, pp. 6 & 7, (Health Conference Issue).

32.) Nancy Hicks, op. cit., p. 24.

33.) "Malpractice Insurance Pushes Fees Up", *The Washington Star,* Washington, DC, October 25, 1976, p. A-6.

34.) *Source Book of Health Insurance Data,* op. cit., p. 12.

35.) "Big Business Digs in Against Rising Health Costs", op. cit., p. 150.

36.) Executive Office of the President, "The Complex Puzzle of Rising Health Care Costs: Can The Private Sector Fit It Together?", Council On Wage And Price Stability, Washington, D.C., December 1976, p. 159.

37.) Ibid., p. 166.

38.) "Administration Promoting HMOs To Nation's Largest Corporations", *Health Services Information,* Washington, DC, November 7, 1977, p. 3.

39.) "The Complex Puzzle of Rising Health Care Costs: Can The Private Sector Fit It Together?", op. cit., p. 152.

40.) "Crisis and Health Insurers", op. cit., p. 100.

41.) Ibid., p. 98.

42.) "Aetna Plan to Reduce Unneeded Surgery", *The Washington Post,* Washington, DC, November 30, 1976, pp. A1 & A9.

In addition to commercial insurance carriers, Blue Cross plans, since 1976, in New York, Pennsylvania, New Jersey, Illinois, Massachusetts, Michigan and Ohio have formed second-surgical opinion programs.
(Blue Shield News, "Plans Experiment With Second Opinions", January 1978, p. 4.

CHAPTER 8

1.) Jordan Braverman, "National Health Insurance: Yesterday's Theory–Tomorrow's Reality", *Journal of the American Pharmaceutical Association,* May 1970, p. 266.

2.) Ibid.

3.) "Cautious Phase-In Approach To NHI Seen As Route Carter Will Take", *National Health Insurance Reports,* November 8, 1976, p. 2.

4.) John K. Iglehart, "The Health Policy Squeeze", *National Journal,* November 12, 1977, p. 1776.

5.) Jordan Braverman, op. cit., p. 267.

6.) Louis Harris, "Significant Minority Wants National Health Insurance", *The Washington Post,* Washington, DC, January 3, 1978, p. A6.

7.) Ibid.

8.) "Champion Discusses HEW's Upcoming NHI Plan", *Washington Information: National Health Insurance,* November 28, 1977, p. 3.

9.) Milton I. Roemer, "Health Care Systems In World Perspective", Health Administration Press, Ann Arbor, Michigan, 1976, p. 105.

10.) Ibid.

11.) Ibid., pp. 112 & 113.

12.) Ibid., p. 107.

13.) Ibid., p. 108.

14.) Ibid.

15.) Ibid.

16.) Consumer Commission on the Accreditation of Health Services Inc. "National Health Service III", *Health Perspectives,* May-June 1977, p. 6.

17.) Milton I. Roemer, op. cit., p. 110.

18.) "Britain's 'Free' Care Found Costly" *American Medical News,* January 2, 1978, p. 10.

19.) Ibid.

20.) Ibid.

21.) "Private Handling of NHI Favored in Poll", *American Medical News,* June 27/July 4, 1977, p. 22.

In a 1977 poll carried out on national health insurance by the American Medical Association of its physician membership of which 47.5 percent of the 158,000 questionnaires were returned, the following opinions were noted:

● *more than 80 percent of the AMA members think that national health insurance should be handled through private insurers, rather than the federal government*
● *more than 70 percent of the AMA's members agreed that participation in national health insurance (NHI) should be voluntary*
● *the national health insurance plan preferred by more AMA members than any other is that supported by the AMA in Congress. The plan favored by 41.7 percent of the AMA members is one in which individuals would purchase private insurance policies, with the federal government paying the premiums for the poor, and contributing partial payments (based on each family's taxable income) for other groups. Second choice among AMA members for an NHI plan—preferred by 30.3 percent of the members—is one in which the federal government would only provide catastrophic coverage*
● *less one-third (29.0%) believed that employers should be required to participate in an NHI program; but almost half (46.0%) believed employer participation should not be mandatory*
● *a majority of members (54.5%) believed NHI should include both basic and catastrophic health insurance coverage; while 35.6% preferred catastrophic coverage only*
● *81.8% favored NHI handled through private insurers; 70.7% favored voluntary citizen enrollment*
● *a deductible was favored by 55.5% of members, and 31.1% favored a co-insurance feature (where the insured pays a percentage of all medical costs). About the same proportion (30.6%) were undecided about whether coinsurance was desirable or not*
● *the great majority of members (84.4%) preferred that NHI pay physicians under a usual, customary, and reasonable fee basis*
● *more than one-third (37.6%) preferred that the government pay insurance premiums only for special categories, such as the aged, unemployed, or uninsurable; while 35.3% preferred that the government pay graduated proportions of the premiums, based on family income*

22.) "AMA Reaffirms Support For Its Version of NHI", *National Health Insurance Reports*, December 20, 1976, p. 4.

23.) "Nearly Two-Thirds of Businessmen Oppose Compulsory Federal NHI", *Hospitals*, August 1, 1975, p. 17.

24.) "HEW Holds Hearings on National Insurance", *Forum*, November/December 1977, p. 25.

25.) Ibid., pp. 25 & 26.

26.) Saul Waldman, "National Health Insurance Proposals As of February 1976", Social Security Administration, Washington, DC, March 1976, p. 3.

27.) Robert Watkins, "Major Pending Proposals For National Health Insurance" *National Health Insurance Reports*, Washington, DC, November 1975, p. 3.

28.) John K. Iglehart, "Health Care Cost Explosion Squeezes Government Programs, Insurers", *National Journal*, (Health Conference Issue), April 19-30, 1976, p. 5.

29.) Ibid.

30.) Robert Watkins, op. cit., p. 2.

31.) Ibid., p. 3.

32.) Ibid., p. 20.
On January 13, 1977, Senator Clifford P. Hansen and Congressman Tim Lee Carter introduced the Comprehensive Health Care Insurance Act of 1977. This bill, sponsored by the American Medical Association, is nearly identical to that sponsored by the American Medical Association in the 94th Congress. Essentially the bill is based on the requirement that employers make qualified health insurance protection available to employees. The bill also would make qualified coverage available to low income, unemployed, and self-employed individuals as well as provide tax credits to Medicare eligible individuals who want to improve their level of health insurance protection. The major changes from the bill that was introduced in the 94th Congress include the following:
● *the concept of reimbursement for physicians' services at usual, customary and reasonable charges was modified to specify that reimbursement will be based on*

"current" charges that are calculated at least twice each year (on January 1 and on July 1), with each calculation being based on the actual charge data from the preceding six month period
- *benefits were expanded to specifically include services for family planning*
- *hospital reimbursement methods were clarified in order to permit hospital costs to be reimbursed through appropriate methods developed after consultation between the insurance carrier and the providers of hospital services, with a specific role for the state agency being eliminated, with no single system of reimbursement being required for all hospitals within a state, and with reimbursement determinations excluding gifts or endowments received by a hospital*
- *the Hospital Insurance Advisory Board was changed by deleting the word "advisory", increasing the majority of health professionals on the board to at least nine members (including at least seven doctors of medicine, one doctor of osteopathy and one dentist), and allowing the board, rather than the Secretary of HEW, to appoint any necessary advisory committees to the board*

(Washington Information: National Health Insurance: *"AMA's NHI Bill Introduced"*, Washington, DC, February 7, 1977; and Washington Report on Health Legislation, *Summary of H.R. 1818 and S. 218 Comprehensive Health Care Insurance Act of 1977,"* Washington, DC, January 26, 1997, p. 3.)

33.) Saul Waldman, op. cit., p.. 5.
On January 4, 1977, Senator Thomas McIntyre and Representative Omar Burleson introduced the National Health Care Act of 1977, S.5 and H.R.5. The measure was drafted in cooperation with the Health Insurance Association of America which represents the commercial insurance industry. Basically, the bill proposes three voluntary health insurance plans which would include: (1) An   employee-employer plan; (2) An individual plan; and (3) A plan for the poor. All of the plans would provide, after a phasing-in period, a broad range of health care services. The plans would all be administered through private insurance carriers, with overall program supervision being performed by the state and federal governments. Qualified employee-employer plans, and qualified individual plans, would be financed by premium contributions, and contributions would receive tax advantages. The plan for the poor would be financed primarily by federal and state general revenues. The bill also includes provisions designed to stimulate the development of ambulatory care centers and increase the supply of health manpower.
   The bill contains some major changes from the measure introduced in the 94th Congress. These include:
- *the benefits structure has been revised to substantially encourage ambulatory and preventive care, especially the use of outpatient facilities for diagnostic x-rays and laboratory tests. To do this, the new bill would prohibit the application of any deductibles or co-payments to outpatient diagnostic x-rays and laboratory tests, well baby care to age six, annual dental exams to age 13 and prenatal checkup for each trimester of pregnancy. Conversely the bill would allow, but not require, a separate hospital deductible equal to room and board charge for the first day of hospitalization and would limit benefits for psychiatric confinements to 90 days per year*
- *the reimbursement provisions have been changed to deny the payment of benefits for services or facilities which are required to have certificate-of-need, but for which no certificates have been issued*
- *the definition of outpatient mental health facilities has been expanded to make more such facilities eligible for benefit payments*
- *the home health services benefit has been expanded by eliminating the 14 day requirement*
- *benefits have been expanded to include the purchase, as well as rental, of durable medical equipment*
- *prenatal benefits, without deductible or co-payments, have been added*
- *a provision has been added to require employers to pay at least one-half of the premium cost of a qualified health plan*
- *the definition of eligible employee has been broadened to include employees who have worked at least 20 hours per week for more than two consecutive calendar months, in addition to full time employees*
- *an assignment of benefits provision has been added which would permit benefits to be assigned to a physician only if the physician agrees to accept assignments for all of his patients all of the time and the names of such participating physicians would be made known to the public*

• *the PSRO program would be expanded to serve all patients, with the costs of PSRO review being included as a valid expense of the provider, rather than as a separate charge to the patient by the PSRO*
• *the National Health Planning and Resources Development Act (P. L.93-641) would be changed to provide that insurers be guaranteed representation on Health Systems Agency boards, that Health Systems Agencies be empowered to recommend the decertification of existing health care facilities, that federal funds be provided to finance the closing of unnecessary hospital facilities, and that ambulatory health care centers and diagnostic centers (but not physicians' offices) be subject to certificate-of-need legislation*
• *the health manpower development section of the bill has been reduced in recognition of the health manpower legislation passed by the 94th Congress*
(Washington Information: National Health Insurance, *"HIAA's NHI Plan Introduced", Washington, DC, February 7, 1977, pp. 3 & 4.)*

34.) Robert Watkins, op. cit., p. 12.
On January 4, 1977, Senator Edward M. Kennedy and Representative James C. Corman introduced the Health Security Act, S.1 and H.R.21. This bill, strongly backed by the AFL-CIO, is virtually identical to that introduced two years ago by Senator Kennedy and Congressman Corman. The only noteworthy change is the addition of clarifying language to Section 83, subsection (a), dealing with hospital reimbursement. (Washington Report on Health Legislation," *Summary of S.1, H.R.21, The Health Security Act", Washington, DC, January 5, 1977, p. 3.)*

35.) Harry Paxton, "Government Controls: Your Prospects Under National Health Insurance", *Medical Economics*, September 29, 1975, p. 144.
On May 18, 1978, Senators Long, Ribicoff, Talmadge and Dole introduced the Catastrophic Health Insurance and Medical Assistance Reform Act. The bill (S.3105) is identical to the measure introduced in the 94th Congress except for changes in effective dates and the income levels for eligibility. The program for low-income persons would be based on annual incomes: under $3,000 for an individual, and under $4,000 for a two-person family, gradually rising to account for increases in family size. The bill would provide catastrophic health insurance, effective January 1, 1980, for all Americans after they had incurred medical expenses of $2,000 or had been hospitalized for 60 days. There is also a medical assistance plan for the poor and a voluntary certification plan. The catastrophic health insurance plan would be financed through a one-percent payroll tax on employers.

36.) The Committee for National Health Insurance, "Why We Need A National Health Security Program", Washington,DC, 1977, p. 25.

37.) Bert Seidman, "Health Security: The Complete RX", *AFL-CIO American Federationist.* October 1975, p. 3 (a reprint).

38.) Harry Paxton, op. cit., pp. 131 & 133.

39.) Ibid., p. 135.

40.) I.S. Falk, "National Health Insurance for the United States", *Public Health Reports,* September/October 1977 p. 405.

41.) "Too Much Surgery by Nonspecialists?", *The Washington Star,* Washington, DC, November 21, 1976, p. A-11; *Rita J. Nickerson et al.,* "Doctors Who Perform Operations", *The New England Journal of Medicine,* October 21, 1976, pp. 921-926 (Part I) and October 28, 1967, pp. 982-988 (Part II).

42.) Saul Waldman, op. cit., pp. 129 & 130.

43.) Harry Schwartz, "Health Insurance: A Fight for Survival", *New York Times,* October 30, 1977, p. 3f.

CHAPTER 9

1.) "Health Cost Rise Pinned To Doctors", *Medical World News,* April 17, 1978, p. 37.

2.) "Doctors Gave Fewer Shots When Watched", *The Washington Star*, Washington, DC, October 11, 1976, p. A-6.

3.) Patrick J. Doyle, "Save Your Health & Your Money", Acropolis Books, Washington, DC, 1971, p. 9.

4.) Deborah Rankin, "Doctors Find Big Expenses Cut Into Their High Incomes", *New York Times,* May 15, 1978, p. 1.

A Glossary of Health Care Terminology

Within recent years, the quality and costs of health care services in this nation has become the subject of a national debate whether the discussions center on hospital costs, physician fees, fraud and abuse in government health programs, private health insurance, medical malpractice lawsuits, national health insurance or prescription drugs. When the discussions take place, they often use terminology which the consumer-patient does not always comprehend, even though he himself is often-times the subject of the debates. This situation is very understandable since health care is a topic that consists of many disciplines. These include economics, political science, sociology, business administration, computer sciences, insurance, law, hospital administration, public administration and many more. Consequently, in order to provide the consumer-patient with such a definitional understanding, the following glossary is presented. The glossary was excerpted from the following publication:

U.S. House of Representatives, "A Discursive Dictionary of Health Care", Subcommittee on Health and the Environment of the Committee on Interstate and Foreign Commerce, Washington, D.C., February, 1976, pp. 1-168.

In the ensuing glossary you will find definitions for such terms as:

antisubstitution laws	generic drugs
catastrophic health insurance	group practice
certificate-of-need	health maintenance
comprehensive health planning	organizations
community rating	health systems agency
copayment	major medical
deductible	prospective reimbursement
defensive medicine	socialized medicine
experience rating	third party payer
first-dollar coverage	vendor payment

The definitions, prepared by the Subcommittee staff, are not considered final nor official nor exhaustive. Nevertheless, the House Subcommittee felt that the definitions are sufficiently complete and accurate throughout to explain the specialized uses these concepts represent. And, with such knowledge, you can participate as a consumer-patient in the national health dialogue being conducted today and contribute to improving the system in a way which will render quality care at reasonable costs not only to yourself, but also to the rest of consumers making up our population.

A

abuse: improper or excessive use of program benefits, resources or services by either providers or consumers. Abuse can occur, intentionally or unintentionally, when services are used which are excessive or unnecessary; which are not the appropriate treatment for the patient's condition; when cheaper treatment would be as effective; or when billing or charging does not conform to requirements. It should be distinguished from *fraud,* in which deliberate deceit is used by providers or consumers to obtain payment for services which were not actually delivered or received, or to claim program eligibility. Abuse is not necessarily either intentional or illegal.

acceptability: an individual's (or group's) overall assessment of medical care available to him. The individual appraises such things as the cost, *quality,* results, and convenience of care, and provider attitudes in determining the acceptability of health services provided.

access: an individual's (or group's) ability to obtain medical care. Access has geographic, financial, social, ethnic and psychic components and is thus very difficult to define and measure operationally. Many government health programs have as their goal improving access to care for specific groups or equity of access in the whole population. Access is also a function of the *availability* of health services, and their *acceptability.* In practice access, availability and acceptability, which collectively describe the things which determine the care people use, are very hard to differentiate.

accident and health insurance: *insurance* under which benefits are payable in case of *disease,* accidental *injury,* or, in some cases, accidental death.

acquisition cost: the immediate cost of selling, underwriting, and issuing a new *insurance policy,* including clerical costs, agents' commissions, advertising, and medical inspection fees. Also refers to the cost paid by a pharmacist or other retailer to a manufacturer or wholesaler for a supply of *drugs.*

actual charge: the amount a physician or other practitioner actually bills a patient for a particular medical service or procedure. The actual *charge* may differ from the *customary, prevailing,* and or *reasonable charges* under *Medicare* and other insurance programs.

actuary: in *insurance,* a person trained in statistics, accounting, and mathematics who determines policy *rates, reserves,* and dividends by deciding what assumptions should be made with respect to each of the risk factors involved (such as the frequency of occurrence of the *peril,* the average benefit that will be payable, the rate of investment earnings, if any, *expenses,* and *persistency* rates), and who endeavors to secure as valid statistics as possible on which to base his assumptions.

acute disease: *a disease* which is characterized by a single episode of a fairly short duration from which the *patient* returns to his normal or previous state and level of activity. While acute diseases are frequently distinguished from *chronic diseases,* there is no standard definition or distinction. It is worth noting that an acute episode of a chronic disease (an episode of diabetic coma in a patient with diabetes) is often treated as an acute disease.

adverse selection: *disproportionate insurance* of *risks* who are poorer or more prone to suffer *loss* or make claims than the average risk. It may result from the tendency for poorer risks or less desirable *insureds* (sick people) to seek or continue insurance to a greater extent than do better risks (healthy people), or from the tendency for the insured to take advantage of favorable options in insurance contracts. Favorable, as compared to adverse, selection, when intentional, is called *skimming*.

affiliation: an agreement (usually formal) between two or more otherwise independent programs or individuals which defines how they will relate to each other. Affiliation agreements may specify: procedures for referring or transferring *patients* from one facility to another; joint faculty and/or medical staff appointments; teaching relationships; sharing of records or services; or provision of *consultation* between programs.

aggregate indemnity: the maximum dollar amount payable for any *disability,* period of disability, or covered service under an *insurance policy.*

allied health personnel: specially trained and *licensed* (when necessary) health workers other than *physicians, dentists, podiatrists* and *nurses.* The term has no constant or agreed upon detailed meaning: sometimes being used synonymously with *para-medical personnel;* sometimes meaning all health workers who perform tasks which must otherwise be performed by a physician; and sometimes referring to health workers who do not usually engage in independent practice.

allocated benefit provision: a provision in an *insurance policy* under which payment for certain *benefits* (such as miscellaneous hospital and medical services like X-rays, dressings and drugs) will be made at a rate for each specified (scheduled) in the provision. Usually there is also a maximum that will be paid for all such expenses. An allocated benefit is one which is subject to such a provision. In an unallocated benefit provision no specification is given of how much will be paid for each type of service although the provision sets a maximum payable for all the listed services.

allowable charge: generic term referring to the maximum fee that a *third party* will use in reimbursing a *provider* for a given service. An allowable charge may not be the same as either a *reasonable, customary* or *prevailing charge* as the terms are used under the *Medicare* program.

allowable costs: items or elements of an institution's costs which are reimbursable under a payment formula. Both *Medicare* and *Medicaid* reimburse hospitals on the basis of certain costs, but do not allow reimbursement for all costs. Allowable costs may exclude for example, uncovered services, luxury accommodations, costs which are not *reasonable,* expenditures which are unnecessary in the efficient delivery of health services to persons covered under the program in question (it would not be allowable to reimburse costs under Medicare involved in providing services to newborn infants), or depreciation on a capital expenditure which was disapproved by a health planning agency.

ambulatory care: all types of health services which are provided on an *outpatient* basis, in contrast to services provided in the home or to persons who are *inpatients.* While many inpatients may be ambulatory, the term ambulatory care usually implies that the patient has come to a location other than his home to receive services and has departed the same day.

ancillary services: hospital, or other inpatient health program, services other than room and board, and *professional* services. They may include X-ray, *drug,* laboratory or other services not separately itemized, but the specific content is quite variable.

annual implementation plan (AIP): a plan, which the National Health Planning and Resources Development Act of 1974 (P. L. 93—641) requires *health systems agencies* to prepare or update annually, specifying, describing how to implement, and giving priority to short-run *objectives* which will achieve the long range *goals* of the agency, detailed in its *health system plan.* Section 1513 of the PHS Act describes the place of AIP's in the larger context of agency functioning.

antibiotic: any *drug* containing any quantity of any chemical substance produced by a microorganism which has the capacity, in dilute solution, to inhibit the growth of, or to destroy, bacteria and other microorganisms (or a chemically synthesized equivalent of such a substance). Antibiotics are used in the *treatment* of infectious diseases.

anti-substitution laws: State laws that require the pharmacist to "dispense as written." The effect is to prohibit a pharmacist from substituting a different *brand name drug* for the one prescribed, or from substituting a *generic equivalent drug* in place of a *drug* prescribed by brand name, even if the drug that would be substituted is considered to be *therapeutically equivalent* to the drug prescribed and perhaps is less expensive. Drug reimbursement programs such as the *Maximum Allowable Cost Program,* which will limit reimbursement to the lowest cost at which a drug is generally available, will be more effective if they override anti-substitution laws.

areawide comprehensive health planning agency (area wide CHP, or 314(b) agency) a sub-state (usually multi-county) agency assisted under section 314(b) of the *PHS Act,* created by the Comprehensive Health Planning and Public Health Service Amendments of 1966 (P. L. 89-749), and charged with the preparation of regional or local plans for the coordination and development of existing and new health services, facilities, and manpower. The agencies were authorized to review and comment upon proposals from hospitals and other institutions for development of programs and expansion of facilities, but had no significant powers of enforcement. Up to three quarters of the operating costs of the 314(b) agencies could be supported by Federal *project grants.* The balance of the costs were obtained from voluntary contributions from any source, including the health care providers affected by the agencies' plans. Under the provisions of the new health planning law, P. L. 93-641, existing 314(b) agencies will be replaced by *health systems agencies* which will have expanded duties and powers.

assessment: in *insurance,* a charge upon *carriers* ro raise funds for a specific purpose (such as meeting the administrative costs of a government required program) made by government (usually State government) or a special organization authorized by government, and provided for in law or regulation. Applied to all carriers handling a specific line of coverage subject to regulation by the government in question and based upon a formula.

assigned risk: a *risk* which *underwriters* do not care to insure (such as a person with hypertension seeking health insurance) but which, because of State law or otherwise must be insured. Insuring assigned risks is usually handled through a group of insurers (such as all companies licensed to issue health insurance in the State) and individual assigned risks are assigned to the companies in turn or in proportion to their share of the State's total health insurance business. Assignments of risks is common in casualty insurance and less common in health insurance. As an approach to providing insurance to such risks, it can be contrasted with pooling of such risks (see *insurance pool*) in which the *losses* rather than the risks are distributed among the group of insurers.

assignment: an agreement in which a *patient* assigns to another party, usually a *provider,* the right to receive payment from a *third-party* for the service the patient has received. Assignment is used instead of a patient paying directly for the service and then receiving reimbursement from public or private insurance programs. In *Medicare,* if a physician accepts assignment from the patient, he must agree to accept the program payment in full (except for specific *coinsurance, copayment* and *deductible* amounts required of the patient). Assignment, then, protects the patient against liability for charges which · the Medicare program will not recognize as *reasonable.* Under some *national health insurance* proposals physicians must agree to assignment for all of their patients or none of them; under Medicare, physicians may choose assignment for some of their patients, but not others, and may do so on a claim by claim basis for some services but not others.

Assisted Health Insurance Plan (AHIP): one of three parts of the Ford administration's proposal for *national health insurance,* the *Comprehensive Health Insurance Plan.* AHIP is designed to provide health insurance coverage for low *income* and high medical risk people. It would be available to anyone electing coverage, at a premium no greater than 150 percent of the average group premium for private health insurance in the State. Premiums and *cost sharing* would be *indexed* to income. AHIP would replace *Medicaid* and would be State administered under contract with fiscal *intermediaries.* Benefits under AHIP would be identical to those under *EHIP* and *FHIP.* The plan would be financed by premiums, and subsidized by State and Federal revenues under a matching formula.

at risk: the state of being subject to some uncertain event occurring which connotes loss or difficulty. In the financial sense, this refers to an individual, organization (like an *HMO*) or insurance company assuming the chance of loss—through running the risk of having to provide or pay for more *services* than paid for through *premiums* of per capita payments. If payments are adjusted after the fact so that no loss can occur, then there is no risk. In fact, losses incurred in one year may be made up by increases in premiums or per capita payments in the next year, so the 'risk' is somewhat tempered. A firm which is at risk for losses also stands to gain from *profits* if costs are less than premiums collected. For a *consumer* being financially at risk usually means being without insurance or at risk for substantial *out-of-pocket* expenses. A second use of the term relates to the special vulnerability of certain populations to certain diseases or conditions; ghetto children are at risk for lead poisoning or rat bite; workers in coal mines are at risk for *black lung* disease.

availability: a measure (in terms of type, volume and location) of the *supply* of health resources and services relative to the *needs* (or *demands*) of a given individual or community. Health care is available to an individual when he can obtain it at the time and place that he *needs* it, from *appropriate* personnel. Availability is a function of the distribution of appropriate resources and services, and the willingness of the *provider* to serve the particular *patient* in need.

B

basic health services: the minimum *supply* of health *services* which should be generally and uniformly *available* in order to assure adequate *health status* and protection of the population from *disease,* or to meet some other *criteria* or *standards.* Given that all possible services cannot be supplied to the entire population, it is surprising how little definition or discussion there has been of what set of services constitutes an *appropriate* minimum and of how to assure its availability. A beginning has been made in Federal *policy* with the definition of *re-*

quired services for *Medicaid* and basic health services required of *HMO's* for Federal assistance or *qualification.* These include: *physician* services, *hospital* services, medically *necessary emergency care, preventive health* services, *home health* services, up to 20 *visits* of *outpatient mental health* services, medical *treatment* and *referral* services for *alcoholism* and *drug abuse,* and laboratory and radiologic services (section 1302(1) of the *PHS Act*). Where a minimum is defined, a higher level of service is usually also defined (*supplemental health* and *optional services* for HMO's and Medicaid, respectively). It is not clear in either case whether the higher level is thought of as all other, all other *needed* or all other *affordable services.*

bed: literally a bed in a *hospital* or other inpatient health facility. Many definitions require that the beds be maintained for continuous (24 hour) use by *inpatients.* Beds are often used as a measure of capacity (hospital sizes are compared by comparing their number of beds). *Licenses* and *certificates-of-need* may be granted for specific numbers or types of beds: e.g. surgical, pediatric, obstetric, or extended care. Facilities may have both licensed and unlicensed beds; and active and licensed but unused beds. Other qualifying adjectives are frequently used to categorize beds: e.g. available, occupied, *acute care* or observation beds.

beneficiary: a person who is eligible to receive, or is receiving, *benefits* from an *insurance policy* (usually) or *health maintenance organization* (occasionally). Usually includes both people who have themselves contracted for benefits and their eligible *dependents.*

benefit: in *insurance,* a sum of money provided in an *insurance policy* payable for certain types of *loss,* or for covered services, under the terms of the policy. The benefits may be paid to the *insured* or on his behalf to others. In *prepayment* programs, like *HMOs,* benefits are the services the program will provide a *member* whenever, and to the extent *needed.*

benefit period: the period of time for which payments for *benefits* covered by an *insurance policy* are available. The availability of certain benefits may be limited over a specified time period, for example two well-baby visits during a one-year period. While the benefit period is usually defined by a set unit of time, such as a year, benefits may also be tied to a *spell of illness.*

bioavailability: the extent and rate of absorption of a dose of a given *drug,* measured by the time-concentration curve for appearance of the administered drug in the blood. The concept is important in attempting to determine whether different *brand name* drugs, a *generic name,* as opposed to a brand name drug, or, in some cases, different batches of the same brand name drug, will produce the same *therapeutic effect.* The same drug made by two different manufacturers or different batches of the same drug made by the same manufacturer may demonstrate differing bioavailability. There is controversy as to whether such differences are therapeutically significant.

bioequivalence: described drug preparations which have the same *bioavailability.* Such *drugs* are *chemically equivalent* (indistinguishable by chemical means) although chemically equivalent preparations are not always bioequivalent. Bioequivalence is a function off bioavailability and the terms are often used synonymously. Chemically equivalent drugs which are bioequivalent are *therapeutically equivalent* (have the same treatment effect), although therapeutically equivalent preparations need not be either chemically or bioequivalent.

blanket medical expense: a provision (usually included as an added feature of a policy primarily providing some other type of coverage, such as loss of income insurance) which entitles the *insured* to collect, up to a maximum established in the policy, for all hospital and medical expenses incurred, without limitations on individual types of medical expenses.

Blue Cross Association (BCA): the national non-profit organization to which the 70 *Blue Cross plans* in the United States voluntarily belong. BCA administers programs of *licensure* and approval for Blue Cross plans, provides specific services related to the writing and administering of health care benefits across the country, and represents the Blue Cross plans in national affairs. Under contract with the *Social Security Administration* (SSA), BCA is *intermediary* in the *Medicare* program for 77 percent of the *participating providers* (90 percent of the participating *hospitals,* 50 percent of the participating *skilled nursing*

facilities, and 76 percent of the participating *home health agencies*).

Blue Cross plan: a nonprofit, tax-exempt health service *prepayment* organization providing coverage for health care and related services. The individual plans should be distinguished from their national association, the *Blue Cross Association.* Historically, the plans were largely the creation of the hospital industry, and designed to provide hospitals with a stable source of revenues, although formal association between the Blue Cross and American Hospital Associations ended in 1972. A Blue Cross plan must be a nonprofit community service organization with a governing body with a membership including a majority of public representatives. Most plans are regulated by State *insurance commissioners* under special enabling legislation. Plans are exempt from Federal income taxes, and, in most States, from State taxes (both property and premium). Unlike most private insurance companies, the plans usually provide *service* rather than *indemnity benefits,* and often pay hospitals on the basis of *reasonable costs* rather than *charges.* There are 70 plans in the United States.

Blue Shield plan: a nonprofit, tax-exempt plan of a type originally established in 1939 which provides coverage of physician's services. The individual plans should be distinguished from the National Association of Blue Shield Plans. Blue Shield coverage is commonly sold in conjunction with *Blue Cross* coverage, although this is not always the case. The relationship between Blue Cross and Blue Shield plans has been a cooperative one; it iss not uncommon for the two organizations to have a common board, one management, and to be located in the same building. Blue Shield plans cover some 65 million Americans through their group and individual business. In addition, plan activities affect some 20 million persons through participation in various government programs, including *Medicare* (32 plans act as *carriers* under part B), *Medicaid, and CHAMPUS.* Most States have enacted special enabling legislation for the Blue plans.

board certified: describes a *physician* or other health *professional* who has passed an examination given by a medical *specialty board* and been *certified* by that board as a specialist in the subject in question. The examination cannot be taken until the professional meets requirements set by the specialty board for *board eligibility.*

brand name: the registered trademark given *to a specific drug* product by its manufacturer. Also known as a *trade name.* As an example, there is a widely-prescribed broad-spectrum antibiotic with the *generic* or *established name* of tetracycline hydrochloride. Its *chemical name* is 4-dimethylamino–1, 4, 4a, 5, 5a, 6, 11, 12a–octahydro–3, 6, 10, 12, 12a–pentahydroxy–6–methyl–11–dioxo–2naphthacenecarboxamide hydrochloride. Its chemical formula is $C_{22}H_{24}N_2O_5HCL$. This drug is marketed by Lederle Laboratories under the brand name "Achromycin", by Bristol-Myers under "Bristacycline", by Robins as "Robitet", by Squibb as "Sumycin", and so on. There are no official rules governing the selection of brand names. According to the Pharmaceutical Manufacturers Association, the objective is to coin a name which is "useful, dignified, easily remembered, and individual or proprietary." Drugs are primarily advertised to practitioners by brand name. When a physician prescribes by brand name, *anti-substitution laws* in most States forbid the pharmacist from substituting either a brand or generic name equivalent made by a different manufacturer, although either may be less expensive than the drug prescribed.

C

capital expenditure review (CER): review of proposed *capital* expenditures of hospitals and/or other health facilities to determine the *need* for, and *appropriateness* of, the proposed expenditures. The review is done by a designated *regulatory* agency such as a *State health planning and development agency* and has a sanction attached which prevents (see *certificate-of-need*) or discourages (see *section 1122*) unneeded expenditures.

capitation: a method of payment for health services in which an individual or institutional provider is paid a fixed, per capita amount for each person served without regard to the actual number or nature of services provided to each person. Capitation is characteristic of *health maintenance organizations* but unusual for physicians (see *fee-for-service*). Also, a method of

Federal support of health professional schools authorized by the Comprehensive Health Manpower Training Act of 1971, P. L. 92-157, and the Nurse Training Act of 1971, P. L. 92-158 (sections 770 and 810 of the PHS Act), in which each eligible school receives a fixed capitation payment from the Federal government for each student enrolled, called a capitation grant.

carrier: a commercial health *insurer,* a government agency, or a *Blue Cross* or *Blue Shield* plan which *underwrites* or administers programs that pay for health services. Under the *Medicare Part B (Supplemental Medical Insurance) Program* and the *Federal Employees Health Benefits Programs,* carriers are agencies and organizations with which the program contacts for administration of various functions, including payment of *claims.*

catastrophic health insurance: health insurance which provides protection against the high cost of treating severe or lengthy *illnesses* or *disabilities.* Generally such policies cover all or a specified percentage of medical expenses above an amount that is the responsibility of the insured himself (or the responsibility of another insurance policy up to a maximum limit of liability). Under pending *NHI* proposals of this type, protection would typically begin after an individual or family unit had incurred medical expenses equal to a specified dollar amount (e.g., $2,000 within a 12-month period) or a specified percentage of *income* (e.g., fifteen percent); or had been in a medical institution for a specified period (e.g., 60 days). Individuals would be liable for all costs up to the specified limits. However, in the absence of any effective prohibition against doing so, they could be expected to obtain health insurance protection for costs below the catastrophic limits. Generally there is no maximum amount of coverage under these plans; however, many include some *coinsurance.*

categorically needy: persons who are both members of certain categories of groups eligible to receive public assistance, and economically needy. As used in *Medicaid,* this means a person who is aged, blind, disabled, or a member of a family with children under 18 (or 21, if in school) where one parent is absent, incapacitated or unemployed and, in addition, meets specified *income* and *resources* requirements which vary by State. In general, categorically needy individuals are persons receiving cash assistance under the AFDC or *SSI* programs. A State must cover all recipients of AFDC payments under Medicaid; however, it is provided certain options (based, in large measure, on its coverage levels under the old Federal/State welfare programs) in determining the extent of coverage for persons receiving Federal SSI and/or State *supplementary SSI payments*. In addition, a State may cover additional specified groups, such as foster children, as categorically needy. A State may restrict its Medicaid coverage to this group or may cover additional persons who meet the categorical requirements as *medically needy*.

categorically related: in the *Medicaid* program, the requirements (other than *income* and *resources*) which an individual must meet in order to be eligible for Medicaid benefits; also individuals who meet these requirements. Specifically, any individual eligible for Medicaid must fall into one of the four main categories of people who are eligible for welfare cash payments. He must be "aged", "blind", or "disabled" (as defined under the *Supplemental Security Income Program*, title XVI of the Social Security Act) or a member of a family with dependent children where one parent is absent, incapacitated, or unemployed (as defined under the Aid to Families with Dependent Children Program, Title IV of the Social Security Act). After the determination is made that an individual is categorically related, than income and resources tests are applied to determine if the individual is poor enough to be eligible for assistance *(categorically needy)*. As a result of this requirement, single persons and childless couples who are not aged, blind or disabled and male-headed families in States which do not cover such groups under their AFDC programs cannot receive Medicaid coverage no matter how poor they are.

categorical program: originally, a health program which concerned itself with research, education, control and/or *treatment* of only one of a few specific *diseases*. Now more generally used for a program concerned with only a part, instead of all, of the population or health system. Even more generally used by the present administration to refer to any existing program which it feels the Federal government should cease to support.

certificate-of-need or necessity: a certificate issued by a governmental body to an individual or organization proposing to construct or modify a *health facility*, or offer a new or different health *service*, which recognizes that such facility or service when available will be *needed* by those for whom it is intended. Where a certificate is required (for instance for all proposals which will involve more than a minimum *capital* investment or change *bed* capacity), it is a condition of *licensure* of the facility or service; and is intended to control expansion of facilities and services in the public interest by preventing excessive or duplicative development of facilities and services. An example of *capital expenditure review*, certificate of need for construction of new *hospitals* is a requirement of law in 23 States and the District of Columbia. Under the National Health Planning and Resources Development Act of 1974, P.L. 93-641, all States are required to have the *State Health planning and development agency* (designated pursuant to the law) administer a State certificate of need program, which must apply to all new *institutional health services* proposed to be offered or developed in the State. The *health systems agencies* (local planning bodies under P.L. 93-641) are required to make recommendations to the State agencies regarding proposed new institutional health services within their areas.

charges: prices assigned to units of medical service, such as a visit to a physician or a day in a hospital. Charges for services may not be related to the actual *costs* of providing the services. Further, the methods by which charges are related to costs vary substantially from service to service and institution to institution. Different *third party* payers may require use of different methods of determining either charges or costs. Charges for one service provided by an institution are often used to subsidize the costs of other services. Charges to one type or group of patients may also be used to subsidize the costs of providing services to other groups.

chemical equivalents: *drug* products from different sources which contain essentially identical amounts of the identical active ingredients in identical dosage forms, meet existing physiochemical *standards* in official *compendia,* and are therefore chemically indistinguishable. See also *bioequivalence.*

chemical name: the exact description of the chemical structure of a *drug*, based on the rules of standard chemical nomenclature, such as the tranquilizer with the chemical name 2–methyl–2–propyl, 3–propenediol dicarbamate. While long and cumbersome, this name is also precise, serving as a complete identification of the compound to any trained chemist. It is related to the chemical formula of the particular drug—

$$H_2NCOO-CH_2-\underset{\underset{CH_2CH_2CH_3}{|}}{\overset{\overset{CH_3}{|}}{C}}-CH_2-OOCNH_2$$

This drug is known *generically* as meprobamate. It is sold under various *brand names* by different firms, such as Miltown, Equanil, Pathibamate, and SK-Bamate.

chronic disease: *diseases* which have one or more of the following characteristics: are permanent; leave residual *disability;* are caused by nonreversible pathological alteration; require special training of the patient for *rehabilitation;* or may be expected to require a long period of supervision, observation or care.

Civilian Health and Medical Program of the Uniformed Services (CHAMPUS): a program, administered by the Department of Defense, without *premium* but with *cost -sharing* provisions, which pays for care delivered by civilian health providers to retired members, and *dependents* of active and retired members, of the seven uniformed services of the United States (Army, Navy, Air Force, Marine Corps, Commissioned Corps of the Public Health Service, Coast Guard, and the National Oceanic and Atmospheric Administration).

claim: a request to an *insurer* by an *insured* person (or, on his behalf, by the provider of a service or good) for payment of benefits under an *insurance policy.*

claims incurred policy: the conventional form of *malpractice insurance*, under which the *insured* is covered for any claims arising from an incident which occurred or is alleged to have occurred during the policy period, regardless of when the claim is made. The only limiting factors are the *statutes of limitations,* which vary from State to State. An alternative type of policy is the *claims made policy.*

claims made policy: a form of *malpractice insurance* gaining increasing popularity among *insurers* because it increases the accuracy of rate-making. In this type of policy the *insured* is covered for any claim made, rather than any *injury* occurring, while the policy is in force. Claims made after the insurance lapses are not covered as they are by a *claims incurred policy.* This type of policy was initially resisted by *providers* because of the nature of medical malpractice claims, which may arise several years after an injury occurs (see *discovery rule*). A retired physician, for example, could be sued and not covered, unless special provisions are made to continue his coverage beyond his years of *practice.* There are also retrospective problems for providers who switch from a conventional policy to a claims made policy, since the latter policy would not cover claims arising from events occurring during the years when the conventional policy was in effect. Insurers marketing such policies are now offering providers the opportunity to purchase insurance for both contingencies.

claims review: review of *claims* by governments, *medical foundations, PSROs, insurers* or others responsible for payment to determine liability and amount of payment. This review may include determination of the eligibility of the claimant or *beneficiary;* of the eligibility of the *provider* of the *benefit;* that the benefit for which payment is claimed is covered; that the benefit is not payable under another policy (see *coordination of benefits*); and that the benefit was *necessary* and of *reasonable cost* and *quality.*

clinic: a *facility,* or part of one, for *diagnosis* and *treatment* of *out-patients.* Clinic is irregularly defined, sometimes either including or excluding physicians' offices, sometimes being limited to facilities in which *graduate* or *undergraduate medical education* is done.

coinsurance: a *cost-sharing* requirement under a health insurance policy which provides that the *insured* will assume a portion or percentage of the costs of covered services. The health insurance policy provides that the *insurer* will reimburse a specified percentage (usually 80 percent) of all, or certain specified covered medical expenses in excess of any *deductible* amounts payable by the insured. The insured is then liable for the remaining percentage of the costs, until the maximum amount payable under the insurance policy, if any, is reached.

community rating: a method of establishing *premiums* for health *insurance* in which the premium is based on the average cost of actual or anticipated health care used by all *subscribers* in a specific geographic area or industry and does not vary for different groups or subgroups of subscribers or with such variables as the group's *claims* experience, age, sex, or *health status.* The *HMO* Act (section 1302(8) of the PHS Act) defines community rating as a system of fixing rates of payments for health services which may be determined on a per person or per family basis "and may vary with the number of persons in a family, but must be equivalent for all individuals and for all families with similar composition." The intent of community rating is to spread the cost of illness evenly over all *subscribers* (the whole community) rather than charging the sick more than the healthy for health insurance. Community rating is the exceptional means of establishing health insurance premiums in the United States today. The *Federal Employee's Health Benefits Program* for example is *experience rated,* not community rated.

comparability provision: a provision in *Medicare* specifying that the *reasonable charge* for a service may not be higher than *charges* payable for comparable services insured under comparable circumstances by a *carrier* for its non-Medicare *beneficiaries* (see section 1842(b)(3)(B) of the Social Security Act).

compendium: a collection of information about *drugs.* Under the Federal Food, Drug, and Cosmetic Act, *standards* for strength, *quality,* and purity of drugs are those which are set forth in one of the three official compendia: the United States Pharmacopeia, the Homeopathic Pharmacopeia of the United States, the National Formulary, or any supplement to any of them. Since the mid-1960s, publication by the FDA of a compendium has been proposed which would compile the *labeling* of all marketed drugs, to improve the amount and quality of information on drugs that is available to physicians or pharmacists as an aid in prescribing or dispensing. The compendium would consist of one or more volumes and would probably resemble an expanded version of the popular *Physicians' Desk Reference,* a private compendium in which drug manufacturers must purchase space and which does not provide information on all drugs.

comprehensive health planning (CHP): health planning which encompasses all factors and programs which impact on people's *health.* Federally assisted CHP was done on a geographic basis by *areawide* and *State CHP agencies* which had authority to concern themselves with environmental and *occupational health,* health education, and personal health behavior as well as medical resources and services. CHP was initiated by the Comprehensive Health Planning and Public Health Services Amendments of 1966, P. L. 89–749, and replaced by the National Health Planning and Resources Development Act of 1974, P. L. 93–641. CHP was also noteworthy for the fact that the planning was guided by a council–a majority of whose members were health services *consumers.*

compulsory: used in connection with coverage under proposed *national health insurance* or other health insurance plans which require coverage to be offered or taken. A plan may be compulsory only for an employer (coverage must be offered to employees and a specified portion of the *premium* paid, if they opt to take itt) or for individuals as well. Any universal public plan is necessarily compulsory in that the payment of taxes to support the plan is not optional with the individual.

concurrent review: review of the medical *necessity* of *hospital* or other health facility *admissions* upon or within a short period following an admission and the periodic review of services provided during the course of *treatment.* The initial review usually assigns an appropriate *length of stay* to the admission (using *diagnosis* specific *criteria*) which may also be reassessed periodically. Where concurrent review is required, payment for unneeded hospitalizations or services is usually denied, HEW recently issued *utilization review rules* which would have required concurrent review (defined as review within one working day of admission) of all *Medicare* and

Medicaid cases after July 1, 1975. Admissions which were found unnecessary would not have been reimbursed under either Medicare or Medicaid beyond three days after this finding. As a result of suit by the AMA against implementation of certain portions of these regulations, particularly the concurrent review requirement, implementation of the requirements was enjoined by temporary injunction. HEW is rewriting the regulations. Under the enjoined regulations, review was to be conducted by a physician member or by a qualified nonphysician member of the committee or group assigned the utilization review responsibility in each hospital. Such individual was to be appropriately trained and qualified to perform the assigned review functions, and the review was to use criteria selected or developed by the hospital *utilization review committee* or group. Concurrent review should be contrasted with a retrospective *medical audit,* which is done for *quality* purposes and does not relate to payment, and *claims review,* which occurs after the hospitalization is over.

Consumer Price Index (CPI): an economic index prepared by the Bureau of Labor Statistics of the U. S. Department of Labor. It measures the change in average prices of the goods and services purchased by urban wage earners and clerical workers and their families. It is widely used as an indicator of changes in the cost of living, as a measure of inflation (and deflation, if any) in the economy, and as a means for studying trends in prices of various goods and services. The CPI is made up of several components which measure prices in different sectors of the economy. One of these, the medical care component, gives trends in medical care *charges* based on specific indicators of hospital, medical, dental and drug prices. The medical care component of the CPI characteristically rises faster than the CPI itself as do some other service components of the index. However, since the CPI measures charges, which are not always related to *costs,* the CPI may fail to accurately reflect changes in medical care costs.

contingency fees: fees based or conditioned on future occurrences or conclusions, or on the results of services to be performed. Contingency fees are used by lawyers representing patients as plaintiffs in *malpractice* cases and are usually a set fraction (commonly a third) of any settlement awarded the patient. If no settlement is awarded, the lawyer is not paid. Such fees are said to give the lawyer incentives to try the case with full vigor, choose only cases which are likely to succeed, choose not only cases which will have large settlements, and increase the amount of settlements sought.

contributory insurance: *group insurance* in which all or part of the *premium* is paid by the employee, the remainder, if any, being paid by the employer or union. In this context, noncontributory insurance is insurance in which the employer pays all the premium. So called because the *risk,* or employee, contributes to the cost of the insurance as well as the *insured.*

conversion privilege: in *group* health *insurance,* the right given the *insured* to change his *group insurance* to some form of individual insurance, without medical examination, upon termination of his group insurance (usually upon termination of employment or other source of membership in the group). Group insurance does not always offer a conversion privilege and, when it does, the available individual insurance is generally not of comparable scope of benefits or cost (usually being more expensive).

coordination of benefits (COB): provisions and procedures used by *insurers* to avoid duplicate payment for *losses* insured under more than one *insurance policy.* For example, some people have a *duplication of benefits,* for their medical costs arising from an automobile accident, in their automobile and health insurance policies. A coordination of benefits or antiduplication clause in one or the other policy will prevent double payment for the expenses by making one of the insurers the *primary payer,* and assuring that no more than 100 percent of the costs are covered. There are standard rules for determining which of two or more plans, each having COB provisions, pays its benefits in full and which pays a sufficiently reduced benefit to prevent the claimant from making a *profit.*

copayment: a type of *cost sharing* whereby *insured* or covered persons pay a specified flat amount per unit of service or unit of time (e.g., $2 per visit, $10 per inpatient hospital day), their *insurer* paying the rest of the cost. The copayment is incurred at the time the service is used. The amount paid does not vary with the cost of the service (unlike *coinsurance,* which is payment of some percentage of the cost).

cost of insurance: the amount which a policyholder pays to the *insurer* minus what he gets back from it. This should be distinguished from the *rate* for a given unit of insurance ($10 for a $1000 life insurance policy). Such costs, which may be difficult to obtain and are rarely compared, are roughly approximated by the *loading* or the ratio of amounts paid in benefits to income produced from premiums. See also *expenses.*

cost-related or cost-based reimbursement: one method of payment of medical care programs by *third parties,* typically *Blue Cross* plans or government agencies, for services delivered to patients. In cost-related systems, the amount of the payment is based on the *costs* to the provider of delivering the service. The actual payment may be based on any one of several different formulae, such as full cost, full cost plus an additional percentage, *allowable costs,* or a fraction of costs. Other reimbursement schemes are based on the *charges* for the services delivered, or on budgeted or anticipated costs for a future time period (*prospective reimbursement*). *Medicare, Medicaid,* and some *Blue Cross* plans reimburse hospitals on the basis of costs; most private insurance plans pay charges.

costs: expenses incurred in the provision of services or goods. Many different kinds of costs are defined and used *(actual, allowable, direct, indirect, life, marginal and opportunity costs). Charges,* the price of a service or amount billed an individual or third party, may or may not be the same as, or based on, costs. Hospitals often charge more for a given service than it actually costs in order to recoup losses from providing other services where costs exceed feasible charges. Despite the terminology, cost control programs are often directed to controlling increases in charges rather than in real costs.

cost sharing: provisions of a health *insurance policy* which require the *insured* or otherwise covered individual to pay some portion of his covered medical expenses. Several forms of cost-sharing are employed, particularly *deductibles, coinsurance* and

copayments. A deductible is a set amount which a person must pay before any payment of *benefits* occurs. A co-payment is usually a fixed amount to be paid with each service. Co-insurance is payment of a set portion of the cost of each service. Cost-sharing does not refer to or include the amounts paid in *premiums* for the *coverage.* The amount of the premium is directly related to the benefits provided and hence reflects the amount of cost-sharing required. For a given set of benefits, premiums increase as cost-sharing requirements decrease. In addition to being used to reduce premiums, cost sharing is used to control *utilization* of covered services, for example, by requiring a large copayment for a service which is likely to be overused.

coverage: the guarantee against specific *losses* provided under the terms of an *insurance policy.* Frequently used interchangeably with *benefits* or protection. The extent of the insurance afforded by a policy. Often used to mean insurance or an insurance contract.

customary charge: *generally, the amount which a physician normally or usually charges* the majority of his patients. Under *Medicare,* it is the median charge used by a particular physician for a specified type of service during the calendar year preceding the *fiscal year* in which a *claim* is processed. There is, therefore, an average delay of a year and a half in recognizing any increase in actual charges. Customary charges in addition to *actual* and *prevailing charges* are taken into account in determining *reasonable charges* under Medicare.

D

deductible: the amount of loss or expense that must be incurred by an *insured* or otherwise covered individual before an *insurer* will assume any liability for all or part of the remaining cost of covered services. Deductibles may be either fixed dollar amounts or the value of specified services (such as two days of hospital care or one physician visit). Deductibles are usually tied to some reference period over which they must be incurred, e.g. $100 per calendar year, *benefit period,* or *spell of illness.* Deductibles in existing policies are generally of two types: (1) static deductibles which are fixed dollar amounts, and (2) dynamic deductibles which are adjusted from time to time to reflect increasing medical prices. A third type of deductible is proposed in some *national health insurance* plans; a *sliding scale deductible,* in which the deductible is related to *income* and increases as income increases.

defensive medicine: alteration of modes of medical *practice,* induced by the threat of liability, for the principal purposes of forestalling the possibility of *malpractice* suits by patients and providing a good legal defense in the event of such lawsuits. While surveys have shown that 50 to 70 percent of physicians say they practice defensive medicine, it is difficult to define and measure specifically and, except for increasing the costs of care, unclear what effects it has.

delegation: in the *PSRO* program, the formal process by which a PSRO, based upon an assessment of the willingness and capability of a hospital or other health program to effectively perform PSRO review functions, assigns the performance of some (partial delegation) or all (full delegation) PSRO review functions to the program. Delegation must be agreed upon in a written memorandum of understanding signed by both the PSRO and the program. The PSRO monitors the program's performance of the delgated functions without itself conducting them, and retains responsibility for the effectiveness of the review.

diagnosis: the art and science of determining the nature and *cause* of a *disease,* and of differentiating among *diseases.*

disability income insurance: a form of health insurance that provides periodic payments to replace *income* when the *insured* is unable to work as a result of *injury* or *disease.*

discovery rule: in *malpractice,* a rule in use in some jurisdictions under which the statute of limitations does not commence to run until the wrongful act is discovered or, with reasonable diligence, should have been discovered. The statute of limitations is the period of time, ordinarily beginning with the wrongful act, during which an *injured* party may sue for recovery of damages arising from the act. In some jurisdictions application of the discovery rule is limited to cases involving a foreign object left in the body of a patient. Some States have

adopted statutory rules in malpractice cases which impose double time limits within which an action for malpractice may be brought. Typically these statutes provide that the action must be brought within a limited time after its discovery as well as within a limited time from the date the negligent act occurred.

disease: literally "without case", may be defined as a failure of the adaptive mechanisms of an organism to counteract adequately, normally or appropriately the stimuli and stresses to which it is subject, resulting in a disturbance in the function or structure of some part of the organism. This definition emphasizes that disease is multifactorial and may be prevented or treated by changing any of the factors. Disease is a very elusive and difficult concept to define, being largely socially defined. Thus, criminality and *drug dependence* presently tend to be seen as diseases, when they were previously considered to be moral or legal problems.

dispensing fee: a fee charged by a pharmacist for filling a *prescription.* One of two ways that *pharmacists* charge for the service of filling a prescription, the other being a standard percentage markup on the *acquisition cost* of the *drug* involved. A dispensing fee is the same for all prescriptions, thus representing a larger mark-up on the cost of an inexpensive drug or a small prescription than on an expensive drug or large prescription. However, it reflects the fact that a pharmacist's service is the same whatever the cost of the drug. Some pharmacists combine the two approaches, using a percentage mark-up with a minimum fee.

doctor: usually used synonymously with *physician,* but actually means any person with a doctoral degree.

drug: any substance intended for use in the diagnosis, cure, mitigation, treatment or prevention of disease, or intended to affect the structure or function of the body (not including food), or components of these substances. Substances recognized in the official U. S. Pharmacopeia, the official Homeopathic Pharmacopeia of the U. S., or the official National Formulary are drugs.

druggist: somebody who operates a *drug* store. Sometimes considered synonymous with *pharmacist,* but is not always limited to people with a pharmacy degree (or even to operators of drug stores in which *prescription drugs* are dispensed) and is usually applied only to pharmacists who operate, or at least work in, drug stores.

E

effectiveness: the degree to which diagnostic, preventive, therapeutic or other action or actions achieves the intended result. Effectiveness requires a consideration of *outcomes* to measure. It does not require consideration of the cost of the action, although one way of comparing the effectiveness of actions with the same or similar intended results is to compare the ratios of their effectiveness to their costs. The Federal Food, Drug, and Cosmetic Act requires prior demonstration of effectiveness for most drugs marketed for human use. No similar requirement exists for most other medical action paid for or *regulated* under Federal or State law. Usually synonymous with *efficacy* in common use.

efficacy: commonly used synonymously with *effectiveness,* but may usefully be distinguished from it by using efficacy for the results of actions undertaken under ideal circumstances and effectiveness for their results under usual or normal circumstances. Actions can thus be efficacious and effective, or efficacious and ineffective, but not the reverse.

emergency care: care for *patients* with severe, life-threatening, or potentially *disabling* conditions that require intervention within minutes or hours. Most hospitals and programs providing emergency care are also asked to provide care for many conditions which *providers* would not consider as emergencies, suggesting that *consumers* define the term more nearly synonymously with *primary care* and use such programs as *screening clinics.*

enroll: to agree to participate in a contract for *benefits*from an *insurance* company or *health maintenance organization.* A person who enrolls is an enrolee or *subscriber.* The number of people (and their *dependents)* enrolled with an insurance company or HMO is its enrollment.

enrollment period: period during which individuals may *enroll* for *insurance* or *health maintenance organization* benefits. There are two kinds of enrollment periods, for example, for *supplementary medical insurance* of *Medicare:* the initial enrollment period (the seven months beginning three months before and ending three months after the month a person first becomes eligible, usually by turning 65); and the general enrollment period (the first three months of each year). Most *contributory group insurance* has an annual enrollment period when members of the group may elect to begin contributing and become covered.

equivalency testing: testing intended to equate an individual's knowledge, experience and skill, however acquired, with the knowledge, experience and skill acquired by formal education or training. Successful completion of equivalency tests may be used to obtain course credits toward an academic degree without taking the courses, or a *license* which requires academic training without having the training.

established name: name given to a *drug* or pharmaceutical product by the United States Adopted Names Council (USAN). This name is usually shorter and simpler than the *chemical name,* and is the one most commonly used in the scientific literature. It is the name by which most physicians and pharmacists learn about a particular drug product in their professional training. An example would be penicillin, a well-known antibiotic. Also known as the *generic name* or official name. An established name for drugs is required by section 502(e) of the Federal Food, Drug, and Cosmetic Act.

ethical drug: a *drug* which is advertised only to physicians and other *prescribing* health *professionals.* Drug manufacturers which make only or primarily such drugs are referred to as the ethical drug industry.

exclusions: specific hazards, perils or conditions listed in an *insurance* or medical care coverage policy for which the policy will not provide benefit payments. Common exclusions may include *preexisting conditions,* such as heart disease, diabetes, hypertension or a pregnancy which began before the policy was in effect. Because of such exclusions, persons who have a serious condition or disease are often unable to secure insurance coverage, either for the particular disease or in general. Sometimes excluded conditions are excluded only for a defined period after coverage begins, such as nine months for pregnancy or one year for all exclusions. Exclusions are often permanent in *individual health insurance*, temporary (e.g., one year) for small groups in *group insurance*, and uncommon for large groups capable of absorbing the extra risk involved.

expenses: in *insurance*, the cost to the *insurer* of conducting its business other than paying *losses*, including *acquisition* and administrative costs. Expenses are included in the *loading*.

experience rating: a method of establishing *premiums* for health insurance in which the premium is based on the average cost of actual or anticipated health care used by various groups and subgroups of *subscribers* and thus varies with the health experience of groups and subgroups or with such variables as age, sex, or health status. It is the most common method of establishing premiums for health insurance in private programs.

F

factoring: the practice of one individual or organization selling its accounts receivable (unpaid bills) to a second at a discount. The latter organization, called the 'factor,' usually, but not always, assumes full risk of loss if the accounts prove uncollectible. In health services delivery, the expression generally refers to a hospital's or physician's sale of unpaid bills to a collection agent. Factoring has sometimes been used in *Medicaid* because of the delays that hospitals and physicians experience collecting from the State Medicaid agency. In these cases, the improved cash flow is worth the discount in the amount received by the *provider*. Because factoring is subject to *fraud* and *abuse*, Congress has sought to prohibit some of its uses.

family physician: a *physician* who assumes continuing responsibility for supervising the health and coordinating the care of all *family* members, regardless of age. Often viewed as low-level generalists, such physicians are now trained as *specialists* whose work demands specific skills. These skills include functioning as medical managers, advocates, educators and counselors for their patients.

Federal Register: an official, daily publication of the Federal government providing a uniform system for making available to the public proposed and final *rules*, legal notices, and similar proclamations, orders and documents having general applicability and legal effect. The Register publishes material from all Federal agencies.

fee for service: method of *charging* whereby a physician or other practitioner bills for each *encounter* or service rendered. This is the usual method of billing by the majority of the country's physicians. Under a fee for service payment system, expenditures increase not only if the fees themselves increase but also if more units of service are charged for or more expensive services are substituted for less expensive ones. This system contrasts with salary, per capita or *prepayment* systems, where the payment is not changed with the number of services actually used or if none are used. While the fee-for-service system is now generally limited to physicians, dentists, podiatrists and optometrists, a number of other practitioners, such as *physician assistants*, have sought reimbursement on a fee for service basis.

fee schedule: a listing of accepted *charges* or established allowances for specified medical or dental procedures. It usually represents either a physician's or *third party's* standard or maximum charges for the listed procedures.

first-dollar coverage: *coverage* under an *insurance* policy which begins with the first dollar of expense incurred by the *insured* for the covered benefits. Such coverage, therefore, has no *deductibles* although it may have *copayments* or *coinsurance*.

fiscal agent or intermediary: a contractor that processes and pays *provider claims* on behalf of a State *Medicaid* agency. Fiscal agents are rarely *at risk*, but rather serve as an *administrative* unit for the State, handling the payment of bills. Fiscal agents may be insurance companies, management firms, or other private contractors. Medicaid fiscal agents are sometimes also *Medicare carriers* or *intermediaries*.

fiscal year: any twelve month period for which annual accounts are kept. Sometimes, but by no means necessarily, the same as a calendar year. The Federal government's fiscal year has been from July 1 to the following June 30 for years, but changed in 1976 to be from October 1 to the following September 30.

formulary: a listing of *drugs*, usually by

their *generic names*. A formulary is intended to include a sufficient range of medicines to enable physicians or dentists to *prescribe* medically *appropriate* treatment for all reasonably common *illnesses*. A hospital formulary normally lists all the drugs routinely stocked by the hospital pharmacy. *Substitution* of a *chemically equivalent* drug in filling a prescription by *brand name* for a drug in the formulary is often permitted. A formulary may also be used to list drugs for which a *third party* will or will not pay, or drugs which are considered appropriate for treating specified illnesses.

fraud: intentional misrepresentation by either *providers* or *consumers* to obtain services, obtain payment for services, or claim program eligibility. Fraud may include the receipt of services which are obtained through deliberate misrepresentation of need or eligibility; providing false information concerning costs or conditions to obtain reimbursement or certification; or claiming payment for services which were never delivered or received. Fraud is illegal and carries a penalty when proven.

G

general practitioner (GP): a *practicing physician* who does not specialize in any particular field of *medicine* (e.g. is not a *specialist*). Should be contrasted with a *family physician* who has specialized (not all do), and is subject to *specialty board* examination, in the care of families, and a *primary care* physician who may be a *specialist* in any of several specialties.

general revenue: government revenues raised without regard to the specific purpose for which they might be used. Federal general revenues come principally from personal and corporate *income* taxes and some *excise* taxes. State general revenues come primarily from personal income and sales taxes. Most proposed *national health insurance* programs would be financed in part from general revenues in addition to whatever financing might be obtained from *premiums, cost-sharing,* and *payroll taxes* whose revenues are used only for the program. The expenditure of general revenues is determined by legislative *authorizations* and *appropriations*.

generic equivalents: drug produces with the same active chemical ingredients sold under the same *generic name* but often with different *brand names*. Generic equivalents are often assumed to be, but are not necessarily, *therapeutic equivalents*. The term has such inconsistent meaning that it must be used with care or avoided.

generic name: the *established,* official, or non-proprietary, name by which a drug is known as an isolated substance, irrespective of its manufacturer. Each drug is *licensed* under a generic name, and also may be given a *brand name* by its manufacturer. The generic name is assigned by the United States Adopted Names Council (USAN), a private group of representatives of the American Medical Association, American Pharmaceutical Association, United States Pharmacopeia and Food and Drug Administration, plus one public member. There have been recent attempts to encourage *physicians* to *prescribe* drugs by generic names whenver possible instead of by brand names. This is said to allow considerable cost savings. Considerable controversy has arisen over whether drugs sold by generic name are in fact *therapeutically equivalent* to their brand-name counterparts. In some cases, two versions of the same drug, manufactured by the same or different manufacturers, may not, usually for reasons of *bioavailability,* be therapeutically equivalent. Advocates of generic prescribing question whether such differences are universal or always significant.

group: in *group insurance,* a body of *subscribers* eligible for group insurance by virtue of some common identifying attribute, such as common employment by an employer, or membership in a union, association or other organization. Groups considered for insurance are usually larger than nine persons.

group insurance: any *insurance* plan by which a number of employees of an employer (and their *dependents*), or members of a similar homogeneous *group,* are *insured* under a single policy, issued to their employer or the *group* with individual *certificates of insurance* given to each insured individual or *family*. Individual employees may be insured automatically by virtue of employment, only on meeting certain conditions (employment for over a month), or only when they elect to be insured (and usually to make a contribution to the cost of the insurance). Group health insurance is usually *experience rated* (except for small groups, all of which insured by an individual company in the same area are given the same rate by that company) and less expensive for the insured than comparable individual insurance (partly because an employed population is generally healthier than the general population, and partly because of lower administrative costs, especially in marketing and billing). Note that the policyholder or *insured* is the employer not the employees.

group practice: a formal association of three or more physicians or other health *professionals* providing services with income from medical *practice* pooled and redistributed to the members of the group according to some prearranged plan (often, but not necessarily, through partnership).

H

health insurance: *insurance* against loss by *disease* or accidental bodily *injury*. Such insurance usually covers some of the medical costs of treating the disease or injury, may cover other losses (such a loss of present or future earnings) associated with them and may be either *individual* or *group* insurance.

Health Insurance for the Aged and Disabled: the *social insurance* program authorized by title XVIII of the Social Security Act and known as *Medicare*.

health maintenance organization (HMO): an entity with four essential attributes:

(1) an organized system for providing health care in a geographic area, which entity accepts the responsibility to provide or otherwide assure the delivery of

(2) an agreed upon set of *basic* and *supplemental health* maintenance and treatment *services* to

(3) a voluntarily enrolled group of persons, and

(4) for which services the HMO is reimbursed through a predetermined, fixed, periodic *prepayment* made by or on behalf of each person or family unit *enrolled* in the HMO without regard to the amounts of actual services provided. (From the report of the Committee on Interstate and Foreign Commerce on the HMO Act of 1973, P. L. 93-222, in which the term is legally defined,

section 1301 of the *PHS Act.)* The HMO is responsible for providing most health and medical care services required by enrolled individuals or *families.* These services are specified in the contract between the HMO and the enrollees. The HMO must employ or contract with health care providers who undertake a continuing responsibility to provide services to its enrolees. The prototype HMO is the Kaiser-Permamente system, a *prepaid group practice* located on the West Coast. However, *medical foundations* sponsored by groups of physicians are included under the definition. HMOs are of public policy interest because the prototypes appear to have demonstrated the potential for providing high *quality* medical services for less money than the rest of the medical system. Specifically, rates of hospitalization and surgery are considerably less in HMOs than occurs in the system outside such prepaid groups, although some feel that earlier care, *skimping* or *skimming* may be a better explanation.

health planning: *planning* concerned with improving health, whether undertaken comprehensively for a whole community (see *CHP*) or for a particular population, type of health service, or health program. Some definitions clearly include all activities undertaken for the purpose of improving health (such as education, traffic and environmental control and nutrition) within the scope of responsibility of the planning process; others are limited to including conventional health services and programs, *public health, or personal health services.* See also *State health planning and development agency,* and *health systems agency.*

health systems agency (HSA): *a health planning* and resources development agency designated under the terms of the National Health Planning and Resources Development Act of 1974, P. L. 93-641. P. L. 93-641 requires the designation of an HSA in each of the *health service areas* in the United States. HSAs are to be non-profit private corporations, public regional planning bodies, or single units of local government, and are charged with performing the health planning and resources development functions listed in section 1513 of the *PHS* Act. The legal structure, size, composition and operation of HSAs are specified in section 1512 of the Act. HSA functions include preparation of a *health* system plan (HSP) and an *annual implementation plan* (AIP), the issuance of grants and contracts, the review and approval or disapproval of proposed uses of a wide range of Federal funds in the agency's health service area, and review of proposed new and existing *institutional health services* and making of recommendations respecting them to *State health planning and development agencies.* HSAs will replace existing *areawide CHP agencies* but with expanded duties and powers.

health system plan (HSP): a long range health plan prepared by a *health systems agency* for its *health service area* specifying the health *goals* considered appropriate by the agency for the area. The HSPs are to be prepared after consideration of national guidelines issued by HEW and study of the characteristics, resources and special needs of the health service area. Section 1513 of the PHS Act requires and specifies the nature of an HSP.

Hill-Burton: legislation, and the programs operated under that legislation, for Federal support of construction and *modernization* of hospitals and other *health facilities,* beginning with P. L. 79-725, the Hospital Survey and Construction Act of 1946. The original law, which has been amended frequently, provided for surveying State *needs,* developing plans for construction of hospitals and public health centers, and assisting in constructing and equipping them. Until the late 1960s, most of the amendments expanded the program in dollar amounts and scope. More recently, the administration has attempted to terminate the program.

hospital: an institution whose primary function is to provide *inpatient* services, *diagnostic* and *therapeutic,* for a variety of medical conditions, both surgical and non-surgical. In addition, most hospitals provide some *outpatient* services, particularly *emergency* care. Hospitals are classified by *length of stay* (short-term or long-term); as teaching or nonteaching; by major type of service (psychiatric, tuberculosis, general and other specialties, such as maternity, childrens' or ear, nose and throat); and by control (government, Federal, State or local, for-*profit* (or *proprietary*), and non profit). The hospital system is dominated by the short-term, general, non-profit community hospital, often called ? *voluntary* hospital.

Hospital Insurance Program (Part A, HI): the *compulsory* portion of *Medicare* which automatically enrolls all persons aged 65 and over, entitled to benefits under *OASDHI* or railroad retirement, persons under 65 who have been eligible for *disability* for over two years, and insured workers (and their *dependents*) requiring renal dialysis or kidney transplantation. The program pays, after various *cost-sharing* requirements are met, for *inpatient* hospital care and care in *skilled nursing facilities* and *home health agencies* following a period of hospitalization. The program is financed from a separate *trust fund* funded with a contributory tax *(payroll tax)* levied on employers, employees and the self-employed. In 1976 the tax was 0.9 percent of the first $15,300 of covered yearly earnings. Under the program each hospital nominates an *intermediary* which reviews and pays *claims* from that hospital for the program.

I

indemnity, indemnity benefits: under health *insurance* policies, *benefits* in the form of cash payments rather than services. The indemnity insurance contract usually defines the maximum amounts which will be paid for the covered services. In most cases, after the provider of service has billed the patient in the usual way the insured person submits to the insurance company proof that he has paid the bills and is then reimbursed by the company in the amount of the covered costs, making up the difference himself. In some instances, the provider of service may complete the necessary forms and submit them to the insurance company directly for reimbursement, billing the patient for costs which are not covered. Indemnity benefits are contrasted with *service benefits.*

individual health insurance: health *insurance* covering an individual (and usually his *dependents*) rather than a group. Individual insurance usually offers *indemnity benefits* and has higher *loadings* than *group insurance.*

individual insurance: insurance policies which provide protection to the policyholder and/or his *family* (as distinct from *group insurance*). Sometimes called personal insurance.

individual practice association (IPA): a partnership, corporation, association, or other legal entity which has entered into an arrangement for provision of their services with persons who are *licensed* to *practice medicine, osteopathy, dentistry,* or with other *health manpower* (a majority of whom are licensed to practice medicine or osteopathy), which arrangement provides: that such persons provide their professional services in accordance with a compensation arrangement established by the entity; and to the extent feasible (i) that such persons use such additional professional personnel, allied health professions personnel, and other health personnel as are available and appropriate for the *effective* and *efficient* delivery of the services, (ii) for the sharing by such persons of *medical* and other *records,* equipment, and professional, technical and administrative staff, and (iii) for the arrangement and encouragement of the *continuing education* of such persons in the field of clinical medicine and related areas. The term originated and is defined in the Health Maintenance Organization Act of 1973. P. L. 93-222, section 1302(5) of the *PHS Act.* IPAs are one source of professional services for *HMOs* and are modeled after *medical foundations.*

individual practice plan: usually synonymous with a *medical foundation.* Sometimes used to refer specifically to a *health maintenance organization* which obtains its professional services from an *individual practice association.*

inpatient: a *patient* who has been *admitted* at least overnight to a hospital or other *health facility* (which is therefore responsible for his room and board) for the purpose of receiving diagnostic treatment or other health services. Inpatient care means the care given inpatients.

institutional health services: health services delivered on an *inpatient* basis in *hospitals, nursing homes,* or other inpatient institutions, and by *health maintenance organizations;* but may also refer to services delivered on an *outpatient* basis by departments or other organizational units of or sponsored by such institutions. The National Health Planning and Resources Development Act of 1974, P. L. 93-641 (section 1531(5) of the *PHS Act*) defines them as services and facilities subject under HEW *rules* to *section 1122* review, and requires

that all institutional, but not non-institutional, health services be subject to *certificate-of-need* review and periodic review for *appropriateness.*

insurable risk: a *risk* which has the following attributes: it is one of a large homogeneous group of similar risks; the *loss* produced by the risk is definable and quantifiable; the occurence of loss in individual cases is accidental or fortuitous; the potential loss is large enough to cause hardship; the cost of insuring is economically feasible; the chance of loss is calculable; and it is sufficiently unlikely that loss will occur in many individual cases at the same time.

insurance: the contractual relationship which exists when one party, for a consideration, agrees to reimburse another for loss to a person or thing caused by designated contingencies. The first party is the *insurer;* the second, the *insured;* the contract, the *insurance policy;* the consideration, the *premium;* the person or thing, the *risk;* and the contingency, the *hazard* or *peril.* Generally, a formal social device for reducing the risk of losses for individuals by spreading the risk over groups. Insurance characteristically, but not necessarily, involves equitable contributions by the insured, pooling of risks, and the transfer of risks by contract. Insurance may be offered on either a *profit* or nonprofit basis, to *groups* or individuals.

insurance commissioner: the State official charged with the enforcement of laws pertaining to *insurance* in the respective States. The commissioner's title, status in government and responsibilities differ somewhat from State to State but all States have an official having such responsibilities regardless of his title. Sometimes called superintendent or director.

insurance pool: an organization of *insurers* or *reinsurers* through which particular types of *risks* are shared or pooled. The *risk* of high *loss* by any particular insurance company is transferred to the group as a whole (the insurance pool) with *premiums,* losses, and *expenses* shared in agreed amounts. The advantage of a pool is that the size of expected losses can be predicted for the pool with much more certainty than for any individual party to it. Pooling arrangements are often used for *catastrophic coverage* or for certain high risk populations like the *disabled.* Pooling may also be done within a single company by pooling the risks insured under various different policies so that high losses incurred by one policy are shared with others.

insurer: the party to an *insurance policy* who contracts to pay *losses* or render services.

intermediary: a public or private agency or organization selected by *providers* of health care which enters into an agreement with the Secretary of HEW under the *Hospital Insurance Program* (PART A) of *Medicare,* to pay *claims* and perform other functions for the Secretary with respect to such providers. Usually, but not necessarily, a *Blue Cross plan* or private insurance company.

J

joint underwriting association (JUA): an association consisting of all *insurers* authorized by a State to write a certain kind of *insurance,* usually some form of liability insurance such as *malpractice insurance.* Such associations may be required or voluntarily agreed to write malpractice insurance on a self-supporting basis.. They may write such insurance on an exclusive basis, which means individual carriers cannot write such insurance, or on a non-exclusive basis. The JUA approach has been used in State legislation to assure the availability of malpractice insurance. Examples of the powers given to such associations are included in the medical malpractice insurance legislation recently enacted in New York. There, the JUA can issue policies, develop rates, employ a service company to handle the insurance (including claims adjustment), assume *reinsurance* from its members, and cede reinsurance.

L

last dollar coverage: *insurance* coverage without upper limits or maximums no matter how great the *benefits* payable.

legend: the statement, "Caution: Federal law prohibits dispensing without prescription," required by section 503(b)(4) of the Federal Food, Drug, and Cosmetic Act as a part of the *labeling* of all *prescription drugs* (and only such drugs). Legend drug is thus

synonymous with prescription drug.

length of stay (LOS): the length of an *inpatient's* stay in a hospital or other *health facility.* It is one measure of use of health facilities, reported as an average number of days spent in a facility per *admission* or discharge. It is calculated as follows: total number of days in the facility for all discharges and *deaths* occurring during a period divided by the number of discharges and deaths during the same period. In *concurrent review* an appropriate length of stay may be assigned each patient upon admission. Average lengths of stay vary and are measured for people with various ages, specific diagnoses, or sources of payment.

liability: something one is bound to do, or an obligation one is bound to fulfill, by law and justice. A liability may be enforced in court. Liabilities are usually financial or can be expressed in financial terms. Also, the probably cost of meeting such an obligation.

loss: in *insurance,* the basis for a *claim* under the terms of an *insurance policy.* Any diminution of quantity, quality or value of property, resulting from the occurrence of some *peril* or *hazard.*

M

major medical: *insurance* designed to offset the heavy medical expenses resulting from catastrophic or prolonged *illness* or *injuries.* Generally, such policies do not provide *first dollar coverage,* but do provide benefit payments of 75 to 80 percent of all types of medical expenses above a certain base amount paid by the *insured.* Most major medical policies sold as private insurance contain maximums on the total amount that will be paid (such as $50,000); thus, they do not provide *last dollar coverage* or complete protection against catastrophic costs. However, there is a trend toward $250,000 limits or even unlimited plans. In addition, benefit payments are often 100 percent of expenses after the individual has incurred some large amount ($500 to $2,000) of *out-of-pocket* expenses.

malpractice: *professional* misconduct or lack of ordinary skill in the performance of a professional act. A practitioner is *liable* for damages or injuries caused by malpractice. Such liability, for some professions like medicine, can be covered by *malpractice* *insurance* against the costs of defending suits instituted against the professional and/or any damages assessed by the court, usually up to a maximum limit. Malpractice requires that the patient demonstrate some *injury* and that the injury be negligently caused.

malpractice insurance: *insurance* against the *risk* of suffering financial damage because of *malpractice.*

maternal and child health services (MCH): organized health and social services for mothers (particularly as they *need family planning* and pregnancy related services), their children, and (rarely) fathers. Mothers and children are often considered particularly vulnerable populations with special health needs; their health to be a matter of high public priority; and particularly benefited by *preventive medicine.* Therefore such services are sometimes separately organized and funded from other health services. One example is the Maternal and Child Health Program operated by the Federal Government under the authority of title V of the Social Security Act.

Maximum Allowable Cost Program (MAC): a Federal program which will limit reimbursement for *prescription drugs* under the *Medicare* and *Medicaid* programs, and Public Health Service projects to the lowest cost at which the drug is generally available. Specifically, the program limits reimbursement for drugs under programs administered by HEW to the lowest of the maximum allowable cost (MAC) of the drug, if any, plus a reasonable *dispensing fee,* the *acquisition cost* of the drug plus a dispensing fee, or the providers' *usual* and *customary charge* to the general public for the drug. The MAC is the lowest unit price at which a drug available from several sources or manufacturers can be purchased on a national basis.

Medicaid (Title XIX): a Federally-aided, State operated and administered program which provides medical *benefits* for certain low-income persons in need of health and medical care. The program, authorized by title XIX of the Social Security Act, is basically for the *poor.* It does not cover all of the poor, however, but only persons who are members of one of the categories of people who can be covered under the welfare cash payment programs—the aged, the blind, the disabled, and members of

families with dependent children where one parent is absent, incapacitated or unemployed. Under certain circumstances States may provide Medicaid coverage for children under 21 who are not *categorically related.* Subject to broad Federal guidelines, States determine the benefits covered, program eligibility, rates of payment for *providers,* and methods of administering the program.

Medicaid mill: a health program which serves, solely or primarily, *Medicaid* beneficiaries, typically on an *ambulatory* basis. The mills originated in the ghettos of New York City and are still found primarily in urban slums with few other medical *services.* They are usually organized on a for *profit* basis, characterized by their great productivity, and frequently accused of a variety of *abuses* (such as *ping-ponging* and *family ganging*).

Medical Assistance Program: the health care program for the *poor* authorized by title XIX of the Social Security Act, known as *Medicaid.*

medical care evaluation studies (MCE studies): retrospective medical care review in which an in-depth assessment of the *quality* and/or nature   of the use of selected health services or programs is made. Restudy of an MCE study assesses the *effectiveness* of corrective actions taken to correct deficiencies identified in the original study, but doess not necessarily repeat or replicate the original study. *Utilization review* requirements under *Medicare* and *Medicaid* require *utilization review committees* in hospitals and skilled nursing facilities to have at least one such study in progress at all times. Such studies are also required by the *PSRO* program.

medical foundation: an organization of *physicians,* generally sponsored by a State or local medical association. Sometimes called a foundation for medical care. It is a separate and antonomous corporation with its own board of directors. Every physician member of the medical society may apply for membership in the foundation and, upon acceptance, participate in all its activities. A foundation is concerned with the delivery of medical services at reasonable cost. It believes in the free choice of a physician and hospital by the patient, *fee-for-service* reimbursement and local *peer review.* Many foundations operate as *prepaid group practices* or as an *individual* *practice association* for an *HMO*. While these are prepaid on a *capitation* basis for services to some or all of their patients, they still pay their individual members on a fee-for-service basis for the services they give. Some foundations are organized only for peer review purposes or other specific functions.

medical indigency: the condition of having insufficient *income* to pay for adequate medical care without depriving oneself or *dependents* of food, clothing, shelter, and other essentials of living. Medical indigency may occur when a self-supporting individual, able under ordinary conditions to provide basic maintenance for himself and his *family,* is, in time of catastrophic illness, unable to finance the total cost of medical care.

medically indigent: a person who is too impoverished to meet his medical expenses. It may refer to either persons whose *income* is low enough that they can pay for their basic living costs but not their routine medical care, or alternately, to persons with generally adequate income who suddenly face catastrophically large medical bills.

medically needy: in the *Medicaid* program, persons who have enough *income* and *resources* to pay for their basic living expenses (and so do not need welfare) but not enough to pay for their medical care. Medicaid law requires that the standard for income used by a State to determine if someone is medically needy cannot exceed 133 percent of the maximum amount paid to a family of similar size under the welfare program for families with dependent children (AFDC). In order to be eligible as medically needy, people must fall into one of the categories of people who are covered under the welfare cash assistance programs; i.e., be aged, blind, disabled, or members of families with dependent children where one parent is absent, incapacitated or unemployed. They receive benefits if their income after deducting medical expenses is low enough to meet the eligibility standard.

medically underserved area: a geographic location (i.e., an urban or rural area) which has insufficient *health resources* (manpower and/or facilities) to meet the medical *needs* of the resident population. *Physician shortage area* applies to a medically underserved area which is particularly short of physicians. Such areas are also sometimes defined by measuring the *health status* of the resident population rather than the supply of resources, an area with an unhealthy population being considered underserved. The term is defined and used several places in the *PHS Act* in order to give priority to such areas for Federal assistance.

medically underserved population: the population of an urban or rural area with a shortage of personal health services or another population group having a shortage of such services. A medically underserved population may not reside in a particular *medically* underserved area, or be defined by its place of residence. Thus migrants, Native Americans or the inmates of a prison or mental hospital may constitute such a population. The term is defined and used several places in the *PHS Act* in order to give such populations priority for Federal assistance, e.g., in the *HMO* and *NHSC* programs.

Medicare (Title XVIII): a nationwide health insurance program for people aged 65 and over, for persons eligible for social security disability payments for over two years, and for certain workers and their dependents who need kidney transplantation or dialysis. Health insurance protection is available to *insured* persons without regard to *income*. Monies from *payroll taxes* and *premiums* from *beneficiaries* are deposited in special *trust funds* for use in meeting the expenses incurred by the insured. The program was enacted July 30, 1965, as title XVIII–Health Insurance for the Aged–of the Social Security Act, and became effective on July 1, 1966. It consists of two separate but coordinated programs: *hospital insurance* (Part A), and *supplementary medical insurance* (Part B).

medicine: the art and science of promoting, maintaining and restoring individual *health,* and of *diagnosing* and *treating disease.*

multi-source drug: a *drug* that is available from more than one manufacturer or distributor, often under different *brand names.* Limits on reimbursement are more likely to be feasible for multi-source drugs than drugs available from only a single source. A drug may not be available from more than one source because it is protected by a patent; only one company has obtained FDA marketing approval; or the demand for it is such that only one *supplier* has entered the market.

N

National Formulary (NF): a *compendium* of standards for certain *drugs* and preparations that are not included in the United States Pharmacopeia (USP). It is revised every five years, and recognized as a book of official *standards* by the Pure Food and Drugs Act of 1906.

O

occupancy rate: a measure of *inpatient health facility* use, determined by dividing *available* bed days by *patient days*. It measures the average percentage of a hospital's *beds* occupied and may be institutionwide, or specific for one *department* or service.

open enrollment: *a period when new subscribers* may elect to *enroll* in a health *insurance* plan or *prepaid group practice*. Open enrollment periods may be used in the sale of either *group* or *individual insurance* and be the only period of a year when insurance is available. Individuals perceived as high-risk (perhaps because of a *pre-existing condition*) may be subjected to high *premiums* or *exclusions* during open enrollment periods. In the Health Maintenance Organization Act of 1973 (P. L. 93-222) the term refers to periodic opportunities for the general public, on a first come, first served basis, to join an *HMO*. The law presently requires that HMOs have at least one annual open enrollment period during which an HMO accepts, "up to its capacity, individuals in the order that they apply" unless the HMO can demonstrate to HEW that open enrollment would threaten its economic viability. In such cases, HEW can waive the open enrollment requirement for a period of up to three years.

out-of-pocket payments or costs: those borne directly by a *patient* without benefit of *insurance*, sometimes called direct costs. Unless *insured*, these include patient payments, under *cost-sharing* provisions.

outpatient: a *patient* who is receiving *ambulatory care* at a hospital or other *health facility* without being *admitted* to the facility. Usually does not mean people receiving services from a *physician's* office or other program which does not also give *inpatient* care. Outpatient care refers to care given outpatients, often in organized programs.

outpatient medical facility: a facility designed to provide a limited or full spectrum of *health* and medical services (including health education and maintenance, *preventive* services, *diagnosis, treatment,* and *rehabilitation*) to individuals who do not require hospitalization or institutionalization *(outpatients)*.

P

Partnership for Health: a synonym for the *comprehensive health planning* program. The first set of amendments to the program were made in 1967 by P. L. 90-174 which was given the *short title*. Partnership for Health Amendments of 1967, and hence the name.

patient: one who is receiving health services; sometimes used synonymously with *consumer*.

patient days: a measure of institutional use, usually measured as the number of *inpatients* at a specified time (e.g., midnight).

peer review: generally, the evaluation by *practicing physicians* or other *professionals* of the *effectiveness* and *efficiency* of services ordered or performed by other practicing physicians or other members of the profession whose work is being reviewed (peers). Frequently refers to the activities of the *Professional Standards Review Organizations* (PSRO) which in 1972 were required by P. L. 92-603 to review services provided under the *Medicare, Medicaid,* and *Maternal and Child Health* programs. Local PSROs, which receive Federal guidance and funding from HEW are staffed by local physicians, osteopaths, and non-physicians. Their duties include the establishment of *criteria norms* and *standards* for *diagnosis* and *treatment* of *diseases* encountered in the local PSRO jurisdiction, and review of services that are inconsistent with the established norms, e.g., hospital stays longer than the normal *length of stay*. The norms may be *input,* *process,* or *outcome measures.* Peer review has been advocated as the only possible form of *quality* control for medical services because it is said that only a physician's professional peers can judge his work. It has been criticized as having inherent conflict of interest, since, it is said, a physician will not properly judge those who will judge him, and also as not adequately reflecting *patient* objectives and points of view.

per diem cost: literally, *cost* per day. Refers, in general, to hospital or other *inpatient* institutional costs per day or for a day of care. Hospitals occasionally *charge* for their services on the basis of a per diem rate derived by dividing their total costs by the number of inpatient days of care given. Per diem costs are therefore averages and do not reflect true cost for each patient. With this approach patients who use few hospital services (typically those at the end of a long stay) subsidize those who need much care (those just *admitted*). Thus the per diem approach is said to give hospitals an incentive to prolong hospital stays.

personal physician: the *physician* who assumes responsibility for the comprehensive medical care of an individual on a continuing basis. The physician obtains *professional* assistance when needed for services he is not qualified to provide, and coordinates the care provided by other professional personnel in light of his knowledge and understanding of the *patient* as a whole. While personal physicians will have an interest in the patient's *family* as they affect his patient, the personal physician may not serve the entire family directly, e.g., a pediatrician may serve as a personal physician for children, while an internist or other *specialist* may serve in this capacity for adults. Personal physician is sometimes more simply defined for any given patient as the one the patient designates as his personal or principal physician.

pharmacist: a *professional* person qualified by education and authorized by law (usually by obtaining a *license*) to *practice pharmacy.*

pharmacy: the science, art and *practice* of preparing, preserving, compounding, dispensing and giving *appropriate* instruction in the use of *drugs;* a place where pharmacy is practiced.

physician: a *professional* person qualified by education and authorized by laws (usually by having obtained a *license*) to *practice medicine.*

ping-ponging: the practice of passing a *patient* from one *physician* to another in a health program for unnecessary cursory examinations so that the program can charge the patient's *third-party* for a physician *visit* to each physician. The practice and term originated and is most common in *Medicaid mills.*

planning: the conscious design of desired future states (described in a plan by its *goals* and *objectives,* and description and selection among alternative means of achieving the goals and objectives), and the conduct of the activities necessary to the designing (such as data gathering and analysis) and the activities necessary to assure that the plan is achieved. There are many different definitions of planning and descriptions of different types, including: long-range or perspective (covering 15 or more years); mid-range or strategic (5-15 years); short-term or tactical (1-3 years) planning *health facilities* or *manpower;* community or program; *categorical* or *comprehensive health;* normative (based on *norms* or *standards* with legal basis); and inductive or deductive (used when the planning is done locally and consolidated and used at State and Federal levels (bubbled up), or vice versa (trickled down), respectively). The extent to which planning is responsible by definition for implementation of the plans is controversial, as is its relation to *management.*

pre-existing condition: an *injury* occurring, *disease* contracted, or physical condition which existed prior to the issuance of a health insurance policy. Usually results in an *exclusion* from coverage under the policy forr costs resulting from the condition.

premium: the amount of money or consideration which is paid by an *insured* person or policyholder (or on his behalf) to an *insurer* or *third party* for insurance coverage under an *insurance policy.* The premium is generally paid in periodic amounts. It is related to the actuarial value of the *benefits* provided by the policy, plus a *loading* to cover administrative costs, *profit,* etc. Premium amounts for employment related insurance are often split between employers and employees; under current tax law, one-half of the amount spent on premiums by employees up to a maximum of $150 is deductible for income tax purposes for those who itemize deductions. Premiums paid by the employer are non-taxable *income* for the employee. Premiums are paid for coverage whether benefits are actually used or not; they should not be confused with *cost-sharing;* like *copayments* and *deductibles* which are paid only if benefits are actually used.

prepaid group practice: an arrangement where a formal association of three or more physicians provides a defined set of services to persons over a specified time period in return for a fixed periodic *prepayment* made in advance of the use of service.

prepaid health plan (PHP): generically, a contract between an *insurer* and a *subscriber* or group of subscribers whereby the PHP provides a specified set of health *benefits* in return for a periodic *premium.* The term now usually means organizational entities in California which provide services to Medi-Cal (the name for California's *Medicaid* program) beneficiaries under contract with the State of California. In the latter instance, provision was made under the Medi-Cal Reform Program of 1971 for Medi-Cal administrators to contract with groups of medical providers to supply specified services on a prepaid, per capita basis. These entities have been the subject of much controversy regarding the *cost* and *quality* of their services.

prepayment: inconsistently used, sometimes synonymous with *insurance,* sometimes refers to any payment ahead of time to a *provider* for anticipated *services* (such as an expectant mother paying in advance for maternity care), sometimes distinguished from insurance as referring to payment to organizations (such as *HMOs, prepaid group practices* and *medical foundations)* which, unlike an insurance company, take responsibility for arranging for and providing needed services as well as paying for them.

prescription: a written direction or order for the preparation and administration of a *drug* or other remedy by a *physician, dentist* or other practitioner licensed by law to administer such drug. Prescriptions may be written as orders in hospitals and other institutions for drugs to be given *inpatients,* or given to *outpatients* to be filled by a *pharmacist.* The prescription properly specifies the drug to be given, the amount of the drug to be dispensed, and the directions necessary for the patient to use the drug.

prescription drug: a *drug* available to the public only upon *prescription.* The availability of such drugs is thus limited because the drug is considered dangerous if used without a *physician's* supervision.

prevailing charge: a *charge* which falls within the range of charges most frequently used in a *locality* for a particular medical *service* or procedure. The top of this range establishes an over-all limitation on the charges which a *carrier,* which considers prevailing charges in reimbursement, will accept as *reasonable* for a given service, without adequate special justification. Current *Medicare rules* state that the limit of an area's prevailing charge is to be the 75th percentile of the *customary charges* for a given service by the *physicians* in a given area. For example, if customary charges for an appendectomy in a locality were distributed so that 10 percent of the services were rendered by physicians whose customary charge was $150, 40 percent by physicians who charged $200, 40 percent who charged $250, and 10 percent who charged $300 or more, then the prevailing charge would be $250, since this is the level that, under Medicare regulations, would cover at least 75 percent of the cases.

preventive medicine: care which has the aim of preventing *disease* or its consequences. It includes health care programs aimed at warding off illnesses (e.g., immunizations), early detection of disease (e.g., Pap smears), and inhibiting further deterioration of the body (e.g., exercise or prophylactic surgery). Preventive *medicine* developed subsequent to bacteriology, and was concerned in its early history with specific medical control measures taken against the agents of infectious diseases. With increasing knowledge of nutritional, malignant and other *chronic diseases,* the scope of preventive medicine has been extended. It is now operatively assumed that most if not all problems are preventable at some stage of their development. Preventive medicine is also concerned with general preventive measures aimed at improving the healthfulness of our environment and our relations with it through such things as avoidance of hazardous substances, modified diet, and *family planning.* In particular, the promotion of health through altering behavior, especially by health education, is gaining prominence as a component of preventive care.

primary care: basic or general health care which emphasizes the point when the *patient* first seeks assistance from the medical care system and the care of the simpler and more common *illnesses*. The primary care *provider* usually also assumes ongoing responsibility for the patient in both *health* maintenance and *therapy* of illness. It is comprehensive in the sense that it takes responsibility for the overall coordination of the care of the patient's health problems, be they biological, behavioral or social. The appropriate use of *consultants* and community resources is an important part of effective primary care. Such care is generally provided by *physicians*, but is increasingly provided by other personnel such as family *nurse practitioners*.

prior authorizaton: requirement imposed by a *third party*, under some systems of *utilization review*, that a *provider* must justify before a *peer review* committee, insurance company representative, or State agent the *need* for delivering a particular *service* to a *patient* before actually providing the service in order to receive reimbursement. Generally, prior authorization is required for non-emergency services which are expensive (involving a hospital stay, *preadmission certification*, for example) or particularly likely to be overused or *abused* (many State *Medicaid* programs require prior authorization of all *dental* services, for instance).

private patient: a *patient* whose care is the responsibility of an identifiable, individual health *professional*, (usually a *physician*) who is paid directly (by the patient or a *third-party*) for his *service* to the patient. The physician is called a *personal physician* and the patient is his private patient. Private patients are contrasted with public, service or ward patients whose care is the responsibility of a health program or institution. Public patients are often cared for by an individual practitioner paid by the program (such as a member of the *house staff*) but the program, rather than the individual, is paid for the care. The distinction is important to third-party payers (including *Medicare*) because situations arise in which payment is made to both a program and an individual practitioner for the same ser-

vices. The term occasionally refers to a patient occupying a room in an institution by himself (a private room).

private practice: medical *practice* in which the practitioner and his practice are independent of any external *policy* control. It usually requires that the practitioner be self-employed, except when he is salaried by a partnership in which he is a partner with similar practitioners. It is sometimes wrongly used synonymously with either *fee-for-service* practice (the practitioner may sell his services by another method: i.e., *capitation*); or *solo practice (group practice* may be private). Note that physicians practice in many different settings and there is no agreement as to which of these does or does not constitute private practice. *Regulation*, which does not exert external control, is not generally felt to make all practice public. The opposite of private practice is not necessarily public, in the sense of employment by government. Practitioners salaried by private *hospitals* are not usually thought to be in private practice.

professional liability: obligation of *providers* or their professional liability *insurers* to pay for damages resulting from the providers acts of omission or commission in *treating patients*. The term is sometimes preferred by providers to medical *malpractice* because it does not necessarily imply negligence. It is also a term which more adequately describes the obligations of all types of *professionals*, e.g. lawyers, architects and other health providers, as well as physicians.

Professional Standards Review Organization (PSRO): a physician-sponsored organization charged with comprehensive and ongoing review of *services* provided under the *Medicare, Medicaid* and *Maternal and Child Health* programs. The purpose of this review is to determine for purposes of reimbursement under these programs whether services are: medically *necessary;* provided in accordance with professional *criteria, norms* and *standards:* and, in the case of institutional services, rendered in an *appropriate* setting. The requirement for the establishment of PSROs was added by the Social Security Amendments of 1972, P. L. 92-603, to the Social Security Act as part B of title XI. PSRO areas have been designated throughout the country and organizations in many of these areas are at various stages of implementing the required review functions.

progressive tax: a tax which takes an increasing proportion of *income* as income rises, such as the Federal personal income tax. Incremental increases in taxable income are subject to an increased *marginal tax rate.*

proprietary: *profit* making; owned and operated for the purposes of making a profit, whether or not made.

prospective reimbursement: any method of paying *hospitals* or other health programs in which amounts or rates of payment are established in advance for the coming year and the programs are paid these amounts regardless of the costs they actually incur. These systems of reimbursement are designed to introduce a degree of constraint on *charge* or *cost* increases by setting limits on amounts paid during a future period. In some cases, such systems provide incentives for improved *efficiency* by sharing savings with institutions that perform at lower than anticipated costs. Prospective reimbursement contrasts with the method of payment presently used under *Medicare* and *Medicaid* where institutions are reimbursed for actual expenses incurred, i.e., on a *retrospective* basis.

provider: an individual or institution which gives medical care. In *Medicare,* an institutional provider is a *hospital, skilled nursing facility, home health agency,* or certain providers of outpatient *physical therapy services.* These providers receive *cost-related reimbursement.* Other Medicare providers, paid on a *charge* basis, are called *suppliers.* Individual providers include individuals who *practice* independently of institutional providers. The term must sometimes be distinguished from *consumer,* for instance when requiring consumer representation in a health program. For these purposes P. L. 93-641 defines the term for individuals as follows (section 1531(3) of the PHS Act):

(3) The term "provider of health care" means an individual—

(A) who is a direct provider of health care (including a *physician, dentist, nurse, podiatrist,* or *physician assistant*) in that the individual's primary current activity is the provision of health care to individuals or the *administration* of facilities or institutions (including hospitals, *long-term care facilities, outpatient facilities* and *health maintenance organizations*) in which such care is provided and, when required by State law, the individual has received *professional* training in the provision of such care or in such administration and is *licensed* or *certified* for such provision or administration; or

(B) who is an indirect provider of health care in that the individual—

(i) holds a *fiduciary* position with, or has a fiduciary interest in, any entity described in subclause (II) or (IV) of clause (ii);

(ii) receives (either directly or through his spouse) more than one-tenth of his gross annual *income* from any one or combination of the following:

(I) fees or other compensation for research into or instruction in the provision of health care.

(II) entities engaged in the provision of health care or in such research or instruction.

(III) producing or supplying *drugs* or other articles for individuals or entities for use in the provision of, research into or instruction in the provision of health care.

(IV) entities engaged in producing drugs or such other articles.

(iii) is a member of the immediate *family* of an individual described in subparagraph (A) or in clause (i), (ii), or (iv) of subparagraph (B): or

(iv) is engaged in issuing any policy or contract of individual or group health *insurance* or hospital or medical service benefits.

prudent buyer principle: the principle that *Medicare* should not reimburse a *provider* for a *cost* that is not a *reasonable cost* because it is in excess of the amount that a prudent and cost-conscious buyer would be expected to pay. For example, an organization that does not seek the customary discount on bulk purchases could, through the operation of this principle, be reimbursed for less than the full purchase price.

public health: the science dealing with the protection and improvement of community *health* by organized community effort. Public health activities are generally those which are less amendable to being undertaken or less *effective* when undertaken on an individual basis, and do not typically include direct *personal health services.* Immunizations, sanitation, *preventive medicine, quarantine* and other *disease* control activities, *occupational health* and safety programs, assurance of the healthfulness of air, water and food, health education, and *epidemiology* are recognized public health activities.

Q

quality: the nature, kind or character of someone or something; hence, the degree or grade of excellence possessed by the person or thing. Quality may be measured: with respect to individual medical *services,* the various services received by individual or groups of *patients,* individual or groups of *providers,* or health programs or *facilities;* in terms of technical competence, humanity, *need, acceptability appropriateness, inputs,* structure, *process,* or *outcomes;* using *standards, criteria, norms,* or direct quantitative or qualitative measures. To avoid the frequent vagueness of the term it is thus necessary to specify who or what is being considered, what aspect of it is being measured, and how it is being assessed. See *efficacy, effectiveness, PSRO, peer* and *utilization review.*

quality assurance: activities and programs intended to assure the *quality* of care in a defined medical setting or program. Such programs must include educational or other components intended to remedy identified deficiencies in quality, as well as the components necessary to identify such deficiencies (such as *peer* or *utilization review* components) and assess the program's own *effectiveness.* A program which identifies quality deficiencies and responds only with negative sanctions, such as denial of reimbursement, is not usually considered as a quality assurance program, although the latter may include use of such sanctions. Such programs are required of *HMOs* and other health programs assisted under author-

ity of the *PHS ACT* (e.g., section 1301(c)(8)).

R

rating: in *insurance,* the process of determing rates, or the cost of insurance, for individuals, *groups* or classes of *risks.*

reasonable charge: for any specific *service* covered under *Medicare,* the lower of the *customary charge* by a particular *physician* for that service and the *prevailing charge* by physicians in the geographic area for that service. Reimbursement is based on the lower of the *reasonable* and *actual charges.* For example, suppose the prevailing charge for a fistulectomy is $100 in a certain *locality,* i.e., this is the 75th percentile of the customary charges for that service by the physicians in that locality. Dr. A's actual charge is $75, although he customarily $80 for the procedure; Dr. B's actual charge is his customary charge of $85; Dr. C's is his customary charge of $125; Dr. D's is $100, although he customarily charges $80; and there are no special circumstances in any case. The reasonable charge for Dr. A would be $75 since the reasonable charge cannot exceed the actual   charge, even if it is lower than his customary charge and below the prevailing charge for the locality. The reasonable charge for Dr. B would be $85, because his customary charge is lower than the prevailing charge for that locality. The reasonable charge for Dr. C would be $100, the prevailing charge for his locality. The reasonable charge for Dr. D would be $80, because that is his customary charge which is lower than the actual charge in this particular case. His reasonable charge cannot exceed his customary charge in the absence of special circumstances, even though his actual charge of $100 is the same as the prevailing charge. Generically, the term is used for any charge payable by an *insurance* program which is determined in a similar, but not necessarily identical fashion.

reasonable cost: generally the amount which a *third party* using *cost-related reimbursement* will actually reimburse.. Under *Medicare* reasonable costs are costs actually incurred in delivering health *services* excluding any part of such incurred costs found to be unnecessary for the *efficient* delivery of *needed* health services (see section 1861 of the Social Security Act). The law stipulates that, except for certain *deductible* and *coinsurance* amounts that must be paid by *beneficiaries*, payments to hospitals shall be made on the basis of the reasonable cost of providing the covered services. The Secretary of HEW has prescribed *rules* setting forth the method or methods to be used and the items to be included in determining the reasonable cost of covered care. The regulations require that costs be apportioned between Medicare beneficiaries and other hospital *patients* so that neither group subsidizes the costs of the other. The items or elements of cost, both *direct* and *indirect*, which the regulations specify as reimbursable are known as *allowable costs.* Such costs are reimbursable on the basis of a hospital's actual costs to the extent that they are reasonable and are related to patient care. Under certain conditions the following items may be included as allowable costs: *capital depreciation;* interest expenses; educational activities; research costs related to patient care; unrestricted grants, gifts and income from endowments; value of services of non-paid workers, compensation of owners; payments to related organizations; return on equity *capital* of *proprietary* providers; and the *inpatient* routine *nursing differential. Bad debts* may only be included to the extent institutions fail in good faith efforts to collect the debts.

Regional Medical Program (RMP): a program of Federal support for regional organizations, called regional medical programs, which seek in their regions to improve the care for heart *disease,* cancer, strokes and related diseases. The legislative authority, created by P. L. 89-239, is found in title IX of the *PHS Act.* Thee programs were heavily oriented towards initiating and improving *continuing education, nursing services,* and *intensive care units.* Some features of the RMP program were combined into the new *health planning* program authorized by P. L. 93-641.

regressive tax: a tax which takes a decreasing proportion of *income* as income rises, such as sales taxes and the social security *payroll tax* on earnings above the maximum to which the tax applies. This tax is a constant percentage of income up to the maximum level (wage base), or a *proportional tax* up to that level.

regulation: the intervention of government in the health care or health *insurance* market to control entry into or change the behavior of participants in that marketplace through specification of rules for the participants. This does not usually include programs which seek to change behavior through financing mechanisms or incentives. It also does not include private *accreditation* programs although they may be relied upon by government regulatory programs, as is the *Joint Commission on Accreditation of Hospitals* under *Medicare.* Regulatory programs can be described in terms of their purpose (control *charges*), who is regulated (*hospitals*), who regulates (State government), and method (prospective rate review). Regulatory programs include some *certification,* some *registration, licensure, certificate of need,* and the *ESP, MAC* and *PSRO* programs. Also, a synonym for a *rule* published by the executive branch of the Federal government implementing a law.

reinsurance: the practice of one insurance company buying *insurance* from a second company for the purpose of protecting itself against part or all of the *losses* it might incur in the process of honoring the *claims* of its policyholders. The original company is called the ceding company; the second is the assuming company or reinsurer. Reinsurance may be sought by the ceding company for several reasons: to protect itself against losses in individual cases beyond a certain amount, where competition requires it to offer policies providing coverage in excess of these amounts; to offer protection against catastrophic losses in a certain line of insurance, such as aviation accident or polio insurance; or to protect against mistakes in *rating* and *underwriting* in entering a new line of insurance such as *major medical.*

relative value scale or schedule (RVS): a coded listing of *physician* or other *professional services* using units which indicate the relative value of the various services they perform; taking into account the time, skill and overhead cost required for each service; but not usually considering the relative cost-effectiveness of the services, the relative *need* or *demand* for them, or their importance to people's *health.* The units in this scale are based on median *charges* by physicians. Appropriate conversion factors are used to translate the abstract units in the scale to dollar fees for each service. Given individual and local variations in *practice,* the relative value scale can be used voluntarily as a guide to physicians in establishing *fees for services,* and as a guide for insurance *carriers* and government agencies in determining appropriate reimbursement (e.g., use of relative value scales under *Medicare* where there is no *customary* or *prevailing charge* for a covered service). An example is the scale prepared and revised periodically by the California Medical Association which includes independent scales for medicine, anesthesia, surgery, radiology and pathology. Relative value scales can contain biases favoring certain specialties (such as surgery) or types of services (highly technical or specialized) over others.

required services: *services* which must be offered by a health program in order to meet some external *standard.* Under *title XIX* of the Social Security Act, each state must offer certain *basic health services* before it can quality as having a *Medicaid* program (and thus for eligibility for Federal matching funds). The required services are: *hospital* services; laboratory and x-ray services; *skilled nursing facility* services for individuals 21 and over; *early and periodic screening, diagnosis and treatment* services for individuals under 21; *family planning* services; *physicians'* services; and *home health care* services for all persons eligible for skilled nursing facility services. It is important to note that, within these requirements, States may determine the scope and extent of *benefits* (limiting hospital care to 30 days a year, etc.). States may offer additional services in their Medicaid program; called *optional services* because they are offered at the option of the State.

residency: a prolonged (usually one or more complete years) period of on the job training which may either be a part of a formal educational program or be undertaken separately after completion of a formal program, sometimes in fulfillment of a requirement for *credentialing.* In *medicine, dentistry, podiatry* and some other health *professions* residencies are the principal part of *graduate medical education,* beginning either after graduation (increasingly) or *internship* (traditionally), lasting two to seven years, and providing

specialty training. Most *physicians* now take residencies in one of the 23 specialties in which they are offered, although they are not required for *licensure.* Residencies are needed for *board eligibility.*

res ipsa loquitur: literally, "the facts speak for themselves." In *malpractice,* a legal doctrine or presumption that, when an *injury* occurs to a plaintiff through a situation where the sole and exclusive control of the defendant and where such injury would not normally occur if the one in control had used due care, then it is presumed the defendent is negligent. Applies, for example, in the classic case of a surgeon who leaves a sponge in the abdomen.

respondeat superior: in *malpractice,* a form of vicarious *liability* whereby an employer is held liable for the wrongful acts of an employee even though the employer's conduct is without fault. Before liability predicated on *respondeat superior* may be imposed upon an employer, it is necessary that a master servant (i.e., controlling) relationship exist between the employer and employee and that the wrongful act of the employee occur within the scope of his employment. The doctrine of *respondeat superior* does not absolve the original wrongdoer, the employee, of liability for his wrongful act. Not only may the *injured* party sue the employee directly, but the employer may seek indemnification from him.

retrospective reimbursement: payment to *providers* by a *third party carrier* for *costs* or *charges* actually incurred by *subscribers* in a previous time period. This is the method of payment used under *Medicare* and *Medicaid.*

risk: generally, any chance of *loss.* In *insurance,* designates the individual or property *insured* by an *insurance policy* against loss from some *peril* or *hazard.* Also used to refer to the probability that the loss will occur.

rule: in the executive branch of the Federal Government, an agency statement of general or particular applicability and future effect designed to implement, interpret or prescribe law or *policy,* or describing the organization, procedure or practice requirements of an agency. Commonly also called a regulation. Rules are published in the

Federal Register. The process of writing a rule is called a rule-making. A rule, once adopted in accordance with the procedures specified in the Administrative Procedure Act (Title V, U. S. C.), has the force of law.

S

section 1122: a section of the Social Security Act added by P. L. 92-603. The section provides that payments will not be made under *Medicare* or *Medicaid* with respect to certain disapproved *capital* expenditures determined to be inconsistent with State or local health plans. P. L. 93-641, the National Health Planning and Resources Development Act of 1974, requires States participating in the section 1122 program to have the new *State health planning and development agency* serve as the section 1122 agency for purposes of the required review.

self-insure: the practice of an individual, group of individuals, employer, or organization assuming complete responsibility for *losses* which might be *insured* against, such as *malpractice* losses, or medical expenses and other losses due to *illness.* In such cases, medical expenses would most likely be financed out of current *income,* personal savings, a fund developed for the purpose, and/or some other combination of personal assets. Self-insurance is contrasted to the practice of purchasing *insurance,* by the payment of a *premium,* from some *third party* (an insurance company or government agency).

service benefits: those received as a result of *prepayment* or *insurance,* whereby payment is made directly to the *provider* of *services* or the hospital or other medical care programs for covered services provided by them to eligible persons. Service benefits may be full service benefits, meaning that the plan fully reimburses the hospital, for example, for all services provided during a period so that the patient has no *out-of-pocket* expenses. Full service benefits may also be available when the program itself provides the service as in a *prepaid group practice.* Partial service benefits cover only part of the expenses, the remainder to be paid by the beneficiary through some form of *cost-sharing.*

skimming: the practice in health programs paid on a *prepayment* or *capitation* basis,

and in health insurance, of seeking to *enroll* only the healthiest people as a way of controlling program *costs* (since income is constant whether or not services are actually used). Contrast with *adverse selection.* Sometimes known as creaming.

sliding scale deductible: a *deductible* which is not set at a fixed amount but rather varies according to *income.* A family is usually required to spend all (a *spend-down*) on a set percentage of their income above some base amount (for example, all or 25 percent of any income over $5,000) as deductible before a member can receive medical care benefits. There may be a maximum amount on the deductible. The sliding scale concept can also be applied to *coinsurance* and *copayments.*

social insurance: a device for the pooling of *risks* by their transfer to an organization, usually governmental, that is required by law to provide *indemnity* (cash) or *service benefits* to or on behalf of covered persons upon the occurrence of certain pre-designaged *losses.* Social insurance is usually characterized by all of the following conditions: coverage is *compulsory* by law; except during a transition period following its introduction, eligibility for benefits is derived, in fact or in effect, from contributions having been made to the program by or in respect of the claimant or the person as to whom the claimant is a *dependent;* there is no requirement that the individual demonstrate inadequate financial *resources,* although a *qualified* status may need to be established; the methods for determining the benefits are prescribed by law; the benefits for any individual are not usually directly related to contributions made by or in respect of him but instead usually redistribute *income* so as to favor certain groups such as those with low former wages or a large number of dependents; there is a definite plan for financing the benefits that is designed to be adequate in terms of long-range consideration; the cost is borne primarily by contributors which are usually made by covered persons, their employers, or both; the plan is administered or at least supervised by the government; and the plan is not established by the government solely for its present or former employees. Examples in this country include social security, railroad retirement, and *workman's* and *unemployment compensation.* In other countries, health insurance is often a government sponsored social insurance program.

socialized medicine: a medical care system where the organization and provision of medical care *services* are under direct government control, and *providers* are employed by or contract for the provision of services directly with the government; also a term used more generally, without recognized or constant definition, referring to any existing or proposed medical care system believed to be subject to excessive governmental control.

solo practice: lawful *practice* of a health occupation as a self-employed individual. Solo practice is thus by definition *private practice* but is not necessarily *general practice* or *fee-for-service* practice (solo practitioners may be paid by *capitation*, although fee for service is far more common). Solo practice is common among *physicians, dentists, podiatrists, optometrists* and *pharmacists;* less common and sometimes illegal in other professions (are all solo practitioners *professionals?).*

specialist: a *physician, dentist* or other health *professional* who limits his *practice* to a certain branch of medicine or dentistry related to: specific *services* or procedures, e.g., *surgery,* radiology, pathology; certain age categories of *patients,* e.g., pediatrics, geriatrics; certain body systems, e.g., dermatology, orthopedics, cardiology; or certain types of *diseases,* e.g., allergy, psychiatry, periodontics. Specialists, usually have special education and training related to their practice and may or may not be *certified* as specialists by the related *specialty board.*

specialty boards: organizations that *certify physicians* and *dentists* as *specialists* or subspecialists in various fields of medical and dental practice. The standards for certification relate to length and type of training and experience and include written and oral examination of applicants for specialty certification. The boards are not educational institutions and the certificate of a board is not considered a degree. Specialties and their boards are recognized and approved by the American Board of Medical Specialties in conjunction with the AMA Council on Medical Education.

specified disease insurance: *insurance* which provides *benefits,* usually in large amounts or with high maximums, toward the expense of the *treatment* of the specific *disease* or diseases named in the policy. Such policies are rarely written these days, being more common in the past for such diseases as polio and spinal meningitis, but coverage of end-stage renal disease under *Medicare* can be thought of as an example.

spend down: a method by which an individual establishes eligibility for a medical care program by reducing gross *income* through incurring medical expenses until net income (after medical expenses) becomes low enough to make him eligible for the program. The individual, in effect, spends income down to a specified eligibility standard by paying for medical care until his bills become high enough in relation to income to allow him to quality under the program's *standard* of *need,* at which point the program *benefits* begin. The spend-down is the same as a *sliding scale deductible* related to the over-all income level of the individual. ·For example, if persons are eligible for program benefits if their income is $200/month or less, a person with $300/month income would be covered after spending $100 *out-of-pocket* on medical care; a person with an income of $350 would not be eligible until he incurred medical expenses of $150. The term spend-down originated in the *Medicaid* program. An individual whose income makes him ineligible for welfare but is insufficient to pay for medical care, can become Medicaid-eligible as a *medically needy* individual by spending some income on medical care. Medicaid only covers an individual if aged, blind, disabled, or a member of a family where one patient is absent, incapacitated, or unemployed—that is, fitting one of the categories of individuals who are covered under the welfare cash payment programs.

sponsored malpractice insurance: a *malpractice insurance* plan which involves an agreement by a *professional* society (such as a State medical society) to sponsor a particular *insurer's* medical *malpractice* insurance coverage, and to cooperate with the insurer in the *administration* of the coverage. The cooperation may include participation in marketing, claims review, and review of ratemaking. Until 1975, this was the predominant approach to coverage. In 1975, a number of *carriers* with such arrangements announced they were withdrawing from them. They have been replaced by professional society operated plans, *joint underwriting associations,* State insurance funds and other arrangements.

staff privilege: the privilege, granted by a *hospital*, or other *inpatient* health program, to a *physician*, or other independent practitioner, to join the hospital's *medical staff* and hospitalize *private patients* in the hospital. A practitioner is usually granted privileges after meeting certain *standards*, being accepted by the medical staff and board of trustees of the hospital, and committing himself to carry out certain duties for the hospital such as teaching without pay, or providing emergency or *clinic services*. Most community and other private hospitals in this country are staffed by physicians who are private practitioners and obtain access to hospital facilities in this manner. It is common for a physician to have staff privileges at more than one hospital. On the other hand, since hospitals accept a limited number of physicians, some practitioners are excluded and end up with no access to hospital facilities, having no staff privileges. The standards used to determine staff privileges sometimes include evaluation by the county medical society, which may give preference to or require membership in that society, which in turn may require membership in the American Medical Association. This practice is formally opposed by the A.M.A. Some hospitals limit privileges for certain services to *board eligible* or *certified* physicians. Full time, or *hospital-based physicians,* and physicians working in a system such as a *prepaid group practice* with its own hospital are not usually thought of as having staff privileges. Sometimes called admitting, hospital, practice, or clinical privilege. Many hospitals have several different types or grades of staff privileges with names like active, associate, courtesy or limited. However, these names have irregular and unsystemized meaning, although the real differences between the different types of privileges deserve a decent nomenclature.

State cost commissions: State agencies assigned various health *services cost* and *charge regulation* or review responsibilities. The duties of a commission may include assuring that: total hospital costs are reasonably related to total services offered; aggregate rates bear a reasonable relationship to aggregate costs; and rates are applied equitably to preclude any possibility of discriminatory pricing among various services and patients of a hospital.

State health planning and development agency (SHPDA): section 1521 of the *PHS Act,* added by P. L. 93-641, requires the establishment of State health planning and development agencies in each State. As a replacement for existing *State CHP agencies,* SHPDAs will prepare an annual preliminary State health plan and ̄ the State medical facilities plan (*Hill-Burton*). The agency will also serve as the designated review agency for purposes of *section 1122* of the Social Security Act and administer a *certificate-of-need* program.

Statewide health coordinating council (SHCC): a State council of *providers* and *consumers* (who shall be in the majority) required by section 1524 of the *PHS Act,* added by P. L. 93-641. Each SHCC generally will supervise the work of the *State Health planning and development agency,* and review and coordinate the plans and *budgets* of the State's *health systems agencies* (HSA). It will also annually prepare a State health plan from HSA plans and the preliminary plans of the State agency. The SHCC will also review applications for HSA planning and resource development assistance.

subrogation: a provision of an *insurance policy* which requires an *insured* individual to turn over any rights he may have to recover damage from another party to the *insurer,* to the extent to which he has been reimbursed by the insurer. Some experts have argued that private health insurance (including *Blue Cross* or *group insurance*) should have subrogation rights similar to those in most property insurance policies, e.g., auto, fire. Having paid the *hospital* bill of a policyholder, the health insurance company could assume his right to sue the party whose negligence might have caused the hospitalization, and be reimbursed for its outlay to the policyholder. Subrogation rights could help insure prompt payment of medical expenses without *duplication of benefits.* (Refer to *Michigan Hospital Service* v. *Sharpe,* 339 Mich. 357, 63 N. W. 2d., 638, 1954 for ruling on subrogation by Michigan Supreme Court.) Others respond that subrogation is time consuming, expensive and may not offer companies adequate protection against loss. Few insurers use it voluntarily and some *insurance commissioners* forbid its use.

subscriber: often used synonymously with either *member* or *beneficiary* but in a strict sense means only the individual *(family* head or employee) who has elected to contract for, or participate in (subscribe to) an *insurance* or *HMO* plan for either himself or himself and his eligible *dependents.*

substitution: the filling of a *prescription* by a *pharmacist* with a *drug* product *therapeutically* and *chemically equivalent* to, but not, the one prescribed. Many States have *anti-substitution laws* which prohibit the pharmacist from filling a prescription with any product other than the specific product of the manufacturer whose *brand name* is used on the prescription.

supplemental health insurance: health *insurance* which covers medical expenses not covered by separate health insurance already held by the *insured,* e.g. which supplements another insurance policy. For example, many insurance companies sell insurance to people covered under *Medicare* which covers either the costs of *cost-sharing* required by Medicare, services not covered, or both. Where *cost-sharing* is intended to control *utilization,* the availability of supplemental health insurance covering cost-sharing limits its *effectiveness.*

supplemental health services: the *optional services* which *HMOs* may provide in addition to *basic health services* and still *qualify* for Federal assistance. They are defined in section 1302(2) of the *PHS Act.*

supplemental security income (SSI): a program of *income* support for low-income aged, blind and disabled persons, established by title XVI of the Social Security Act. SSI replaced State welfare programs for the aged, blind and disabled on January 1, 1972, with a Federally-administered program now paying a monthly basic *benefit* nationwide for an individual and for a couple. States may supplement this basic benefit amount. Approximately 4 million people currently receive benefits under the program. Receipt of a Federal SSI benefit or a State supplement under the program is often used to establish *Medicaid* eligibility.

Supplementary Medical Insurance Program (Part B, SMI): the voluntary portion of *Medicare* in which all persons entitled to the *hospital insurance program* (Part A) may *enroll.* The program is financed on a current basis from monthly *premiums* ($8.20 in 1978) paid by persons insured under the program and a matching amount from Federal *general revenues.* About 95 percent of eligible people are enrolled. During any calendar year, the program willl pay (with certain exceptions) 80 percent of the *reasonable charge* (as determined by the program) for all covered *services* after the *insured* pays a $60 *deductible* on the costs of such services. Covered services include *physician* services, *home health care* (up to 100 visits), medical and other health services, *outpatient* hospital services, and laboratory, pathology and radiologic services. Any individual over 65 may elect to enroll in Part B. However individuals not eligible for Part A who elect to buy into Part A must also buy into Part B. State welfare agencies may buy Part B coverage for elderly and disabled public assistance recipients and pay the premiums on their behalf. The program contracts with *carriers* to process *claims* under the program. The carriers determine amounts to be paid for claims based on reasonable charges. The name, Part B, refers to part B of title XVIII of the Social Security Act, the legislative authority for the program.

surgery: any operative or manual procedure undertaken for the *diagnosis* or *treatment* of a *disease* or other disorder; the branch of *medicine* concerned with diseases which require or are responsive to such treatment; or the work done by a surgeon (one who practices surgery).

surgicenter: a *facility* which serves *outpatients* requiring surgical *treatment* exceeding the capability of the *physician's* office but not requiring hospitalization as an *inpatient.* Also known as ambulatory surgery, day surgery, and in-and-out surgery.

T

tertiary care: *services* provided by highly specialized *providers* (e.g., neurologists, neurosurgeons, thoracic surgeons, *intensive care units).* Such services frequently require highly sophisticated technological and support facilities. The development of these services has largely been a function of diagnostic and therapeutic advances attained through basic and clinical *biomedical research.*

therapeutic equivalents: *drug* products with essentially identical effects in *treatment* of some *disease* or condition. Such products are sometimes, but not necessarily, *chemically equivalent* or *bioequivalent*. Therapeutic equivalents are sometimes defined as chemically equivalent, and drugs with the same treatment effect, which are not chemically equivalent, called clinically equivalent. This is a useful distinction but inconsistently used.

third-party payer: any organization, public or private, that pays or *insures* health or medical expenses on behalf of *beneficiaries* or recipients (e.g. *Blue Cross* and *Shield*, commercial insurance companies, *Medicare*, and *Medicaid*). The individual generally pays a *premium* for such coverage in all private and some public programs. The organization then pays bills on his behalf; such payments are called third party payments and are distinguished by the separation between the individual receiving the *service* (the first party), the individual or institution providing it (the second party) and the organization paying for it (the third party).

Title XVIII: the title of the Social Security Act which contains the principal legislative authority for the *Medicare* program, and therefore a common name for the program.

Title XIX: the title of the Social Security Act which contains the principal legislative authority for the *Medicaid* program, and therefore a common name for the program.

treatment: the *management* and care of a *patient* for the purpose of combating *disease* or disorder.

triage: commonly used to describe the sorting out or screening of *patients* seeking care, to determine which *service* is initially required and with what priority. A *patient* coming to a *facility* for care may be seen in a triage, screening or walk-in *clinic*. Here it will be determined, possibly by a triage *nurse*, whether, for example, the patient has a medical or surgical problem, or requires some non-physician service such as *social work* consultation. Such rapid assessment units may merely refer patients to the most appropriate treatment service, or may also give treatment for minor problems. Originally used to describe the sorting of battle casualties into groups who could wait for care, would benefit from immediate care, and were beyond care.

trust funds: funds collected and used by the Federal government for carrying out specific purposes and programs according to terms of a trust agreement or statute, such as the social security and unemployment trust funds. Trust funds are administered by the government in a *fiduciary* capacity for those benefitted and are not available for the general purposes of the government. Trust fund receipts whose use is not anticipated in the immediate future are generally invested in interest bearing government securities and earn interest for the trust fund. The *Medicare* program is financed through two trust funds–the Federal Hospital Insurance Fund which finances Part A, and the Federal Supplementary Medical Insurance Trust Fund which finances Part B.

U

underwriting: in *insurance,* the process of selecting, classifying, evaluating and assuming *risks* according to their *insurability*. Its fundamental purpose is to make sure that the group insured has the same probability of *loss* and probable amount of loss, within reasonable limits, as the universe on which *premium* rates were based. Since *premium* rates are based on an expectation of loss, the underwriting process must classify risks into classes with about the same expectation of loss.

uniform cost accounting: the use of a common set of accounting definitions, procedures, terms, and methods for the accumulation and communication of quantitative data relating to the financial activities of several enterprises. The American Hospital Association, for example, encourages the use of its Chart of Accounts as a system which can be employed by *hospitals* in the United States.

United States Pharmacopeia (USP): a legally recognized *compendium* of *standards* for *drugs,* published by the United States Pharmacopeial Convention, Inc., and revised periodically. It includes also assays and tests for the determination of strength, *quality* and purity.

usual, customary and reasonable plans (UCR): health *insurance* plans that pay a *physician's* full *charge* if: it does not exceed his usual charge; it does not exceed the amount customarily charged for the service by other physicians in the area (often defined as the 90 or 95 percentile of all charges in the community), or it is otherwise *reasonable*. In this context, usual and customary charges are similar, but not identical, to *customary* and *prevailing charges*, respectively, under *Medicare*. Most private health insurance plans, except for a few *Blue Shield plans*, use the UCR approach.

utilization: use. Utilization is commonly examined in terms of patterns or rates of use of a single *service* or type of service, e.g., *hospital care, physician visits, prescription drugs*. Measurement of utilization of all medical services in combination is usually done in terms of dollar expenditures. Use is expressed in rates per unit of population at *risk* for a given period, e.g., number of *admissions* to hospital per 1,000 per persons over 65 per year, or number of visits to a physician per person per year for *family planning* services.

utilization review (UR): evaluation of the *necessity, appropriateness* and *efficiency* of the use of medical *services*, procedures and *facilities*. In a hospital this includes review of the appropriateness of *admissions*, services ordered and provided, *length of stay*, and discharge practices, both on a concurrent and retrospective basis. Utilization review can be done by a *utilization review committee, PSRO, peer review* group, or public agency.

utilization review committee: a staff committee of an institution or a group outside the institution responsible for conducting *utilization review* activities for that institution. *Medicare* and *Medicaid* require as a *condition of participation* that *hospitals* have a utilization review committee in operation.

V

vendor: a *provider;* an institution, agency, organization or individual practitioner who provides health or medical *services. Vendor payments* are those payments which go directly to such institutions or providers from a *third party* program like *Medicaid*.

vendor payment: used in public assistance programs to distinguish those payments made directly to *vendors* of service from those cash income payments made directly to assistance recipients. The vendors, or providers of health services, are reimbursed directly by the program for services they provide to eligible recipients. Vendor payments are essentially the same as *service benefits* provided under health *insurance* and *prepayment* plans.

W

Wagner-Murray-Dingell Bill: one of the original *national health insurance* proposals, first introduced by Congressmen Wagner, Murray and Dingell in the 1940s.. It is still updated and introduced in each Congress by Congressman John Dingell of Michigan who succeeded his father, the original sponsor, in office.

waiting period: a period of time an individual must wait either to become eligible for *insurance* coverage, or to become eligible for a given *benefit* after overall coverage has commenced (see *exclusions*). This does not generally refer to the amount of time it takes to process an application for insurance, but rather is a defined period before benefits become payable. Some policies will not pay *maternity benefits*, for example, until nine months after the policy has been in force. Another common waiting period occurs in *group insurance* offered through a place of employment where coverage may not start until an employee has been with a firm over 30 days. For disabled persons to be covered under *Medicare*, there is a waiting period of two years; a person must be entitled to social security *disability* benefits for two years before medical benefits start.

warranty: in *malpractice*, actions against *physicians* are normally based on negligence, but in certain circumstances the plaintiff can bring his action on the basis of a warranty. A warranty arises if the physician promises or seems to promise that the medical procedure to be used is *safe* or will be *effective*. One of the advantages to bringing an action on warranty grounds, rather than for negligence, is that the statute of limitations is usually longer. A warranty action may be brought and maintained if there is an express warranty offered by the physician to the *patient*.

workmen's compensation programs: State *social insurance* programs which provide cash *benefits* to workers or their *dependents injured, disabled,* or deceased in the course, and as a result, of employment.. The employee is also entitled to benefits for some or all of the medical services necessary for treatment and restoration to a useful life and possibly a productive job. These programs are mandatory under State laws in all States.

Source: U.S. House of Representatives, "A Discursive Dictionary of Health Care", Committee on Interstate and Foreign Commerce, Subcommittee on Health and the Environment, Washington, D.C., February, 1976, pp. 1-168.

The Author

Jordan Braverman has served as the Director of Policy Analysis, Health Policy Center, Georgetown University. His prior affiliations include the Pharmaceutical Manufacturers Association, the Blue Cross Association, and the American Pharmaceutical Association.

A graduate of Harvard College, he received a M.P.H. degree from Yale University Medical School, and a M.S. degree from Georgetown University's Graduate School of Foreign Service and held the William Stoughton Scholarship at the Harvard University Graduate School of Design.

In addition to journal articles, he is the author of several books including *Nursing Home Standards: A Tragic Dilemma in American Health; Pharmaceutical Payment Plans-An Overview;* and the editor of *State Health Insurance Plans: Is Anyone Listening?*

The author resides in Washington, D.C.

Index

Readers desiring additional information either in purchasing or seeking health care services should refer to the following citations in the Index—*business corporations, health insurance, health maintenance organizations, medical malpractice, physicians,* and *prescription drugs.*